Fundamentals of **Human**

Nutrition

D1380027

Commissioning Editor: Mairi McCubbin
Development Editor: Catherine Jackson
Project Manager: Frances Affleck
Designer/Design Direction: Charles Gray
Illustration Manager: Merlyn Harvey
Illustrator: Peters & Zabransky

Fundamentals of Human Nutrition

For students and practitioners in the health sciences

Catherine A. Geissler BDS MS PhD RNutr

Professor Emerita of Human Nutrition, Department of Human Nutrition and Dietetics, and Director, Health Sciences and Practice Subject Centre, Higher Education Academy, King's College London, London, UK

Hilary J. Powers BSc PhD RNutr

Professor of Nutritional Biochemistry and Head of Human Nutrition Unit, University of Sheffield, Sheffield, UK

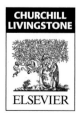

CHURCHILL
LIVINGSTONE

ELSEVIER

EDINBURGH LONDON NEW YORK OXFORD PHILADELPHIA ST LOUIS SYDNEY TORONTO 2009

CHURCHILL
LIVINGSTONE
ELSEVIER

First published 2009, © Elsevier Limited. All rights reserved.

ISBN 978 0 443 06972 7

British Library Cataloguing in Publication Data
A catalogue record for this book is available from the British Library

Library of Congress Cataloging in Publication Data
A catalog record for this book is available from the Library of Congress

Notice

Knowledge and best practice in this field are constantly changing. As new research and experience broaden our knowledge, changes in practice, treatment and drug therapy may become necessary or appropriate. Readers are advised to check the most current information provided (i) on procedures featured or (ii) by the manufacturer of each product to be administered, to verify the recommended dose or formula, the method and duration of administration, and contraindications. It is the responsibility of the practitioner, relying on their own experience and knowledge of the patient, to make diagnoses, to determine dosages and the best treatment for each individual patient, and to take all appropriate safety precautions. To the fullest extent of the law, neither the Publisher nor the Authors assume any liability for any injury and/or damage to persons or property arising out of or related to any use of the material contained in this book.

The Publisher

ELSEVIER your source for books,
journals and multimedia
in the health sciences

www.elsevierhealth.com

Working together to grow
libraries in developing countries

www.elsevier.com | www.bookaid.org | www.sabre.org

ELSEVIER   **BOOK AID** International   Sabre Foundation

The Publisher's policy is to use **paper manufactured from sustainable forests**

Printed in China

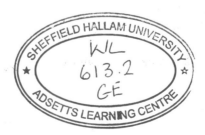

CONTENTS

PREFACE

Few would argue with the statement that a diet adequate in vitamins, minerals and energy, whilst not supplying energy in excess of needs, is central to health and wellbeing. Equally, most people living in high-income countries will be aware of the failing of much of the population in these countries to consume a healthy diet. The ever-increasing incidence of obesity and associated diseases has been key to the extraordinary increase in public and corporate interest in diet. But the importance of diet is not confined to obesity. The more we learn about the role of nutrients in cellular processes, the clearer it becomes that an adequate diet can play a critically important role in protecting against other public health diseases of importance, including cancer, and, in poorer countries in particular, infectious diseases.

In recent times, there has been great preoccupation with health in Western countries. Food-based products are increasingly marketed on the basis of health and vitality-giving properties, and sportsmen and women are encouraged to consume performance-enhancing snacks. For these reasons it is not surprising that, in many different sectors of life, individuals are recognizing the benefits of a reasonable grasp of the principles of human nutrition.

Of course, human nutrition is a very broad subject. It covers topics as diverse as the role of nutrients in gene expression and effects of international trade on the nutritional status of populations. This book provides the interested layperson and the student of many disciplines (sports science, pharmacology, nursing, dentistry and medicine) with up-to-date concise instruction in human nutrition in its broadest sense. The book is a digest of material in the highly successful *Human Nutrition, 11th edition*, edited by Geissler and Powers. The chapters in the original textbook have been condensed with due regard to the anticipated broad readership, but without compromising scientific rigour. To address the needs of the non-specialist, *Fundamentals* pays more attention to explaining technical terms; it also includes a comprehensive glossary. The interested reader wishing to access more detailed information is directed to *Human Nutrition* and then to various textbooks, reviews and websites, as appropriate. The authors of *Fundamentals* are indebted to the authors of the original textbook chapters for producing the material on which this is based.

Catherine A. Geissler
Hilary J. Powers
London and Sheffield, 2009

ACKNOWLEDGEMENTS

The authors sincerely acknowledge the authors of chapters in *Human Nutrition, 11th Edition*, on which this book is based. In chapter order, they are: Chapter 2, John Garrow, Abdul Dulloo, Yves Schutz; Chapter 3, Michael H. Gordon, Lawrence Haddad, John M. Kearney, Tom A.B. Sanders, Jane Thomas; Chapter 4, Nils-Georg Asp, David A. Bender, D. Joe Millward, Anne Marie Minihane, Ross Hunter, Timothy J. Peters, Victor Preedy, Christine M. Williams, Parveen Yaqoob; Chapter 5, David Bender, Paul Sharp, David Thurnham; Chapter 6, Robert Fraser, Salah Gariballa, Jane Morgan, Elizabeth Poskitt, Alan Sinclair; Chapter 7, Luc J.C. Van Loon, Wim H.M. Saris; Chapter 8, Arne Astrup, B. Capaldo, Maureen B. Duggan, Barbara Golden, Andrew J. Hill, Christopher G. Fairburn, Timothy J. Key, Jim I. Mann, Gabrielle Riccardi, A.A. Rivallese; Chapter 9, Margo E Barker, Aubrey Blumsohn, Paula Moynihan; Chapter 10, V.A. Chudleigh, George Grimble, J.O. Hunter, Stephan Strobel, A.M. Tomkins, The Late Anne Ferguson; Chapter 11, Paul Trayhurn, Stuart Wood; Chapter 12, Christopher Bates, Eric Brunner, Michael Nelson, Stanley J. Ulijaszek, Annhild Mosdøl; Chapter 13, Marc J. Cohen, Catherine Geissler, Lawrence Haddad.

CHAPTER 1

The Importance of Nutrition

1.1 INTRODUCTION

The term 'nutrition' incorporates the concepts of nutrient supply, utilization and effects on health. The subject therefore has a very broad range and includes a consideration of the politics and economics of food and drink availability, the ability of populations and individuals to access that food, the biochemical processes involved in the metabolism of the nutrients and their interactions, the genes that affect these processes, and the effects of different levels of intake on health. It is therefore a subject that embraces politics, agriculture, economics, sociology, public health, psychology, physiology, biochemistry, genetics and other disciplines. Nutritionists may have a broad view across these areas or specialize in a particular area. Whilst it cannot be disputed that food and nutrients are essential for good health, the habits and rituals of food consumption have also always made an important contribution to cultures and to the psychological wellbeing of individuals, friends and families.

Nutrition is a subject that is of interest to a wide range of people, and in almost every newspaper and magazine there are articles on nutrition and food. Much of what is written in the press is responsible and well researched, but there is also much that is based on no evidence, with suggestions of 'superfoods' that have implausible effects on health, or diets that guarantee rapid weight loss. With the increasing prevalence of obesity and concern for health these are of great interest but it is difficult for the general public to distinguish between advice that is given by a properly qualified nutritionist who understands the science and the quality of the evidence and those who have very little training and whose advice lacks a robust evidence base.

1.2 THE IMPORTANCE OF NUTRITION FOR HEALTH

In developing countries, poverty and disease result in a significant proportion of the population consuming diets deficient in energy (overall calories from food whether fat, protein or carbohydrate) and specific vitamins and minerals. These diets have many adverse effects both in the short term and the long term. Growth in infancy and childhood is very often impaired, and this can affect education, ability to work, and childbearing, so that the long-term consequences are manifold. Additionally, vitamin or mineral deficiencies can lead to a range of conditions such as anaemia, bone abnormalities, increased susceptibility to infection, even blindness. Levels of child and maternal mortality in these countries are high.

In the developed countries, such as the UK, the prevalence of specific nutrient deficiencies is generally low, although there are groups of the population in which nutrient deficiencies are still evident. For example, vitamin B_{12} and D deficiencies are a problem among the elderly and folate and vitamin B_2 status are often poor in young women. In association with changes in dietary intake and physical activity over the last few decades, there has been an increase in the prevalence of obesity and related pathologies in middle- and high-income countries, so that chronic diseases such as diabetes, coronary heart disease and stroke have taken the place of classic nutrient deficiency diseases. A very important task for nutritionists is to conduct research that contributes to our understanding of the role of diet and physical inactivity in the development of these diseases, and to help inform the public and politicians of ways of addressing these problems. Self restraint is exceedingly difficult in a society where, for most people, there is access to a huge variety of tempting foods, often not well balanced nutritionally, and at a relatively low price, and where work and leisure pursuits are usually sedentary.

1.3 NUTRITIONAL CONTROVERSY

The general public is often given the impression that disagreement exists between nutritional scientists, as the press highlights new findings. In the press, discrepancies in research findings are generally given prominence, often giving the impression that nutritionists are not consistent in the advice they give, and so the reader asks, why not eat what I like and ignore the advice?

However, advances in scientific knowledge are made through a variety of research studies at different levels – molecular, cellular, clinical, and epidemiological – all providing different elements of evidence which have to be integrated into a portfolio of the available evidence in its entirety. Lack of agreement between studies can arise for a variety of reasons. The age and gender of the subjects under study, the season in which a study is carried out, dietary intake of the study sample, or simply errors associated with estimates of dietary intake or other measurements, are all factors that can lead to different findings in different studies. Also, studies that examine the effect of a single nutrient on some health outcome can give results that are very different from studies that examine interactions between a number of nutrients.

A particular difficulty of nutrition research is that people consume diets, not single nutrients, and diets are complex combinations of different foods, each with its own particular profile of nutrients and non-nutrients. In experimental studies, changing one dietary component inevitably changes the relative levels of other components. For example, devising a low fat diet whilst maintaining the same calorific value automatically increases the carbohydrate and/or protein content and this needs to be appreciated and taken into account. Finally, some discrepancies in research findings between different studies is now known to be partly explained by differences in the genotype of certain individuals, leading to different responses to various dietary factors.

1.4 APPLICATION TO DIFFERENT PROFESSIONS

Nutritionists and dietitians are the main practitioners of the science of nutrition, but many others in the health professions and food professions may be asked for advice and for this reason require access to reliable condensed information. The general public may also wish this for their own interest. The number of qualified nutritionists is small compared with other professionals who have contact with the public and require some background in nutritional science, such as nurses, pharmacists and sports and exercise advisers. Others, such as food technologists and food distributors, may need to know the nutritional value of the foods they produce and distribute, and the interested general public may want an understandable but reliable source of information across the breadth of nutrition.

It is the intention of the authors that this book provides a reliable, concise source of information for these interested groups.

1.5 IMPORTANCE OF EVIDENCE BASE

For information to be valid it has to be supported by reliable evidence that has been tested and replicated in epidemiological, laboratory and clinical studies. The information in this book has been summarized from detailed chapters written by scientists who have specialized in particular areas of nutrition and who therefore have in depth knowledge of the evidence base. In a short book it is not possible to present the evidence, and what is included here are the conclusions from these specialist reviews. For people who would like more detailed background, further reading is suggested, and the original chapters from which this digest is drawn can be read in *Human Nutrition* (Geissler & Powers 2005) as well as in the further reading suggestions at the end of each chapter. The original authors are not responsible for the summarizing of their contributions.

REFERENCE

Geissler C, Powers H J (eds) 2005 Human nutrition, 11th edn. Elsevier Churchill Livingstone, Edinburgh; and 2010, 12th edn (in press)

CHAPTER 2

Body Composition and Energy Balance

OBJECTIVES

By the end of this chapter you should be able to:

- define terms for components of body composition
- describe their relative size and variation
- describe their main characteristics and functions
- summarize the use of composition information in nutrition
- define energy balance
- explain the laws of thermodynamics
- define types and units of energy
- identify and quantify the food sources of energy
- describe the main factors affecting energy intake
- explain the components of energy expenditure, their relative size and variability
- describe the methods of measurement of energy expenditure for different purposes
- describe the assessment of energy needs
- identify the main types of signals in relation to hunger and satiety
- describe the changes in energy expenditure that occur in response to undernutrition and overnutrition

2.1 INTRODUCTION

This chapter is concerned with composition of the body throughout the life span, as well as how body weight is regulated.

2.2 BODY COMPOSITION AND FUNCTION

The percentage of body weight made up of the main tissues is typically: adipose tissue 28, 35; muscle 37, 33; bone 14, 13; and skin 6, 6, *for men and women respectively*.

Fat-free mass or lean body mass

Fat and *fat-free mass* together make up total body weight. These terms should be distinguished from adipose tissue and lean body mass which also together make up total body weight. The terms fat-free mass and lean body mass are often used interchangeably but this is not appropriate. Adipose tissue is not pure fat, but approximately 79% fat, 3% protein and 18% water. Also, tissue other than adipose tissue is not totally fat-free, since there is lipid in cell membranes and in nervous tissue. Our understanding of body composition in human subjects is based on the chemical analyses of six cadavers (five male and one female), performed between 1945 and 1956. On average fat-free tissue contains about 72.5% water, 20.5% protein and 69 mmol K/kg. However, individual tissues and organs vary in their protein, water and mineral content.

Water and electrolytes

A typical normal young adult male who weighs 70 kg with an assumed fat content of 12 kg (17%), would have fat-free mass of 58 kg (83%). By far the largest component of fat-free mass is water, on average 72.5%. Approximately two-thirds of this water is inside cells, ie intracellular fluid (ICF), and the remaining third is extracellular, ie extracellular fluid (ECF).

The total amount of water in the body, and the partition of body water between ICF and ECF, is closely regulated (see chapter 4). Body stores of protein, energy, vitamins and minerals ensure survival for many weeks without dietary intake, but deprivation of water causes death in a few days. The principal anion in ICF is K, with a small amount of Na and Mg. The principal anion in ECF is Na, and Cl is the principal cation.

Bone

An adult body contains approximately 1 kg of Ca, of which 99% is in bone. This acts as a reservoir to maintain an appropriate plasma concentration of calcium. The skeleton also contains approximately 500 g of P and more than half the collagen in the body, the remaining collagen being in skin, tendons, and fascial sheaths. For more details see chapter 9.

Muscle

There are three types of muscle: skeletal, smooth and cardiac. In a typical adult, skeletal muscle accounts for approximately 35% of body weight, and another 10% is smooth muscle. Resting skeletal muscle has a lower energy consumption per unit weight than tissues such as heart, liver, kidneys or brain, but during vigorous physical exercise the energy consumption in muscle greatly exceeds the total of all other body tissues. Skeletal muscle consists of bundles of individual muscle fibres, each constituting a muscle cell and containing hundreds to thousands of myofibrils which each contains about 1500 myosin filaments overlapping with around 3000 actin filaments. When the muscle contracts the overlap between the actin and myosin fibres increases and the bones to which these ends are attached are pulled towards each other.

Skeletal muscle has two types of muscle fibres: red and white fibres. Red muscle sustains posture for long periods, while white muscle is for rapid movement. In human subjects most muscles contain a mixture of red and white fibres. The process of muscle contraction is considered in chapter 7.

Smooth muscle fibres are far smaller and lie in the walls of blood vessels, gut, bile ducts, ureters, and uterus. Contraction and relaxation of the smooth muscle in the walls of these organs alters the diameter of the tubes, or may be organized in peristaltic waves so as to move forwards the contents of the tube.

Cardiac muscle forms the chambers of the heart. Unlike skeletal muscle it is not organized as bundles of individually innervated muscle fibres, but is a syncytium of cells fused end-to-end in a latticework. The electrical potential that causes one cell to contract passes to adjacent cells so that the whole mass of muscle contracts and relaxes synchronously. Contraction expels the blood within the chamber through an exit valve, and then as it relaxes the chamber refills with blood that flows in through an entry valve.

Blood

Blood consists of plasma and cells – red blood cells (RBCs), white blood cells (WBCs) and platelets. Its main function is to transport oxygen, nutrients, and hormones to the tissues, and to remove carbon dioxide and other waste products from tissues. In a typical adult the volume of blood is approximately 5 L, of which about 55% of the volume is plasma and 45% packed cells (the haematocrit). In a glass test tube blood solidifies as a web of the protein fibrin forms and contracts, trapping the cells to form a blood clot and a clear yellowish supernatant fluid (serum). Serum is plasma from which the blood clotting proteins have been removed. To obtain plasma fresh blood is put into a tube with an anticoagulant, and then separated from the cells by centrifugation.

RBCs contain haemoglobin in a biconcave cell wall which is freely permeable to oxygen. They enable blood to transport large amounts of oxygen. RBCs develop in the bone marrow from stem cells to reticulocytes which contain remnants of nucleic acid and are the most immature form of red cell normally seen in the peripheral circulation. Normally 99% of RBCs are fully mature, with no nucleic acid or nucleus, and survive in the circulation for about 120 days, then are destroyed in the reticulo-endothelial system. The haemoglobin is broken down to bilirubin, and the iron is recycled for the synthesis of new haemoglobin for new RBCs.

WBCs are approximately a thousand times less common than RBCs in the blood. The commonest type of WBC is the polymorph, or neutrophil granulocyte, which, like RBCs, is formed in bone marrow and rapidly increases in number in response to infection or tissue injury, surviving in the peripheral circulation for a very short time; their half-life is estimated at 6–8 hours. The next commonest WBC is the lymphocyte, which is formed in lymphoid tissue and is involved in immune responses. The remaining WBCs (monocytes, basophil and eosinophil granulocytes) occur still more rarely. Platelets are very small cells that are involved in blood clotting and the repair of damaged blood vessels.

Body fat

Body fat is a valuable store of energy during times of famine, and a thermal insulator against cold, but in affluent countries (and increasingly in developing countries) the need for protection from famine and cold is less often required, and excessive fatness is increasingly common.

The typical 70 kg adult male contains 12 kg of fat, which is 17% of body weight. This degree of fatness is within the healthy range (15–18%). Usually 90% of this fat is under the skin, but some is within the abdominal cavity, and a small amount between muscles. Not all body fat is available for energy; even in people who have died of starvation about 2 kg of fat remains. A reserve of 10 kg of fat can provide 375 MJ (90,000 kcal) of energy, which is equivalent to about 4 weeks of normal energy requirements. In fact people of normal weight undergoing total starvation survive for about 10 weeks, because energy expenditure decreases. In severely obese people the fat stores may reach 80 kg; such people could survive a year of starvation, although this is not appropriate treatment for severe obesity. The amount and distribution of body fat differs between men and women, women having a higher % body fat, the healthy range being 22–25%. At puberty, women tend to store fat around breast, hip and thigh regions, whereas men tend to accumulate fat in and on the abdomen.

Body fat is synthesized by, and stored in, fat cells, or adipocytes. There are two types, white (the majority) and brown. White adipocytes can develop at any age if the amount of fat to be stored increases. They contain a single central droplet of triacylglycerol, surrounded by a thin layer of cytoplasm containing the nucleus. White adipose tissue is a source of hormones, at least two of which, oestrogen and leptin, have important functions related to energy balance and reproductive function. In post-menopausal women adipose tissue is the only route of oestrogen production. Leptin is the product of the *ob* gene, which is involved in the control of both food intake and energy expenditure. Obese mice which lack this gene are deficient in leptin and infertile; administration of leptin corrects both obesity and infertility in these animals. Unfortunately obese human subjects usually have abnormally high circulating leptin concentrations, and the administration of leptin is not an effective therapy.

The brown fat cell differs from white adipocytes in having only small fat droplets in a cytoplasm rich in mitochondria. Brown fat cells are particularly important to small mammals including human babies because they generate heat, which helps to maintain body temperature in cold environments.

2.3 CHANGES IN BODY SIZE AND COMPOSITION

Throughout the lifespan

On the first day after fertilization the human embryo is a single cell, approximately 0.15 mm in diameter. After two months of intrauterine life it is about 30 mm long with recognizable head, trunk and limbs; the head accounts for half the total body length. By the end of normal gestation at 9 months, the fetus is 500 mm long and weighs about 3.5 kg, the head being one-quarter of total length. After two decades of extrauterine life the average adult weighs about 70 kg and is 1.7–1.8 m tall, with the head accounting for only one-eighth of total height.

Table 2.1 Effect of growth, malnutrition and obesity on the composition of the body

	Fetus 20–25 weeks	Full-term baby	Infant (1 year)	Malnourished infant	Adult man	Obese man
Body weight (kg)	0.3	3.5	20	5	70	100
Water (%)	88	69	62	74	60	47
Protein (%)	9.5	12	14	14	17	13
Fat (%)	0.5	16	20	10	17	35
Remainder (%)	2	3	4	2	6	5

During growth there are changes in the composition of the tissues (Table 2.1). The embryo contains a very high percentage of water, but with maturation during childhood and adolescence the proportion of water in the body, and the proportion of extracellular to intracellular water, decreases. Fat-free mass remains fairly constant in both men and women between the ages of 20 and 65 years, but then decreases by about 15% in the next two decades. Throughout adult life there is a trend for fat mass to increase in both men and women, but the increase is more rapid in post-menopausal women.

Through diet and exercise

Over a given period, if the energy intake of an individual is less than energy output, then the energy stored in the body is reduced by the same amount, by losing fat, fat-free tissue, or (more probably) a mixture of both lean and fat tissue. However as weight is lost, resting energy expenditure also decreases, so for a given energy intake the energy deficit, and hence the rate of weight loss, also decreases. Weight loss is significantly faster during the first week than during the next 2 weeks because during the first week on a diet glycogen and its associated water (see chapter 4) is lost, especially on very low carbohydrate diets. During total starvation weight loss is even more rapid, partly because the energy deficit is greater, and partly because a higher proportion of the weight loss is fat-free mass to provide amino acids for glucose synthesis (see chapter 4). Total starvation has ceased to be an acceptable treatment for gross obesity because several patients died unexpectedly, due to damage to heart muscle.

Strenuous exercise causes muscle hypertrophy, and immobilization causes atrophy of muscle. Exercise also increases energy expenditure, so a combination of a low energy diet and exercise should achieve more fat loss, and less loss of fat-free mass, than diet alone.

Bone density is affected by diet, exercise, genetic and other factors (see chapter 9).

Through changes in hydration

Regulation of body water is discussed in chapter 4. Dehydration may occur if water losses are very high, as in severe diarrhoea, or with sweat loss in high ambient temperature or during prolonged vigorous exercise. Dehydration may also occur with abuse of diuretic drugs to achieve weight loss, or during the recovery phase of diabetic coma.

Water excess, indicated by oedema, is much more common than dehydration. The commonest cause in elderly people is congestive heart failure: the heart is unable to pump blood out as fast as it returns from the veins, the veins become engorged and leak fluid into the tissues. Another cause is when the kidney leaks albumin into the urine, so decreasing the plasma oncotic pressure allowing fluid to pass from the vascular system into the extracellular spaces.

Oedema is also a feature of certain types of malnutrition. It is a striking feature of kwashiorkor (see chapter 8). A marasmic child does not show obvious oedema; however in such children water accounts for an abnormally high proportion of body weight.

2.4 USE OF BODY SIZE AND COMPOSITION DATA IN NUTRITION

Body size and composition is useful for the assessment of current nutritional status, and serial measurements for changes in status, and also for standardization of physiological measurements and drug dosage. Measurements of the size and composition of a body are made for nutrition assessment to estimate the extent of obesity, thinness, muscle wasting and stunting (see chapter 12), osteoporosis (see chapter 9) and anaemia (see chapter 5). Many physiological measurements give results that are related to body size or composition and so have to be standardized for comparisons. For example larger people expend more total energy than smaller people for the same activity but if the energy expended is expressed per unit body weight or per unit fat-free mass, this may not be the case. It is sometimes necessary to adjust for body size or composition, for example to calculate the dose of drugs given to small children.

KEY POINTS

- A healthy adult male contains about 60% water, 17% protein and 17% fat
- Total body water, the partition between intracellular and extracellular water, and its electrolyte composition are normally tightly regulated
- The skeleton accounts for 14% of total body weight; 99% of total body calcium is in bone; this acts as a reservoir to maintain an appropriate plasma calcium concentration
- Skeletal muscle accounts for 35% of body weight, and smooth muscle 10%
- The healthy range for fat in males is 15–18% of body weight, of which about 80% can be considered to be energy reserves; in females the healthy range is 22–25%
- Fat reserves are in white adipose tissue whilst the main function of brown fat is thermogenesis

- Males tend to accumulate fat in the abdomen, while women accumulate subcutaneous fat stores around the breast, hip and thigh
- Adipose tissue has endocrine functions concerned with fertility and regulation of food intake and energy balance
- Body composition changes throughout life. The water content of the body decreases, and the content of protein and fat increases, through gestation, infancy and into adolescence
- Fat-free mass remains relatively constant from age 20–65 y, but then decreases; fat mass increases throughout adult life
- Food restriction and starvation result in loss of fat-free mass as well as adipose tissue
- Excessive water losses can lead to dehydration
- Several conditions can lead to excessive accumulation of body water, resulting in oedema. Even severely wasted undernourished people may be oedematous
- Body composition can be used to assess current nutritional status; serial measurements assess changes in status

2.5 INTRODUCTION TO ENERGY BALANCE AND BODY WEIGHT REGULATION

Understanding how body weight is regulated is still challenging. Failure of this regulation leads either to obesity or to protein-energy malnutrition An understanding of how energy balance and weight homeostasis are achieved requires an appreciation of the following:

- the basic concepts and principles of energy transformations through which body weight is regulated
- factors affecting food intake and energy expenditure, which represent the input and output of energy
- the methods for assessing energy expenditure and energy requirements
- models proposed to explain the regulation of body weight and body composition in humans.

2.6 BASIC CONCEPTS AND PRINCIPLES IN HUMAN ENERGETICS

Energy balance and the laws of thermodynamics

Energy is the capacity to perform work and has various forms – light, chemical, mechanical, electrical – all of which can be completely converted to heat. According to the *first law of thermodynamics*, energy cannot be created or destroyed but can only be transformed from one form into another. Plants depend on light energy captured from the sun to perform the work of synthesizing molecules like carbohydrates, proteins and fats, while animals meet their energy needs from chemical energy stored in plants or in other animals, which is used to perform a variety of work, such as the synthesis of new macromolecules (*chemical work*), in muscular contraction (*mechanical work*) or in the maintenance of ionic gradients across membranes (*electrical work*).

Overall energy balance is given by the following equation:

$$\text{Energy intake} = \text{Energy expenditure} + \Delta\text{Energy stores}$$

Thus, if the total energy contained in the body (as fat, protein and glycogen) is not altered (ie ΔEnergy stores $= 0$), then energy expenditure must be equal to energy intake and the individual is said to be in a state of *energy balance*. If the intake is less than expenditure the *negative energy balance* results in a decrease of the body's energy stores (glycogen, fat and protein) or if intake is more than expenditure the *positive energy balance* results in an increase in body energy stores, primarily as fat.

The *second law of thermodynamics* states that when food is utilized in the body, there is an inevitable loss of energy as heat. The conversion of available food energy is therefore not a perfectly efficient process, and about 75% of the chemical energy contained in foods may be ultimately dissipated as heat. The energy in food is converted into discrete amounts of chemical energy, usually as adenosine triphosphate (ATP), which can be used for useful work, whether it is the internal work required to maintain structure and function or external physical work.

Units of energy

Since all the energy used by the body at rest is ultimately lost as heat, the energy that is consumed, stored and expended is expressed as its heat equivalent. The calorie was originally adopted as the unit of energy in nutrition; it is defined as the amount of heat required to raise the temperature of 1 gram of water by 1°C (from 14.5°C to 15.5°C); nutritionally the kilocalorie (= 1000 calories) is used. With the introduction of the SI system, energy is expressed as joule (J). One joule is the energy used when a mass of 1 kilogram (kg) is moved through 1 metre (m) by a force of 1 Newton (N). Because one joule is a very small unit of energy, it is more convenient to use kilojoule (kJ) or megajoule (MJ) in nutrition. Rates of energy expenditure (often referred to as metabolic rate) are expressed in kJ or MJ per unit time (kJ/min or MJ/day), which correspond to 10^3J and 10^6J, respectively. The conversion of calories to joules is: 1 calorie = 4.18 J, or 1 kilocalorie (kcal) = 4.18 kilojoule (kJ).

Sources of energy and macronutrient balance

The macronutrients (carbohydrate, fat, protein and alcohol) are the sources of energy, so it makes sense to consider energy balance and macronutrient balance together:

$$\text{carbohydrate intake} - \text{carbohydrate oxidation} = \text{carbohydrate balance}$$

$$\text{protein intake} - \text{protein oxidation} = \text{protein balance}$$

$$\text{lipid intake} - \text{lipid oxidation} = \text{lipid balance}$$

$$\text{total energy intake} - \text{total oxidation} = \text{energy balance}$$

Unlike the size of the fat stores, which can increase very considerably, there is a limited capacity for storing protein in fat-free mass and for carbohydrate as glycogen in liver and muscles. Protein and glucose tend to be oxidized more readily than fat, and alcohol, which is not stored in the body, is oxidized rapidly (sparing fat).

2.7 ENERGY INTAKE

Energy value of foods and Atwater factors

The traditional way of measuring the energy content of foodstuffs is to use a 'bomb calorimeter' in which the heat produced when a sample of food is combusted (in presence of oxygen) is measured. When the food is combusted, it is completely oxidized to water, carbon dioxide and oxides of other elements such as sulphur and nitrogen. The total heat liberated (expressed in kilocalories or kilojoules) represents the *gross energy* value or *heat of combustion* of the food. The heat of combustion differs between carbohydrates, proteins, and fats and there are differences within each category of macronutrient.

However, there is less energy available to the body than the gross energy of food consumed. Firstly, none of the foodstuffs is completely absorbed; although on average more than 90% of fat, carbohydrate and protein is absorbed, some is not and therefore some energy is excreted in faeces. Secondly, whilst the tissues are able to oxidize carbohydrate and fat completely to carbon dioxide and water, the oxidation of protein is not complete, and results in the formation of urea and other nitrogenous compounds which are excreted in the urine. This energy represents metabolic loss and must be subtracted from the 'digestible' energy of protein. From these considerations, the 'Atwater factors' for available energy (or metabolizable energy) of the three macronutrients have been derived (Fig. 2.1). These are, in kcal/g, protein 4, carbohydrate 4 and lipid 9. The value for alcohol is 7. It is the metabolizable energy value that is quoted in food composition tables. It is important to remember that these factors make allowance for the energy in the food lost in faeces and urine and they are *approximations*.

Pattern of food intake

In contrast with energy expenditure, which is continuous, human beings eat food in a discontinuous manner and the amount of food eaten can range from zero to up to 21 MJ/day (5000 kcal) in highly active individuals or during acute episodes of overeating (hyperphagia). This lack of regularity of food behaviour occurs both within-day and between-days, which explains the difficulty in assessing food intake in order to obtain a representative picture of 'habitual' food (energy) intake. The various methods used to assess energy intake are described in chapter 12 including factors leading to underestimation or overestimation of energy intake, and hence leading to a bias in the estimation of energy balance.

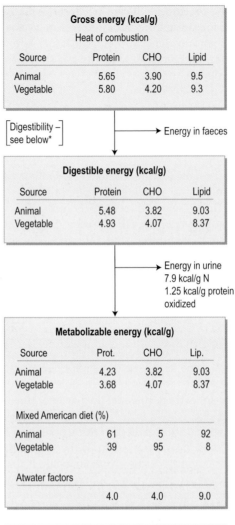

Figure 2.1 Gross, digestible and metabolizable energy values of macronutrients.

Components of energy expenditure

Energy expenditure is made up of three components: basal metabolism (or basal metabolic rate), physical activity, and thermogenesis, which is the response to a variety of stimuli (including food, cold, stress and drugs). These three components are described below.

Basal metabolic rate (BMR)

This is the largest component of energy expenditure for most individuals. Typically, in developed countries BMR accounts for 60–75% of daily energy expenditure, and reflects the energy needed for the work of vital functions (maintaining electrolyte equilibrium across cell membranes, cell and protein turnover, respiratory and cardiovascular functions, etc). By far the most important determinant of BMR is body size, and in particular the fat-free mass, which is influenced by weight, height, gender and age. On average, men have greater fat-free mass and total BMR than women of the same age, weight and height, and older people have lower fat-free mass and total BMR than young adults. Most, but not all, of the differences in BMR between these groups disappear when BMR is expressed per unit of fat-free mass which includes tissues and organs which have high metabolic activities such as liver, kidneys, and heart. In contrast, the contribution of adipose tissue to BMR is small. BMR is greater than the metabolic rate during sleep by 5–20%, the difference between BMR and sleeping metabolic rate being explained by the stimulation of being awake. BMR is known to be depressed during starvation and energy restricted dieting due to the loss in body weight and lean tissues.

Physical activity

The energy spent on physical activity naturally depends on the type and intensity of the physical activity and on the time spent in different activities. There is a wide variation in the energy cost of any activity both within an individual and between individuals, due to differences in body size and in the speed and dexterity with which an activity is performed. To adjust for differences in body size, the energy cost of physical activities is expressed as multiples of BMR, generally ranging from 1–5 for most activities, but reaching values of 10–14 during intense exercise. Physical activity can represent up to 70% of daily energy expenditure in an individual involved in heavy manual work or competition athletics but for most people in industrialized societies physical activity represents only 10–15% of daily energy expenditure.

Thermogenesis

The main forms of thermogenesis are:

1. *Psychological*: Anxiety, anticipation and stress stimulate adrenaline secretion, leading to increased heat production. The best evidence comes from a study on pilots, whose energy expenditure increased when they were under air traffic control, with the rise being inversely related to their level of experience.
2. *Cold-induced*: Human beings rarely need to increase heat production for the purpose of thermal regulation because they are able to seek a warm environment or wear suitable clothing. However at low temperatures,

resting metabolic rate (and hence heat production) increases. For example, normal weight women maintained in identical clothing in a room calorimeter increased their 24h heat production by about 7% when the temperature in the calorimeter room was reduced from 28°C to 22°C. Two forms of cold-induced thermogenesis exist: shivering thermogenesis, which is rhythmic muscle contraction, and non-shivering thermogenesis, which is due to increased sympathetic nervous system activity. This occurs particularly in brown adipose tissue in small mammals but is also demonstrated in adult humans chronically exposed to extreme cold.

3. *Diet-induced*: Heat production increases following the consumption of a meal, and with high levels of food consumption. 'Diet-induced thermogenesis' or DIT, can be divided into an *obligatory* component (related to the energy costs of absorption and metabolic processing of nutrients or the energy cost of tissue synthesis during overfeeding) and a *facultative* component which results from the smell and taste of food, and from stimulation of the sympathetic nervous system as part of the regulation of energy balance.

4. *Drug-induced*: The consumption of caffeine, nicotine and alcohol may form an integral part of daily life for many people, and all three of these drugs stimulate thermogenesis. A cup of coffee (containing 60–80 mg caffeine) can increase BMR by 5–10% over an hour or two. Taking 100 mg caffeine every two hours during the day or smoking a packet of 20 cigarettes increase daily energy expenditure by 5% and 15%, respectively. This may be a factor that contributes to the average weight gain of 7 kg after cessation of smoking.

5. Energy expenditure during involuntary activity, including fidgeting, is referred to as non-exercise activity thermogenesis (NEAT), and this can be important in body weight regulation.

2.9 FUEL METABOLISM AT THE LEVEL OF ORGANS AND TISSUES

Metabolic rate of organs and tissues

The heat production of individual tissues and organs can be calculated from the oxygen consumption by measuring blood flow and the arteriovenous difference in oxygen concentration across tissues and organs. Normalized for body mass, adipose tissue has the lowest metabolic rate and in a non-obese subject contributes to 3–5% of the total resting energy expenditure, although it represents 20–30% of body weight. The majority of the heat production (about 60%) comes from active organs such as the liver, kidney, heart and brain, although they account for only 5–6% of total body weight. The heat production of muscles per unit mass is much lower than that of metabolically active organs, but because of their large size (more than half of the total fat-free mass) they contribute about 20% of total heat production.

The metabolic rate per kg body weight (or per kg fat-free mass) is much greater in young children than in adults. The reduction of metabolic rate with increasing age is mostly due to a change in the proportion of different tissues. The larger proportion of metabolically active tissues (brain, liver, heart, kidneys) in infants and children explains their higher metabolic rates compared with adults (when expressed in relation to fat-free mass).

2.10 MEASUREMENTS OF ENERGY EXPENDITURE

Principles of energy expenditure measurements

The energy expended by an individual can be assessed by *direct* and *indirect* calorimetry. Direct calorimetry is the direct measurement of heat output but is rarely used because in order to measure this, activity needs to be restricted. Indirect calorimetry involves calculating heat production from the rate of oxygen consumption (VO_2). This is because energy expenditure utilizes ATP (adenosine triphosphate) which is directly linked to the oxidation of substrates. It is the rate of ATP utilization that determines the rate of substrate oxidation and therefore oxygen consumption and carbon dioxide production, which can be measured.

Assessment of BMR and energy cost of activity

The measurement of BMR is made under standardized conditions – ie in an awake subject lying in the supine position, in a state of physical and mental rest in a comfortably warm environment, and in the morning in the post-absorptive state, usually 10–12 hours after the last meal. Under these conditions, the expired air (collected in a gas bag over a certain period of time or coming from a ventilated hood system at a constant flow rate) is analysed for changes in O_2 and CO_2 concentrations. The energy cost of activities is measured by a portable indirect calorimeter.

Assessment of energy expenditure in free-living conditions

Various indirect methods have been used to assess total energy expenditure in free-living humans. Early studies estimated energy expenditure using an activity diary, but today the two most commonly employed non-calorimetric methods are the heart rate and the doubly-labelled water technique.

Heart rate

The method involves establishing individual regression lines between heart rate and energy expenditure of a range of activities within the habitual heart rates observed in normal life. Heart rate is recorded minute-by-minute throughout the day, using portable heart rate monitors, to give the number of minutes spent at each heart rate. The energy expenditure at a given heart rate is calculated from the regression line, and integrated throughout the day. However the heart rate method gives much less reliable estimate of energy expenditure for an individual than for a group.

Doubly-labelled water

The stable (non-radioactive) isotope method for estimating energy expenditure by giving the subject a measured dose of doubly-labelled water ($^2H_2$ and ^{18}O)

to drink is based on the subsequent difference in the rates of disappearance of ^2H_2O and $H_2^{18}O$ in body water, which is used to estimate the rate of energy expenditure.

Estimations of energy requirements

The energy requirement of an individual is defined by the World Health Organization (WHO) as 'the level of energy intake that will balance energy expenditure when the individual has a body size and composition, and a level of physical activity, consistent with long-term good health'. The energy requirement should also allow the maintenance of economically necessary and socially desirable physical activity. In children and pregnant or lactating women, the energy requirement includes the energy needs associated with the deposition of tissues or the secretion of milk at rates consistent with good health.

The energy needs of a group represent the *average* value of the individuals making up that group. The term 'requirements' refers to the 'habitual' or 'usual' requirements over a certain period and can best be determined from expenditure rather than intake measurements or estimated by the 'factorial' approach. The BMR is first calculated from equations based on body weight and the physical activities are classified into levels such as *light*, *moderate* or *heavy* and multiplied by the appropriate factor, and the total energy requirement can be calculated by summation. A group with occupational work classified as 'moderate' activity will have an energy requirement calculated over 24 hours of 1.78 × BMR in men and 1.64 × BMR in women.

The rate of total energy expenditure (TEE), directly assessed in a respiration chamber or by doubly-labelled water, can also be expressed as a multiple of BMR. The ratio of TEE and BMR provides a rough index of physical activity (referred to as 'physical activity level' or PAL). Based on double-labelled water measurements in free living non-obese adults, typically the ratio TEE/ BMR ranges from 1.64 to 1.98.

2.11 TIMESCALE OF ENERGY BALANCE AND BODY WEIGHT VARIABILITY

In many individuals, body weight remains relatively constant over many years in spite of large day-to-day variations in the amount of food consumed. There is little doubt that regulation of body weight occurs, with varying degrees of precision, although the timescale over which it occurs is not clear. Three important features of energy balance and weight regulation are:

- human beings do not balance energy intake and energy expenditure on a day-to-day basis but usually over 1–2 weeks
- for most individuals weight remains within a few kg over several decades; matching of long-term energy intake and expenditure must be extremely precise since a persistent difference of only 1% would lead to a gain or loss of about 10 kg per decade
- body weight tends to fluctuate around a constant mean value, with small or large deviations from a 'set' or 'preferred' value being triggered

by events that are seasonal and/or cultural (week-end parties, holiday seasons), psychological (stress, depression, anxiety or emotions) and pathophysiological (ranging from minor health disturbances to serious diseases).

2.12 CONTROL OF FOOD INTAKE

Hunger and satiety

Research into the control of energy intake is very difficult, primarily because habitual intake is not easy to measure and because the intake of foods is altered by the experiments themselves. Because of these difficulties, much of the work carried out in human beings has been concerned with short-term hunger and appetite studies or with short-term satiety and satiation. *Hunger* may be defined as a 'demand for energy' (eg after starvation), while appetite refers to 'a demand for a particular food'. Appetite is a powerful but poorly controlled stimulus to eat even when not hungry. *Satiety* refers to the inhibition of further intake of a food and meal after eating has ended.

Even though subjects may feel satiated by one particular food, they will continue to eat when a new food is presented. Conversely, when presented with a monotonous diet, their intakes are usually low. These observations suggest that when the psychosocial incentives to eat are removed, human beings can control food intake quite precisely. However several other factors contribute to a poor control of food intake in affluent societies, leading to obesity (Box 2.1).

Hunger–satiety control centres in the brain

'Centres' in the hypothalamus are involved in the control of feeding behaviour. People with damage in the hypothalamus, due to trauma or tumour, often show abnormalities in feeding behaviour and weight regulation, although many other extra-hypothalamic areas of the brain also play a role in the control of food intake.

Satiety signals from the periphery

The sensations of hunger and satiety result from integration in the brain of numerous signals originating from a variety of peripheral tissues and organs,

---

Box 2.1 Factors contributing to a poor control of food intake in humans

- Large food diversity and high palatability diets
- Profuse availability of food
- Television watching (reduced activity, pressure of food advertising)
- Snacking rather than meal eating
- Fast rate of eating ('fast foods')
- High-energy-dense diets (eg high-fat diet)
- Eating outside home and unsociable eating
- Technological developments, less activity
- Reduced physical activity level
- Urbanization: more access to energy-dense foods; less need to walk

including the gastrointestinal tract, liver, adipose tissue, and perhaps also skeletal muscle. These include:

Gastrointestinal signals

Signals from stretch- and mechano-receptors or from chemoreceptors in the gastrointestinal tract that respond to the products of digestion (sugars, fatty acids, amino acids and peptides), have a major role in the short-term regulation of food intake by limiting the size of a single meal. For example, cholecystokinin (CCK) decreases meal size.

Aminostatic or protein-static signals

Based on observations that dietary protein induces satiety in the short-term, and consumption of low-protein diets leads to increased appetite for protein-containing foods, the aminostatic theory states that food intake is determined by the concentration of plasma amino acids.

Glucostatic and glycogenostatic signals

A glucostatic theory for the regulation of feeding behaviour proposes that there are chemoreceptors in the hypothalamus sensitive to the arteriovenous differences in glucose or to the availability and utilization of glucose.

Lipostatic or adipostat signals

A lipostatic theory of food intake control postulates that substances released from the fat stores function as satiety signals. For example, leptin is primarily produced by adipocytes, is released into the circulation from adipocytes and acts on hypothalamic receptors to induce satiety. The blood concentration of leptin is proportional to the adipose mass, and its elevation in the obese has led to the hypothesis that resistance to the action of leptin is a factor in obesity.

Integrated models of food intake control

The control of food intake is considered in three phases:

- *short-term* (hour-to-hour) blood glucose homeostasis
- *medium-term* (day-to-day) maintenance of adequate hepatic stores of glycogen
- *long-term* (weeks, months or years) maintenance of the body's fat and protein, ie fat mass and fat-free mass.

The long-term stability of body weight and body composition requires that energy expenditure be equal to energy intake, and that the composition of the fuel used be equal to that ingested. Since the protein and carbohydrate stores in the body are limited, there is an increase in their oxidation in response to an increase in their ingestion. In contrast, an increase in dietary fat does not immediately promote its oxidation and so fat balance is not precisely regulated. This contributes to depletion of glycogen stores by increasing carbohydrate oxidation. When the higher fat intake is eventually matched by higher fat oxidation the individual would then be both in fat balance and in energy balance, but at a higher percentage of body fat. The interpretation of this concept of nutrient balance is that the control of food intake can be viewed as both glycogenic (short-term) and lipostatic (long-term).

2.13 ADJUSTMENTS IN ENERGY EXPENDITURE

In addition to the control of food intake there is also ample evidence that autoregulatory adjustments in energy expenditure play an important role in the regulation of body weight and body composition. Any imbalance between energy intake and expenditure results in a change in body weight which, in turn, will alter the maintenance energy requirements – which tends to counter the original imbalance.

Even after adjusting for changes in body weight and composition subjects maintaining weight 10% below their initial weight have lower daily energy expenditure. These compensatory changes in energy expenditure reflect changes in metabolic efficiency (ie adaptive thermogenesis) that oppose the maintenance of a body weight that is above or below the 'set' or 'preferred' body weight. There is a wide range of individual variability in the amount of weight gained per unit of excess energy consumed which is strongly influenced by the genetic make-up of the individual.

2.14 INTEGRATING INTAKE AND EXPENDITURE

In order to achieve long-term constancy of body weight, compensatory adjustments occur in both energy intake and energy expenditure. Body weight regulation involves physiologically-induced *autoregulatory* adjustments in energy intake and in energy expenditure, ie those beyond voluntary control. However, if there is a change of several kilograms in body weight there will be changes in appearance, the fit of clothes, exercise tolerance, and general wellbeing. The response is to control or attempt to control food intake or energy expenditure via changes in physical activity. In many individuals, the importance of such cognitive (conscious) controls over food intake and energy expenditure can be as important as non-conscious physiological regulations.

KEY POINTS

- Energy in foods is provided by the macronutrients (carbohydrate, proteins, fats) and alcohol. The average metabolizable energy of carbohydrate is 16 kJ/g (4 kcal/g), protein 17 kJ/g (4 kcal/g), fat 37 kJ/g (9 kcal/g) and alcohol 29 kJ/g (7 kcal/g)
- Energy balance is the difference between metabolizable energy intake and total energy expenditure
- The matching between energy intake and expenditure is poor over the short term, but (in most people) it is accurate over the long term

- Because day-to-day variability in energy intake is much greater than that of energy expenditure, the habitual energy requirement is best determined from total energy expenditure
- The mechanisms underlying long-term energy balance and weight regulation are not well known, but involve both involuntary controls as well as conscious alterations in lifestyle to correct unwanted changes in body weight
- Modern lifestyles have led to considerable changes in the foods eaten and in the amount of time spent on physical activity, leading to an environment in which it is more difficult to match energy intake and energy expenditure
- A high-fat (energy-dense) diet promotes weight gain because it promotes increased energy intake
- Undernutrition, including dieting, leads to a decrease in energy expenditure, in part because of the loss in body weight (and metabolically active tissues) and in part because of increased efficiency of metabolism
- Overnutrition leads to gain in body weight which is often less than predicted because of compensatory increases in energy expenditure – the magnitude of which is determined by the composition of the diet, the proportion of lean to fat tissue in the extra weight gained and by capacity of the individual to burn off excess calories through diet-induced thermogenesis

FURTHER READING

DoH 1991 Dietary Reference Values of Food Energy and Nutrients for the UK. Report on Health and Social Subjects, no. 41. Department of Health, London

Flatt JP 1995 Diet, lifestyle and weight maintenance. American Journal of Clinical Nutrition 62:820–836

Murgatroyd PR, Shetty PS, Prentice AM 1993 Techniques for the measurement of human energy expenditure: a practical guide. International Journal of Obesity 17:549–568

WEBSITES

Body composition
http://www.rowett.ac.uk/edu_web/sec_pup/body_comp.pdf
Energy expenditure
http://www.rowett.ac.uk/edu_web/sec_pup/energy_expenditure.pdf

CHAPTER 3

Food Consumption

OBJECTIVES

By the end of this chapter you should be able to:

- list the major food groups
- identify the main sources of nutrients in Western diets
- understand the purpose of additives in food processing
- describe the main types of natural toxins, pollutants and pathogenic agents
- appreciate the similarities and variability in food and nutrient patterns in different population groups and countries
- describe the different types of vegetarian diets
- identify the nutrients most likely to be lacking from vegetarian diets
- understand how the health of vegetarians/vegans differs from those of omnivores
- understand the social, psychological, geographic and economic factors determining food choices and diet patterns
- be aware of changing trends over time including novel foods

3.1 INTRODUCTION TO FOOD CONSUMPTION

In this chapter the major food groups in the diet are presented in terms of their nutrient and non-nutrient content including food additives and food toxins and pollutants. The variability of dietary patterns between countries and between subgroups in the population is discussed, with special reference to vegetarians; the factors that account for dietary variations, and changing trends in food intake patterns (including novel foods) over time are also examined.

3.2 MAJOR FOOD GROUPS IN THE WESTERN DIET

Western diets are composed of several food groups that provide all the nutrients and non-nutrients for optimum health, including cereals and cereal products (eg bread); vegetables and fruit; roots and tubers; milk and other

Table 3.1 Food intakes among British adults

Food group	Foods	g/day
Cereal	White bread	64
	Wholemeal bread	28
	Other bread	13
	Pasta and rice	34
	High-fibre breakfast cereals	15
	Other cereals	5
	Potatoes (not fried)	68
	All starchy foods	227
Dairy	Whole milk	162
	Reduced fat milk	62
	Cheese and dairy desserts	28
	All dairy products	253
Meat, fish, etc	Meat and poultry	165
	Eggs	25
	Fish and shell fish	30
	Nuts and pulses	18
	All meats and alternatives	238
Vegetables and fruit	Vegetables	143
	Fresh fruit	59
	Canned fruit and other fruit	77
	All vegetables and fruit	279

Data from Gregory et al 1990

dairy products; meats, fish, eggs and other sources of protein; fats and oils. The food intake patterns for British adults are shown in Table 3.1. The non-nutrients discussed in this chapter include those for which there is evidence for a beneficial effect on human health, as well as other non-nutrients in foods such as contaminants, allergens and food additives that do not have specific health benefits.

Nutritional importance of major foods and food products in the Western diet
Cereals and cereal products

The major cereals in the human diet are wheat and rice followed by maize, barley, oats and rye. Cereals are the staple foods in almost all populations. Carbohydrates form the major part of the cereal grain and consequently these are often referred to as carbohydrate foods. Cereals represent the most important plant foods in the human diet for their contribution to energy and carbohydrate intake and their micronutrient content. In developed countries, such as the UK, cereals provide approximately 30% of the energy intake whilst in developing countries they contribute as much as 70% or more. In the UK, cereals also provide about 10% of dietary fat, 25% of protein and 50% of available carbohydrates. They also make a significant contribution to dietary fibre as non-starch polysaccharides (NSP). They contribute over 40% and 30% of iron and folate intakes respectively – especially breakfast cereals which contribute 20% and 15% respectively.

Vegetables and fruit

These include a wide range of plant families and consist of any edible portion of the plant including roots, leaves, stems, buds, flowers and fruits. Some fruits (tomatoes, cucumbers, marrows and pumpkins) are commonly classified as vegetables while the fruits that are sweet are classified as fruits. In the context of the human diets, root crops are usually classified separately. Fruits tend to be high in potassium and low in sodium and are the most important source of vitamin C. Although fruits and vegetables are quite low in B vitamins generally, green leafy vegetables are a good source of folates. Vegetables and fruits are important contributors to the intake of dietary fibre. Also, fruits and vegetables are important sources of such non-nutrients as the phytoprotectants, carotenoids and anthocyanins (flavonoids in berries).

Roots and tubers

Roots and tubers are the underground organs of many plants:

- Root crops (eg turnips, beetroots): Most roots have high water content and tend to be rich in carbohydrates as free sugars (with small amounts of starch in mature organs). They are generally low in dietary fibre, protein and micronutrients.
- Tubers (eg potato): Tubers are not true roots but rather underground stems that store large quantities of carbohydrate – usually starch. The potato is a stem tuber native to the Andes. All contain large amounts of starch and significant amounts of vitamin C and their high levels of consumption makes them an important source.

Meat and meat products

Meat has comprised an important part of the human diet for a large part of our history and still is the centrepiece of most meals in developed countries, providing about 15% of total energy intakes. In many developing countries, non-animal-based sources of protein such as legumes are still dominant. In the US and the UK the most important meat sources are pigs, sheep and cattle. In the UK poultry (chicken) has now become the most popular meat source. Meat products such as sausages, salami and pork pies account for almost half of total meat consumption. In developed countries, meats are an important source of protein (contributing about 50% of the UK protein intake), total fat (about 20% of total fat in the UK diet) and saturated fat in the diet.

Fish

While fish catches worldwide are on the increase according to FAO (Food & Agriculture Organization of the UN), fish stocks are being depleted due to over-fishing. The main sea-food consumed is white fish, oily fish and sea-food invertebrates. Fish are an important source of good quality protein and are low in fat (except for the oily fish which provide a very good source of long-chain polyunsaturated fatty acids – PUFA). Fish are also a major source of iodine which has been accumulated from their environment. Also, they may be an important source of calcium (in fish with fine bones) and vitamin D.

Eggs

The most widely consumed eggs in the UK are hens' eggs. Lipids found in eggs are rich in phospholipids and cholesterol. The fatty acid profile shows a high proportion of polyunsaturated fatty acids to saturated fatty acids (high P:S ratio).

Milk (and other dairy products)

Cows provide the bulk of all milk consumed in the UK. Milk is an excellent source of many nutrients. The major protein in milk is casein, while lactalbumin and immunoglobulins are responsible for the transfer of maternal immunity to the young animal for a short period following birth. Milk from ruminant animals, such as the cow, contains a large proportion of short chain fatty acids produced from the fermentation of carbohydrates in the rumen. Milk and its products provide 10% of total energy intake in the UK, about a quarter of the saturated fat intake, and are excellent sources of many inorganic nutrients especially calcium and certain vitamins (both fat-soluble and water-soluble). Other dairy products include cheese, which contains, in a concentrated form, many of milk's nutrients, and yoghurt which is produced from the culturing of a mixture of milk and cream products with the lactic acid-producing bacteria, *Lactobacillus bulgaricus* and *Streptococcus thermophilus* and other bacterial cultures (eg *Lactobacillus acidophilus*, *Bifidobacteria*). The contribution of dairy products to the UK diet (and to that of many other Northern European countries) is very important. They can be an important source of calcium and riboflavin, especially in children and adolescents.

Fats and oils

Fats are solid at room temperature (due to a high relative concentration of saturated fatty acids) while oils are liquid and usually of plant origin, either from the flesh of the fruit (olive oil) or from the seed (sunflower and linseed). They have a higher concentration of unsaturated fatty acids. Lipids that are isolated from animal products tend to be solid fats such butter, lard and suet. Margarine is made from highly unsaturated fats such as sunflower, which have beneficial effects on serum cholesterol. In many countries, including the UK, margarines are required by legislation to be fortified with vitamins A and D so that they are nutritionally equivalent to butter.

Food sources of nutrients and health related non-nutrients

The importance of specific foods to the nutrient intake of a group in the population depends both on the nutrient composition and the frequency and level of consumption. In the UK population cereals and cereal products,

Table 3.2 Typical values for macronutrient content of selected foods (% of wet weight)

Food	Protein	Fat	Carbohydrate
Apple	0.4	0.1	11.8
Runner beans: raw	1.6	0.4	3.2
Runner beans: boiled	1.2	0.5	2.3
Beef	22.5	4.3	0.0
White bread	7.9	1.6	46.1
Hard cheese	24.9	34.5	0.1
Roast chicken	27.3	7.5	0
Baked cod	21.4	1.2	Tr
Sweetcorn	4.2	2.3	19.6
Egg	9.0	Tr	Tr
Haddock, steamed	20.9	0.6	0
Whole milk	3.3	3.9	4.5
Peas	5.8	0.7	13.8
Pork	21.8	4.0	0.0
Potatoes, new boiled	1.5	0.3	17.8
Rice: white, raw	7.3	3.6	85.8
Rice: cooked	2.6	1.3	30.9
Sardines, canned, drained	21.5	9.6	0
White wheat flour	9.4	1.3	77.7

Data with permission from: Food Standards Agency 2002 McCance and Widdowson's The composition of foods, 6th summary edn

including cakes and biscuits, are the important sources of carbohydrate. Meat, fish, eggs and dairy products are the main sources of protein and fat, whilst fruits and vegetables supply dietary fibre and various vitamins and minerals. Table 3.2 summarizes the macronutrient content of selected foods.

Fruits, vegetables, grains, legumes, nuts and teas are rich sources of phytonutrients (see chapter 5). Phytonutrients (also called phytoprotectants), while not regarded strictly as nutrients, may have certain health benefits. They are extremely varied in their chemical composition, the plants in which they are found and their putative beneficial effects. There are tens of thousands of phytonutrients in plants that have not yet been tested for health benefits. A diet rich in a variety of plant foods (of different colours) ensures a good intake of phytonutrients. Polyphenols are a group of phytonutrients present in onion, apple, tea, red wine, red grapes, grape juice, strawberries, raspberries, blueberries, cranberries, and certain nuts; they are also known as secondary plant metabolites. Much of the total antioxidant activity of fruits and vegetables is related to their phenolic content.

Contribution of macronutrients to energy needs

The energy needs of the body are provided by the three macronutrients: carbohydrate, fat and protein. Alcohol is the other energy source. Carbohydrate and fat are the primary fuel sources and for this purpose they can largely be used interchangeably.

Patterns of consumption of the macronutrients have changed radically from our ancient ancestors where the relative contribution to energy of these macronutrients has been estimated as 34% protein, 45% carbohydrate and 21% fat, contrasting to that of a typical current Western diet of 15% protein, 46% carbohydrate and 39% fat. In the developing countries such as in Asia and Africa protein levels are lower (10%), carbohydrates higher (60–70%) and fats considerably lower (20%) (Table 3.3). The currently acceptable (ie healthy) macronutrient distribution ranges (AMDR) are 10–15% of energy from protein, 25–30% of energy from fat and 45–65% of energy from carbohydrate.

KEY POINTS

- Food groups that provide nutrients in the diet are cereals and cereal products; vegetables and fruit; roots and tubers; milk and other dairy products; meats, fish, eggs and other sources of protein; fats and oils
- Non-nutrients in food include those considered to have a potentially beneficial effect on human health such as natural phytoprotectants, as well as food additives that do not have specific health benefits, and toxins and pollutants that are detrimental to health
- In a typical Western diet the percentage of total energy provided by protein is about 15%, carbohydrate 46% and fat 39%
- In developing countries these percentages are typically protein 10%, carbohydrate 60–70% and fat 20%
- Current guidelines for the contribution to energy intake are 10–15% for protein, 45–46% for carbohydrate and 25–30% for fat

3.3 EFFECTS OF FOOD PROCESSING AND STORAGE

Types of food processing

Foods are processed either to improve their palatability and digestibility or to extend their lifetime before deterioration reduces sensory or microbial quality to a level where they can no longer be consumed. The methods vary in the temperatures used and in the contact with water or oil as heat transfer media. Other variables that affect the rate of destruction of nutrients are the presence of oxygen, light and the pH of the aqueous phase.

Cooking processes such as roasting, boiling, baking, frying and fermentation have been used for thousands of years. Preservation processes such as salting or drying in air have also been applied for hundreds of years. Many of these methods result in losses of nutrients through leaching of water soluble vitamins or oxidation, especially of vitamin C. Modern industrial processes have been developed to maintain or improve flavour, texture, and nutritional or other quality aspects. Preservation techniques have been improved so as to increase the shelf life of products, whilst maintaining optimal quality. These include pasteurization, canning, refrigeration and freezing, freeze drying, irradiation and high pressure processing. The modern methods result in less loss of nutrients. Industrial processing techniques are focusing more on producing healthy foods without loss of palatability, such as foods with lower fat or salt content.

Table 3.3 Mean energy intake and macronutrient energy intakes in 14 EU member states

Country	Energy (MJ/day)	% Energy		
		Carbohydrate	Protein	Fat
Northern Europe				
Belgium	13.2	38.7	14.3	41.8
Denmark	10.2	43.5	14.5	37.0
Finland	9.0	47.7	16.1	33.8
France	8.6	38.2	17.4	38.9
Germany	9.6	39.2	15.1	40.7
Ireland	9.4	47.8	14.8	35.2
Netherlands	9.7	43.6	15.4	37.5
Sweden	8.8	46.0	15.0	36.5
UK	8.6	42.3	14.7	38.4
Southern Europe				
Greece	7.6	44.0	14.2	40.3
Italy	8.7	47.5	16.9	32.6
Portugal	9.7	49.1	18.0	28.5
Spain	8.9	40.2	19.6	38.0
Africa developed	12.4	66.0	10.4	23.6
Africa developing	10.1	72.0	10.0	18.0
Asia developed	11.7	58.2	13.3	28.5
Asia developing	11.3	66.2	10.3	23.5

Source: British Journal of Nutrition 1999 Food-based dietary guidelines – a staged approach.
Vol 81 (Suppl 2). Africa & Asia calculated from FAO Food balance sheets 2003

Food additives

The use of additives in food in the UK is strictly controlled by legislation to protect the health of the consumer and to prevent fraud. Additives are allowed for specific functions (antioxidant, colour etc) and are restricted to those listed in the regulations.

Preservatives are substances added to foods to inhibit microbial spoilage. Common foods including meats, cheeses, baked goods, fruit juices and soft drinks are likely to include preservatives. Even if sterile foods are produced initially by thermal processing, infection with bacteria, fungi and yeasts can occur in these foods, which are often not consumed at one sitting, and pre-servatives are required to extend the shelf life of the products. Sorbic acid, benzoic acid, sulfites, thiabendazole, nitrites and biphenyl are amongst the substances approved for use as food preservatives.

Flavours added to food may be natural components derived from raw materials such as spices by physical processes such as extraction or distilla-tion. A range of essential oils, including clove oil and orange oil, are widely used for flavouring foods. Synthetic flavours are also used.

Colours. The classes of natural or nature-identical colourings used for food include carotenoids, chlorophyll, anthocyanins and betalaines. Besides these, some synthetic compounds are allowed for addition to food. Most concern has been expressed about tartrazine.

Sweeteners. Since the sugars present are significant contributors to the calorific content of many foods, the food industry has developed a range of zero-calorie or low-calorie, high-potency sweeteners, including aspartame, saccharin, acesulfame K and cyclamates. Sucralose was developed as a non-nutritive sweetener in the 1970s as a derivative of sucrose with excellent flavour and stability. Sugar alcohols including sorbitol, mannitol and xylitol have comparable sweetness and about the same calorific content as sucrose but they are absorbed more slowly from the digestive tract and do not raise postprandial blood sugar and insulin levels and are therefore suitable for sweetening diabetic foods.

Processing aids facilitate food processing by acting as chelating agents, enzymes, antifoaming agents, catalysts, solvents, lubricants or propellants. They are not consumed as food ingredients by themselves, and are used during food processing. Residues of the processing aids may be present in the finished product. It is a legal requirement that they do not present any risk to human health.

Toxic components formed by processing

Processing may lead to losses of nutrients, and may also lead to the formation of toxic components under certain conditions, such as *acrylamide* (2-propenamide). This is found in fried and baked goods with highest levels in crisps, crisp bread, chips and fried potatoes and is a probable human carcinogen.

3.4 FOOD TOXINS AND POLLUTANTS

Toxins in foods are substances that cause harmful effects when foods are consumed in typical amounts. Food components may cause toxic effects within hours, days or weeks of consumption of the food. They may have mutagenic or carcinogenic effects in which an inheritable change in the genetic information of a cell may lead to cancer or other disease states over a period of years. Close monitoring of foods by Government agencies helps to prevent chemical toxins reaching levels at which harmful effects occur, and pathogenic bacteria are much more common causes of human disease than chemical toxins. A few examples follow:

Natural plant toxins

Solanine is a glycoalkaloid which commonly occurs at low levels in potatoes but may be found at high levels in green potatoes, causing gastric pain followed by nausea, vomiting and respiration difficulties.

Marine toxins

Shellfish such as clams or mussels may feed on dinoflagellate algae, which reach high concentrations in red tides that develop in seawater. The algae produce a toxin that accumulates in the flesh of the shellfish and can cause paralytic shellfish poisoning.

Fungal toxins (Mycotoxins)

Many species of fungi produce metabolites that are toxic. Aflatoxins occur in mouldy grain, soybeans or nuts and are carcinogenic at very low levels of intake. They can be transmitted to humans via animals in meat or eggs. Aflatoxin B_1 is one of the most potent chemical carcinogens known. The toxins remain in the contaminated food even after the mould has been removed or has died and are quite stable during normal food processing operations.

Pollutants

Many pollutants are potentially found in foods but are continually monitored. The maximum levels of many in plant and animal products are specified in regulations to ensure that any residues that occur are unlikely to pose a risk to health. These include pesticides, antibiotics, hormones, heavy metals, polychlorinated and polybrominated biphenyls (PCBs and PBBs) and radioactive fallout.

Pathogenic agents

Pathogenic agents are a very common cause of food poisoning. These include animal infections transmissible to man (zoonoses) by consumption of meat or fish, which can be bacterial, viral, fungal, helminthic and protozoan species; and other contaminants of food, which may cause infections of man, such as *Salmonella*, *Staphylococcus* and *Clostridium botulinum*.

Viral infections

Viruses have no cellular structure and possess only one type of nucleic acid (either RNA or DNA) wrapped in a protein coat. They cannot multiply in foods, but food handlers with dirty hands or utensils may allow foods to become contaminated. Viruses can subsequently multiply in the intestinal tract by using the host cells for replication. Viral infections often have incubation periods of up to several weeks compared to several hours for bacterial infections.

Hepatitis A, of the genus *Enterovirus*, causes symptoms of anorexia, fever, malaise, nausea and vomiting followed after a few days by symptoms of liver damage. Poliomyelitis is another enterovirus that can be transmitted by contaminated food such as milk. However, it is now virtually eradicated in developed countries.

Prions

A prion protein is a small protein molecule that occurs mainly in the brain cell membrane. It differs in conformation from most proteins since it occurs mainly in a flattened form, which is heat and enzyme resistant. Prions are believed to be the infectious agent causing humans to develop new variant Creutzfeldt–Jakob disease (vCJD). Cases of this disease were first reported in the early 1990s. This disease is believed to have developed in humans following consumption of meat from cattle affected by BSE (bovine spongiform encephalopathy), which is a fatal brain disease that affected large numbers of cattle in the UK in the 1980s and 1990s, but was reduced after 1993 by the removal of meat and bone meal from cattle feed concentrates and by the slaughter of large numbers of animals. vCJD presents itself as psychiatric disorders including anxiety, depression, and withdrawal but it develops over a period of months into forgetfulness and memory disturbance. A cerebellar syndrome develops with gait and limb ataxia and eventually death.

Helminths and nematodes

Helminths and nematodes are flatworms and roundworms, which develop as parasites in humans following consumption of contaminated water or food, especially meat or raw salads. Liver flukes and tapeworms are the most common helminths.

KEY POINTS

- Foods are processed to improve palatability and digestibility or to extend their shelf life
- Traditional cooking processes include roasting, boiling, baking, frying, and fermentation and preservation processes include salting and air drying
- Losses of water-soluble vitamins may occur by leaching into processing water. Vitamins may also be lost by reaction with oxygen or by thermal degradation. Vitamin C and thiamin are particularly susceptible to degradation
- Modern industrial processes include pasteurization, canning, refrigeration and freezing, freeze drying, irradiation and high pressure processing, and generally result in fewer losses
- Frying or grilling of foods may lead to the formation of toxic components in some products
- Food additives include preservatives, processing aids, flavours, colours, sweeteners
- Natural plant toxins, marine toxins, fungal toxins and pollutants may contaminate food, but they rarely occur in foods sold in Western Europe at levels which are harmful to health
- Growth of pathogenic organisms including bacteria, yeasts and moulds may cause food poisoning
- Processing of foods, eg heat treatment, reduces the levels of many pathogenic organisms, so that the foods may be consumed safely
- Under certain conditions, processing of foods may cause the formation of potentially toxic compounds, although effects in humans have rarely been demonstrated

Examples of variations in diet
Comparison of developing with developed countries

Diets in the developing world are very different from those in the rich countries, although there is some evidence of convergence between the two. The diets of the former tend to be characterized by lower total calorie intake, more calories from cereals and roots and tubers, less diversity in terms of food groups consumed, less animal source foods (and less fat), less processed food and less food eaten away from home. Many of these differences are explained by socioeconomic factors, but there is considerable variation in consumption patterns even accounting for such factors.

Variation within the UK

There is considerable variation between regions with the lowest and highest levels of consumption of particular foods. For example the highest consumption of fruit is in London and the lowest in Scotland, whereas the highest consumption of meat products, bread, confectionery and sugar and preserves is in Wales and the lowest in London. The low levels of vegetable and fruit consumption recorded in Scotland are the result of a number of historical and economic factors, but this observation is clearly linked to the current high levels of cardiovascular disease.

A number of important variations are also evident in relation to income. Low income households consume less than the all-household average amounts of fresh fruits and fresh vegetables (excluding potatoes) and less skimmed milk, cheese, fish, fruit juices, breakfast cereals, alcoholic drinks and confectionery. They consume more liquid whole milk, eggs, fats and oils, sugar and preserves, fresh potatoes, frozen and canned vegetables, bread and beverages than the average for all households.

Vegetarianism as an example of variation between individuals

Because of the popularity of vegetarianism in the UK, this variation is described more fully here. It can be defined as avoiding the consumption of meat or flesh food. The commonplace use of the term vegetarian is to describe someone who does not eat animal flesh (meat, poultry, fish) but who includes eggs and dairy products in their diet. The terms *ovo-vegetarian*, *lacto-vegetarian* and *ovo-lacto-vegetarian* describe subjects who consume eggs, milk or both respectively. The term *vegan* is used to describe subjects who consume no food of animal origin. Veganism is a way of life that avoids the exploitation of animals. Besides avoiding food of animal origin, vegans will not use products that have been derived from animals, such as leather, wool and vaccines. Fruitarianism is an extreme form of veganism where dietary intake is restricted to raw fruits, nuts and berries, a practice which has resulted in severe malnutrition in children. Macrobiotic diets consist of relatively large amounts of brown rice, accompanied by smaller amounts of fruits, vegetables and pulses.

The risk of nutrient deficiency is greatest in childhood as requirements relative to body weight are greater and children are unable to exert the same degree of control over what they eat compared with adults. There have been several reports of severe protein-energy malnutrition as well as deficiencies of iron, vitamins B_{12} and D in infants and toddlers fed inappropriate vegetarian diets. Older children are less susceptible to the dietary strictures imposed by their parents as they are able to forage for food at home independently. However, children can be brought up healthily on both vegan and vegetarian diets with sufficient care. The health and diet of adult Western vegetarian groups generally appears to be good, and certain aspects of a vegan diet, notably the low saturated fat and high dietary fibre content, may offer certain advantages to the health of adults.

People follow vegetarian diets for religious, health and ethical reasons. Vegetarianism is widely practised by Hindus, Buddhists, Seventh Day Adventists, Jains and Rastafarians. The leading reason currently given in the UK for following a vegetarian diet is the belief that the diet is healthier, reinforced by a series of food scares related to the intensive production of poultry, meat and fish. Other reasons are that it is wrong and cruel to eat animals. Some also argue that it is better for the environment to depend upon plant foods for our nutritional needs because it takes less land to feed a family on food of plant origin. The popularity of vegetarian diets has increased over the last few decades and most international airlines and restaurants now offer vegetarian options. Most of the dietary and nutritional studies of vegans and vegetarians have been carried out on members of the Vegan and Vegetarian Societies and the Seventh Day Adventists Church and they may not be truly representative of all vegetarians.

Dietary diversity is important in maintaining the adequacy of a vegetarian diet as the nutrient density of plant foods is often lower than those of meat, fish, eggs and milk. In practice, there are surprisingly few qualitative differences in the intake of proximate nutrients between vegetarians/vegans compared with omnivores in developed countries (Table 3.4). Energy intakes appear to be similar to non-vegetarians although some reports, which have estimated energy intake by food frequency questionnaire, suggest that energy intakes are lower among vegan and vegetarians.

Protein intakes are slightly lower in vegetarians than in omnivores, typically supplying about 12% of the energy intake as opposed to 15% in omnivores but these intakes support nitrogen balance and the protein quality of vegetarian diets differs little from that of diets containing meat, as the constituent amino acids in the different plant proteins mutually complement each other. The intake of complex carbohydrates and dietary fibre is generally high in vegan/vegetarian diets owing to their higher consumption of cereals compared with omnivores. Sugar intakes on the other hand are similar. The proportion of energy derived from fat is only slightly lower in vegetarians/vegans than in omnivores and is typically in the region of 30–37% of the dietary energy. Saturated fatty acid intakes are slightly lower in vegetarians but markedly lower in vegans. Cholesterol is virtually absent from plant foods, which also provide small amounts of phytosterols ($\sim 0.5\,g/day$) that inhibit the reabsorption of cholesterol from the intestinal tract.

Meat and fish provide several nutrients that are scarce or absent from common foods of plant origin and these include iodine, taurine, vitamin B_{12},

Table 3.4 Proximate nutrient intakes in vegetarians, vegans and omnivores

	Energy (MJ/day)	% energy				
		Protein	Carbohydrate	Sugar	Fat	Fibre (g/d)
European men (UK)						
Omnivores	10.3	14.4	42	19	38	26
Vegetarians	9.4	12	48	21	37	34
Vegans	9.2	11.7	50	21	34	44
European women (UK)						
Omnivores	7.28	15.5	43	20	38	20
Vegetarians	7.67	12.6	46		37	33
Vegans	7.35	10.8	53	21	34	36
South Asian (UK)						
Men	9.3	12.6	47		38	23
Women	6.1	11.7	54	15	37	16

Data derived from: Draper et al 1993, Miller et al 1988, Reddy & Sanders 1992

vitamin D and long-chain polyunsaturated fatty acids. Eggs, dairy food and rice are poor sources of iron and the availability of iron from foods of plant origin is low compared with that from meat. Good sources of iron for vegetarians include wheat, pulses, dark green vegetables (especially low oxalate varieties), fortified cereals, dried fruit and iron cooking equipment. Vegetarians are more prone to iron deficiency than meat eaters. Haemoglobin concentrations are generally normal in vegans and vegetarians but serum ferritin concentrations are low ($<12\mu g/L$).

Vitamin B_{12} deficiency has been reported in both vegans and vegetarians, presenting with neurological signs of deficiency because their high intake of folate masks the megaloblastic anaemia of vitamin B_{12} deficiency. Elevated plasma total homocysteine concentration has been reported in a high proportion of vegan men and in a smaller proportion of vegetarian men, which may increase the risk of cardiovascular disease. Dietary vitamin B_{12} deficiency in an asymptomatic mother can also result in severe neurological signs of deficiency in the offspring. Vegans and vegetarians who only consume small amounts of dairy products and eggs need to be vigilant regarding their intake of vitamin B_{12}. There are a variety of B_{12} fortified foods available including soya milks, textured vegetable protein, margarine and yeast extracts, but some vegans are reluctant to use these products as they regard them as unnatural.

Docosahexaenoic acid (22:6 n-3; DHA) is believed to play an important role in the development of the retina and the central nervous system. Vegan diets are devoid of DHA and the levels of DHA in blood, arterial and breast milk lipids are approximately only one-third of the level of those found in omnivores. Products acceptable to vegans, fortified with an algal source of DHA, are now available.

Vegetarians who consume milk and cheese regularly have relatively high intakes of calcium but vegans tend to have low intakes of calcium and absorption of calcium is inhibited by phytic acid in legumes and unrefined cereals. A high prevalence of rickets has been noted in children reared on macrobiotic diets but not among the white vegetarian population. Vitamin D acceptable to vegetarians can be provided as ergocalciferol in fortified foods and supplements.

Several studies report shorter pregnancies and lower birth weights in vegetarians. According to the fetal origins hypothesis a lower birth weight and head circumference may increase risk the of developing diabetes and cardiovascular disease in later life. Children will grow and develop quite normally on a diet consisting of plenty of bread and vegetables with minimal amounts of milk and meat. Lower rates of growth particularly in the first five years of life have been reported in children reared on vegan and macrobiotic diets because the energy density of some plant foods is very low and some vegetarian diets may be so bulky that they restrict the energy intake of young children, but catch-up growth occurs by the age of about 10 years. The significance of slightly slower rates of growth is debatable, but a small fraction of vegan children do show evidence of impaired growth. It needs to be more widely recognized that severe nutritional deficiencies do occur in children reared on inappropriate vegetarian and vegan diets.

In summary, the health of Western vegetarian groups is generally good. Serum cholesterol is 20% lower in vegans than in omnivores with intermediate values in vegetarians. Blood pressure is lower in vegetarians, attributed to a higher consumption of potassium from fruit and vegetables. Vegetarians and vegans are lighter in weight and have lower age-standardized mortality rates compared with the general population but a large proportion of this variability can be accounted for by lifestyle factors other than diet, such as smoking and alcohol use. The death rate for ischaemic heart disease is significantly lower in vegetarians but cancer incidence is similar between vegetarians and omnivores when other lifestyle factors such as smoking and alcohol intake are taken into account. In contrast, elevated homocysteine has been found in vegetarians and vegans, which may increase the risk of cardiovascular disease.

3.6 FACTORS IN DIETARY VARIATIONS

Of all the animal and plant species that could be safely consumed, humans choose from a relatively narrow range of species. Those which may be considered a delicacy by some groups are rejected as inedible by others. An individual's food choice at any given time will be influenced by what they consider to be 'food', whether it is available (either physically accessible or affordable) and appropriate according to a variety of sociocultural factors, ideas, beliefs and attitudes as well as psychological factors and their level of hunger or satiety. The main factors in dietary variation for developed and developing countries are shown in Figure 3.1.

Biological and physiological factors

Age, gender, pregnancy, lactation and activity patterns all affect nutritional requirements, but humans are often unable to perceive their specific needs and respond appropriately. If the consumption of a particular food is not pleasant this will limit the amount of that food which is eaten. This innate

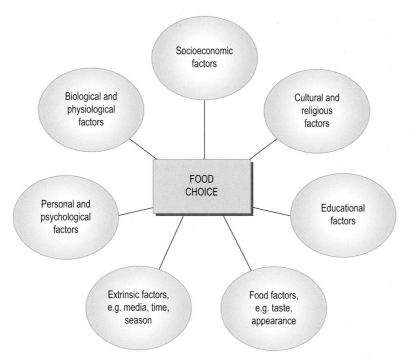

Figure 3.1 The main factors determining dietary variation.

mechanism (sensory specific satiety) ensures that humans eat a varied diet and are therefore more likely to meet their requirements for all nutrients but is more problematic when surrounded by a huge variety of different, highly palatable, food items (see chapter 2).

Economic factors

The availability of food is influenced by (a) geography, season and factors such as food preservation and distribution systems which affect physical availability and (b) the ability of the individual to acquire what is available. As income levels increase, families spend more on food, although as a proportion of overall expenditures food is likely to decline in importance (called Engels' Law). This occurs within a fairly narrow range in an industrialized country, such as the UK, where the range is from 15% to 29% of reported expenditure between low income and high income households. However in developing countries the differences may be far more dramatic. The cost of utilities – fuel, water, clothing, transport, rent – also affects food choices. The budgets of low income households leave very little room for manoeuvre and often food is the most flexible element of expenditure. Income has a marked influence on the type of foods eaten. Internationally, as income levels rise people rely less on cereals and roots/tubers and purchase more animal source foods, fruits and vegetables. Food prices affect food consumption and diets, and paid employment may cause men and women to work outside the home with less food prepared at home and more food consumed away from home, affecting the types of food which are eaten.

Cultural and religious factors

Eating practices, in terms of food types and food preparation, presentation and serving, is strongly influenced by culture and religion. Food appropriate for one occasion or a particular gender or age group, may not be appropriate for others. Food has many important social uses which vary from society to society and over time, and include:

Communication

An invitation to share food or drink, in a range of different settings, is widely used to initiate and maintain personal relationships.

Identity

The saying 'Tell me what you eat, and I will tell you who you are' is attributed to Brillat-Savarin and encapsulates this phenomenon. The existence of clearly defined 'food rules' may play an important role in reinforcing 'in-group' identity, with considerable importance in the context of religion.

Ethics and religion

As food must be eaten every day it serves as a constant reminder of what we believe. In recent years vegetarianism and veganism have become increasingly popular in the UK (see above) and for many people this choice is based on ethical concerns about the exploitation of farm animals. Religious food rules not only enhance the spiritual life of the individual but also enhance allegiance to a community of believers.

To prevent and treat illness

Popular beliefs about the links between diet, health and disease are shaped by their cultural context and consequently vary in different parts of the world. Ideas vary geographically, and also change over time. Despite an enormous growth in the understanding of physiology and the origins of disease, popular advice in the early 19th century in England was still based on the dietetic works of Hippocrates and ideas about the effects of diet on humoral balance attributed to Galen and Avicenna. The concept of 'balance' as a key to health is central to these and in relation to diet focus particularly on the 'heating' and 'cooling' effects attributed to foods, regardless of the actual temperature of the food when eaten. Some conditions and diseases are associated with an excess of 'cold' or 'heat' and treatment includes foods with the opposite characteristic to restore health. These ideas about the heating and cooling effects of foods are found in the classical health systems of the Indian sub-continent (Ayurvedic-Hindu and Unani-Islamic medicine) as well as in traditional Chinese medicine, and are still widely practised in these communities.

Personal and psychological factors

Personal factors, including emotions, personality, self-esteem and self-efficacy, as well as beliefs and attitudes play an important role in shaping eating habits.

Food becomes associated with emotion from the very start of life, when feeding provides a pleasurable experience of comfort, security and well-being, as well as satiety. Throughout childhood, humans learn to associate particular foods with feelings related to the circumstances in which they were eaten. Thus feelings of pleasure may be associated with foods given as a reward, or eaten on special occasions with much-loved people whilst negative feelings may be felt with foods used as a punishment or which had to be eaten because of financial hardship. A response to stress, loneliness and anxiety may be to choose particular foods that provide comfort through positive associations. The hoarding of food for security is often seen as a response to past experiences of food insecurity. Food also provides a useful vehicle for demonstrating emotions such as anger and protest and may elicit very powerful feelings in the bystanders. The refusal to eat is a particularly powerful weapon, whether that is in the context of a child refusing to eat because they are angry or attention-seeking or a politically motivated hunger striker.

Attitude and belief factors

Health beliefs that underpin eating behaviour have focused on three particular aspects:

Perceptions of risk

People find it very difficult to assess the relative risk of different diet-related health threats, particularly in the face of frequent 'food scares'. These risk perceptions are powerful drivers of food choice and are influenced by trust in government, the food industry and scientists, and also by the accuracy of the information contained in food labels and in media reporting.

Perceptions of effectiveness of dietary advice

Coverage of nutritional topics in the popular media is frequently adversarial, where a topic is debated by two 'experts' with opposing views which can confuse people. Dietary advice may change as scientific understanding unfolds.

Belief that benefits outweigh the costs

Perceptions of the behaviour that is considered to be the 'norm' in an individual's particular social group and the extent to which they feel bound to comply with that 'norm' or to go against that norm, may be important determinants of food choice.

Educational factors

People who have more knowledge about nutrition tend to have better diets. However just giving people more information about food and health does not necessarily result in a change to healthier eating habits. The practical difficulties of implementing change (access to affordable, healthy food) and the social barriers to changing eating patterns (lack of support from family, friends and neighbours) will result in apparently insurmountable difficulties when the benefits of making changes are weighed up against the costs.

Food factors (taste and appearance)

People are generally cautious when encountering foods for the first time (neophobic) and repeated exposure and consumption of a range of different foods in early childhood plays an important part in establishing a varied diet in later life. A range of senses (vision, smell, hearing etc) contribute to our perception of the appearance, texture and flavour of foods. Whether or not we like them depends on our expectations of how that food should be, our memories of past experiences, and the context in which the food is served. Finally our level of hunger will determine whether we accept and consume the food item.

There are four basic taste qualities – salty, sweet, sour, bitter – and the experience of taste is also influenced by the smell of food. Infants have an innate preference for sweet tastes, whilst a preference for salty foods does not appear until later in the first year of life and is more susceptible to modification by experience. Ageing is often associated with marked losses in sensitivity to taste which can contribute to a decline in the enjoyment of food by older people. Perception of texture also makes a major contribution to the overall acceptability of the food. Socially and culturally learned expectations play a role in evaluating texture. Awareness of the sensory attributes of food which appeal to consumers is of major importance to food manufacturers.

Extrinsic factors

Advertising is a very powerful influence on food choice, especially for highly processed and packaged foods. Some groups of the population may be much more susceptible to this influence and there has been particular concern about the impact on children. Advertising also contributes to the creation of social norms, projecting images about what 'people do' and offering images of people with whom the audience might want to identify. The types of foods that are advertised are often high in fat and simple sugars and the emphasis on the promotion of these types of foods in contrast to the low level of marketing of fruit and vegetables is also considered to have a distorting effect on food habits.

Seasonality

In parts of the world where food marketing is not well developed, local availability is a key determinant of food consumption. In rich countries, there are fewer and fewer seasonal food items as foods are sourced from all corners of the globe.

3.7 CHANGING DIETARY PATTERNS

Globally diets are changing due to population movements, food trade and employment patterns. The large scale rural–urban and international migration seen around the world in the second half of the 20th century has been accompanied by major changes in eating habits as people have adapted to their new environments. Access to familiar foods, economic factors and food preparation facilities contribute to changes in both the eating habits of international migrants and of the host community. The strength of individual factors may affect their resistance to change. The dietary changes that are made first usually involve the adoption of foods that are convenient, affordable and do not clash with religious or cultural beliefs. Also the more widespread employment of women and increased affluence have led to increased demand for and production of pre-prepared convenience foods.

Over the past 50 years global food supply systems have been transformed, through changes in agriculture, food technology and transport. Throughout history foods have 'migrated' and been incorporated into the diets of people thousands of miles away – the tomato and potato, originally from America, transformed the cuisines of Europe. These dietary changes have sometimes had huge social consequences, as in the case of sugar and the slave trade or the development of the Irish dependence on the potato and subsequent impact of the potato famine. What is different about the changes in the past 50 years is the pace and scale of change. A relatively small number of companies now dominate the world food markets, affecting every aspect of the route from farm to consumer. Supermarkets place contracts with distant suppliers to enable previously seasonal foods to be available all year round. The UK's food manufacturing sector is also highly concentrated. In 1995, three companies (Unilever, Cadbury Schweppes and Associated British Foods) dominated UK food manufacturing, and half the world's top 100 food sector companies are US owned. It has been suggested that sophisticated systems of contracts and specifications and tight managerial control enable the retailer rather than the primary food producer or consumer to control the entire supply chain. Selection of foods which are *acceptable* to an individual increasingly takes place in a context where *availability* is substantially influenced by the food industry and food retailers.

Examples of variation in diets over time
The UK

World War II and its aftermath had a significant effect on the UK diet. While many foods such as fruits and meat were restricted, others such as foods rich in starch including potatoes and wholemeal brown bread (known as national bread) were increased. From 1954, consumers were able to return to their pre-war diets, higher in butter, sugar, fresh meat and white bread. The 50-year trend shows a marked decline in total bread consumption. Recent changes in the pattern of milk products in the UK include a substantial demand for low-fat and skimmed milk, and butter has largely been replaced by margarines and low-fat spreads and vegetable oils since the early 1980s. There has been a huge rise in the consumption of chicken over the last 50 years in the UK and it has become the most common form of dietary protein. Overall, fish, fruit and vegetable consumption have not changed appreciably in the last 50 years in the UK. There has been a decline in intakes of brassica vegetables including cabbage, cauliflower and Brussels sprouts as well as the traditional root vegetables, while there has been an increase in salad vegetables and frozen vegetables.

Novel foods

'Novel foods' are foods or food ingredients that do not have a significant history of consumption in the European Union before 1997. Most of these foods are now known as genetically modified or GM foods. These are crop plants such as corn, canola, potatoes, and soybean that have been genetically modified to improve characteristics such as crop yield, hardiness and uniformity, insect and virus resistance, and herbicide tolerance.

An example of this is a corn plant with a gene that makes it resistant to insect attack. With this technology it is possible to speed up the breeding of new, improved crop varieties, with characteristics such as drought resistance, increased shelf life and higher nutrient content, and to introduce completely new genetic information, for example from bacteria or animals into plants. Despite the potential of this technology lack of trust in government sources with respect to information on food safety has resulted in the slower adoption of GM foods in Europe compared with the US.

Other novel foods include 'functional foods'. A functional food is one claiming to have additional benefits other than nutritional value, for example a margarine that contains a cholesterol-lowering ingredient. A functional food may be a food in which one of the components has been naturally enhanced through special growing conditions; to which a component has been added to provide benefits; from which a component has been removed so that the food has less adverse health effects (eg the reduction of saturated fatty acids); in which the nature of one or more components has been chemically modified to improve health (eg the hydrolysed protein in infant formulas to reduce the likelihood of allergenicity); or in which the bioavailability of one or more components has been increased to provide greater absorption of a beneficial component.

KEY POINTS

- The factors that influence diet are biological and physiological, economic, cultural and religious, personal and psychological, attitude and beliefs, educational, food taste, appearance and texture, advertising, and seasonality
- Vegetarianism is a popular dietary variation that is followed for religious, ethical or health reasons
- Diets high in fruit and vegetables can be bulky and low in energy and so vegetarians tend to have a lower body weight than omnivores

- Vegetarians are at increased risk of iron deficiency anaemia and of vitamin B_{12} deficiency
- Long chain n-3 fatty acids important for the development of the retina and central nervous system are absent from vegan diets
- As intakes of saturated fatty acids are much lower and cholesterol is absent in vegan diets plasma cholesterol concentrations are 20% lower than in meat-eaters
- The incidence of ischaemic heart disease is lower in vegetarians but that of cancer does not differ
- Dietary patterns are different between developing and developed countries, between countries and between regions, and change over time
- While nutrient intakes have remained remarkably constant over the last 50 years, there have been changes in food consumption in the UK and other countries
  These include more low-fat spreads and margarines and less butter, more low fat and skimmed milk and less full fat milk, more fruit juice, a decrease in certain vegetables (eg swedes, turnips and Brussels sprouts) but an increase in salad vegetables and mushrooms
- The production of novel foods, including genetically modified and functional foods, is increasing

FURTHER READING

Fieldhouse P 1995 Food and nutrition: customs and culture. Chapman Hall, London

MacBeth H 1997 Food preferences and taste: continuity and change. Berghahn Books, Oxford

Meiselman H L, Macfie H J H (eds) 1996 Food choice, acceptance and consumption. Blackie Academic and Professional, London

WEBSITES

Department for Environment, Food and Rural Affairs
www.defra.gov.uk
Food Standards Agency
www.food.gov.uk
European Union
http://europa.eu
Food and Agriculture Organization
www.fao.org
UK Vegetarian Society
http://www.vegsoc.org/health/
British Nutrition Foundation
http://www.nutrition.org.uk/information/dietandhealth/vegetarian.html

CHAPTER 4

Main Dietary Components

OBJECTIVES

By the end of this chapter you should be able to:

- describe structure and associated functions of carbohydrates, fats and protein
- summarize the main features of aerobic and anaerobic metabolism of carbohydrate, fat and protein
- explain the regulation of metabolism of these major dietary components
- explain mechanisms for integration of fat, carbohydrate and protein metabolism, and response to specific dietary circumstances
- explain the glycaemic index in the context of health, with reference to specific foods
- discuss the health effects of dietary fibre
- explain what is meant by nitrogen balance
- describe methods for determining protein requirements
- describe what is meant by water balance, how this is usually maintained and the effects of imbalance

4.1 INTRODUCTION

The human body has a remarkable ability to adapt to different dietary circumstances. This is because there are biochemical mechanisms in place to ensure that flux through particular metabolic pathways is the most appropriate for the circumstances at the time. Thus, following a meal there is likely to be a drive towards the storage of fuel, as carbohydrate or as fat, whilst during the overnight fast or during the period between meals the body can mobilize these stores to ensure that all cells receive the fuel they need for normal cellular function. For these processes to occur efficiently there needs to be communication between metabolic pathways occurring in different organs but also interaction between different pathways of metabolism of the major macronutrients. For convenience this chapter examines carbohydrate, fat and protein separately, but the reader should always bear in mind that these pathways have common intermediates and there is considerable inter-action between the various pathways.

4.2 CARBOHYDRATE AND ITS METABOLISM

In Western diet carbohydrate contributes about 40% to energy intake, com-pared with 75% or more in developing countries. Carbohydrate can be clas-sified according to the length of the constituent polysaccharide chain. Monosaccharides are single sugar units; they exist in one of two chemical forms: aldoses, which contain an aldehyde group, as in glucose and galactose; and ketoses, containing a ketone group, as in fructose (Fig 4.1). Monosaccharides can form chemical bonds with one another, to form disaccharides. Sucrose, which is commonly known as table sugar, consists of glucose bound to fruc-tose; lactose, which is found in milk, consists of glucose bound to galactose, and maltose, which is found in sprouting grain, consists of two glucose units. The term oligosaccharide can be used for sugars with 3–9 monosaccharide units, and this group includes maltodextrins and fructo-oligosaccharides. Polysaccharides consist of more than 9 monosaccharide units joined together. This group of sugars includes starch and non-starch polysaccharides.

Starch is a mixture of two polymers, amylose and amylopectin, and is found in foods of plant origin including potatoes and bread. Non-starch polysaccharides include cellulose and pectins, neither of which is digestible by humans. Monosaccharides, disaccharides and maltodextrins are readily digestible in the small intestine and referred to as 'digestible'. Non-starch polysaccharides are 'indigestible' or 'unavailable' and pass to the large intestine, providing substrate for the colonic microflora; this group of carbo-hydrates is also referred to as dietary fibre. There are three classes of carbo-hydrate in dietary fibre: non-starch polysaccharide (NSP), resistant starch (RS) and resistant oligosaccharides (ROS). The main constituent is NSP, which is found in plant cell walls. Resistant oligosaccharides include poly-mers of fructose and galacto-oligosaccharides from legumes.

Dietary carbohydrate can also be classified by the glycaemic index (GI), which is a measure of the extent to which blood glucose concentration is raised compared with an equivalent amount of a reference carbohydrate (glucose or

MAIN DIETARY COMPONENTS

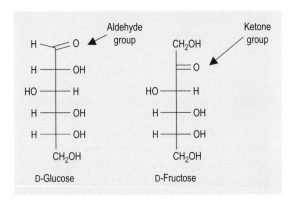

Figure 4.1 Common sugar structures.

white bread). Carbohydrate with a high GI generally provokes a higher secretion of insulin than carbohydrate with a low glycaemic index. The main glycaemic carbohydrates are glucose, fructose, sucrose, lactose and starch. Foods with a low GI generally have a high RS content, but some foods, such as bread and cornflakes, have quite a high GI despite having a high RS content.

Glycaemic carbohydrates function primarily as an energy source because in the fed state most tissues use glucose as their main metabolic fuel. In addition, liver and muscle synthesize the polysaccharide glycogen as a storage form of carbohydrate. Carbohydrate in excess of requirements for immediate metabolism or synthesis of glycogen can be used in the synthesis of fatty acids and triacylglycerol. Carbohydrate also contributes to the synthesis of non-essential amino acids. The metabolism of glucose is a source of pentoses, which are essential components of the nucleic acids RNA and DNA, and of glucuronic acid, which is required for the conjugation of bile salts. Carbohydrate can form complex molecules with fat or protein to form glycolipids, amino sugars such as glucosamine, and glycoproteins such as albumin and collagen.

The metabolism of glycaemic carbohydrates

Figure 4.2 gives an overview of carbohydrate metabolism integrated with fat metabolism. The first stage is glycolysis, which is the anaerobic oxidation of glucose to pyruvic acid (pyruvate), and takes place in the cytoplasm of all

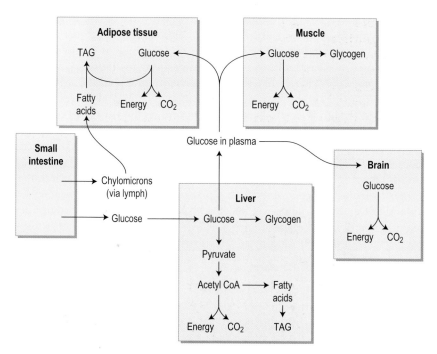

Figure 4.2 Main routes of metabolism of carbohydrate and fat following a meal. Following a meal containing carbohydrate, fat and protein there is a drive to store fuel for later use. Glycogen is stored in liver and muscle whilst fat is stored mainly in adipose tissue, as triacylglycerol (TAG). There will be net protein synthesis.

cells. Glycolysis yields a very modest amount of energy but because it can occur in the absence of oxygen it is important in muscle during intense exercise. Pyruvate formed from glycolysis can be oxidized further by crossing into the mitochondria for entry into the tricarboxylic acid (TCA) cycle, which generates much more energy than glycolysis. The glycolytic pathway also provides a route for the metabolism of fructose, galactose and glycerol. The metabolism of galactose and fructose occurs in the intestinal mucosa and liver, so little fructose or galactose reaches the peripheral circulation. In cells lacking mitochondria, such as red blood cells, or when conditions in a cell become anaerobic (such as in an intensely active muscle), pyruvate is reduced to lactate, which leaves the cell and goes to the liver where it can be reconverted to pyruvate. The pentose phosphate pathway (also known as the hexose monophosphate shunt) is an alternative cytoplasmic pathway for the anaerobic oxidation of glucose. This is important because it yields useful products such as pentoses for RNA and DNA synthesis, and the reduced form of the important compound nicotinamide adenine dinucleotide phosphate (NADPH), which is essential for fatty acid synthesis.

The metabolic fate of pyruvate is determined by metabolic circumstances at the time. It may be reduced to form lactate under anaerobic conditions (described above), oxidized completely via the TCA cycle and the electron transport chain, used as a substrate for glucose synthesis or used as a substrate for fatty acid synthesis. Pyruvate thus fulfils an important role in the integration of the metabolism of fat, carbohydrate and protein. For pyruvate to undergo complete oxidation it passes into the mitochondria where it is initially converted to the compound acetyl CoA in a reaction dependent upon vitamins B_1 (thiamin), B_2 (riboflavin), and niacin, which act as cofactors. Acetyl CoA then enters the TCA cycle, which involves a series of reactions leading to the production of energy. Importantly, as the TCA cycle is an oxidative process it also yields reducing power as the reduced form of the nucleotides nicotinamide adenine dinucleotide (NAD) and flavin adenine dinucleotide (FAD). These molecules are central to the processes of energy generation from the oxidation of fuel molecules, and to the synthesis of complex molecules from simple precursors. The reduced NAD and FAD enter the electron transport chain, which involves the successive reduction and oxidation of intermediates, with the overall production of substantial amounts of energy through a process of oxidative phosphorylation. Thus, the complete oxidation of glucose, fructose or galactose yields energy and important intermediates that link carbohydrate metabolism with fat and protein metabolism.

Glycogen as a carbohydrate store

Glycogen is a branched polymer of glucose. In the fed state, glycogen is synthesized from glucose in both liver (50–150 g) and muscle (350–400 g), through the stepwise addition of glucose to an existing glycogen molecule. The branched structure of glycogen means that it binds a lot of water within the molecule. In the early stages of food restriction, such as during an overnight fast, or between meals, the body uses glycogen as a fuel source (Fig 4.3), and there is an associated excretion of this bound water. This leads to an initial high rate of weight loss but it cannot be sustained because once glycogen has

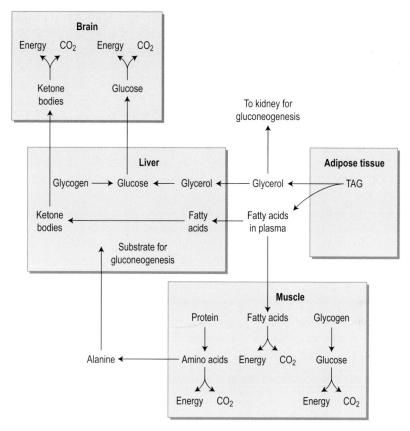

Figure 4.3 Main routes of metabolism in the period between meals and during an overnight fast. In the absence of fuel from the gut the body mobilizes its fuel stores. There is net breakdown of glycogen in liver and muscle and of triacylglycerol (TAG) in adipose tissue. Amino acids from protein turnover will be directed towards glucose synthesis in liver and the renal medulla.

been depleted the rapid loss of water (and weight) will cease. In the fasting state, glycogen is broken down in the muscle and the liver. In the liver this process leads to the formation of glucose, which can be exported to other tissues. In contrast the muscle is unable to carry out the final step in the breakdown of glycogen to glucose, meaning that muscle is unable to export glucose for use by other tissues but can use the phosphorylated glucose it generates in glycolysis.

Gluconeogenesis

Cells in the liver and kidney medulla are able to synthesize glucose in a process called gluconeogenesis. This becomes particularly important during times of fasting or on very low carbohydrate diets. This process is largely a reversal of glycolysis except for three irreversible steps in glycolysis, for which alternative reactions occur. Many of the products of amino acid metabolism can be used for gluconeogenesis, since they are sources of pyruvate or intermediates in the tricarboxylic acid cycle. Substrates that give rise to acetyl CoA directly (alcohol, fatty acids, ketone bodies and ketogenic amino acids) cannot be substrates for gluconeogenesis, but glycerol, which is produced from the hydrolysis of triacylglycerol in the fasting state, can (Fig 4.3).

The control of carbohydrate metabolism

Energy expenditure is relatively constant throughout the day, but in humans most of the daily food intake typically occurs in two or three meals. There is therefore a need for metabolic regulation to ensure that there is a reasonably constant supply of metabolic fuel to tissues, regardless of the variation in intake. There is a particular need to regulate carbohydrate metabolism since the nervous system is largely reliant on glucose as its metabolic fuel, and red blood cells and the kidney cortex are entirely so. The plasma concentration of glucose is maintained in short-term fasting by the mobilization of liver glycogen, and by releasing free fatty acids from adipose tissue. Should the fasting state extend beyond about 12 hours gluconeogenesis becomes very important.

Hormonal control of carbohydrate metabolism in the fed state

Carbohydrate metabolism is regulated by the co-ordinated action of hormones, enzymes and metabolic intermediates, and in a healthy person the concentration of glucose in the peripheral circulation is maintained at about 4–6 mmol/L.

During the 3–4 hours after a meal glucose, galactose and fructose will enter the portal blood following carbohydrate digestion and amino acids will enter the portal blood following protein digestion. Under these conditions glucose is the main fuel for tissues. The increased concentration of glucose and amino acids in the portal blood stimulates the β-cells of the pancreas to secrete the hormone insulin, and suppresses the secretion of the hormone glucagon by the α-cells of the pancreas. Insulin has four main actions:

- increased uptake of glucose into muscle and adipose tissue
- stimulation of the synthesis of glycogen from glucose in both liver and muscle
- stimulation of fatty acid synthesis in adipose tissue
- stimulation of amino acid uptake into tissues, leading to an increased rate of protein synthesis.

Hormonal control of carbohydrate metabolism in the fasting state

In the fasting state (sometimes known as the post-absorptive state, since it begins about 4–5 hours after a meal, when the products of digestion have been absorbed) metabolic fuels enter the circulation from the reserves of glycogen, triacylglycerol and protein laid down in the fed state. The metabolic problem in the fasting state is that the brain is largely dependent on glucose as its metabolic fuel, and red blood cells cannot utilize any metabolic fuel other than glucose. As the concentration of glucose and amino acids in the portal blood falls, so the secretion of insulin by the pancreas decreases and the secretion of glucagon increases. Glucagon has two main actions:

- stimulation of the breakdown of liver glycogen
- stimulation of the synthesis of glucose from amino acids in liver and kidney.

At the same time, the reduced secretion of insulin results in:

- a reduced rate of glucose uptake into muscle and adipose tissue
- a reduced rate of protein synthesis, so that the amino acids arising from protein catabolism are available for gluconeogenesis
- relief of the inhibition of lipid breakdown in adipose tissue, leading to release of free (non-esterified) fatty acids into the circulation.

The net effect is an increase in the provision of glucose for the brain and RBCs and an increased availability of fatty acids for oxidation by other tissues.

Dietary fructose metabolism

High intakes of fructose cause increased plasma concentrations of triacylglycerol. This is because fructose metabolism in the liver bypasses phosphofructokinase, which is the major control point for glycolysis, so that more fructose enters the pathway than is required for energy-yielding metabolism. The resultant acetyl CoA is used for synthesizing lipid.

Functions and metabolism of non-digestible carbohydrates (dietary fibre)

Carbohydrates that are not digested in the small intestine are subject to anaerobic fermentation by the colonic microflora. Fermentation products, mainly short-chain fatty acids, are now known to play an important role in colon health. Short-chain fatty acids (SCFA) such as acetate, propionate and butyrate, and gases, notably hydrogen and methane, are the main fermentation products. Butyrate is a major source of energy for colonocytes with effects on cell differentiation and programmed cell death (apoptosis) that may be protective against cancer. Propionate inhibits liver cholesterol synthesis in experimental animals, but the importance in humans is not yet clear. Viscous types of soluble fibre that have a high water-binding capacity may inhibit gastric emptying, and also have beneficial effects on both lipid and carbohydrate metabolism, including a lowering of plasma total and LDL-cholesterol and a lowering of postprandial glucose and insulin response.

Carbohydrate malabsorption

In certain individuals malabsorption of dietary carbohydrates may cause excessive delivery of fermentable substrate to the large intestine, causing intolerance. Congenital sucrase deficiency is a rare cause of sucrose malabsorption, which can cause gastrointestinal complaints, including diarrhoea, when an increasing amount of sucrose is introduced in the diet. Similarly, congenital lactase deficiency is a rare condition causing severe diarrhoea and malnutrition in the newborn. Breast milk has a high content (7%) of lactose.

Carbohydrate and disease

Blood glucose concentration is determined by three main factors: the rate of intestinal carbohydrate absorption, the net liver uptake or output, and glucose uptake by other tissues, which in turn depends upon blood insulin concentration and the sensitivity of tissues to insulin. With a constant dietary carbohydrate load, there is a range of change in blood glucose concentration in individuals; large increases indicate impaired glucose tolerance. The change in blood glucose after a meal is determined by both the glycaemic index (GI) of the meal and the amount of carbohydrate consumed. The protein and fat content and the amount of water taken with the meal also influence the glycaemic response. Excessive postprandial glycaemia may be related to increased all-cause mortality in diabetics as well as in people with normal fasting blood glucose concentration.

There is evidence from both epidemiological studies and intervention studies that diets rich in dietary fibre are healthy, and may reduce the risk of coronary heart disease and certain cancers, as well as reducing the risk of obesity. Viscous types of dietary fibre, such as pectin, guar gum and oat β-glucans lower serum cholesterol, but it is not known to what extent the protective effects of whole grain cereals and fruits are due to dietary fibre, to other constituents of these foods, or to other diet or lifestyle-related factors associated with the consumption of whole grain foods and fruits and vegetables.

KEY POINTS

- Carbohydrates constitute the main energy source in the diet
- The main monosaccharides are all metabolized to pyruvate, or lactate under anaerobic conditions
- Pyruvate can be converted to acetyl CoA which can be oxidized further in the TCA cycle or used in the synthesis of fatty acids
- The main storage carbohydrate in the body is glycogen; its synthesis in the fed state and utilization in the fasting state are closely regulated by insulin and glucagon
- The brain has a particular requirement for glucose, and during fasting glucose can be synthesized from non-carbohydrate precursors
- The glycaemic index denotes the potential of a food to elevate blood glucose. Low glycaemic index foods may confer benefits in metabolic control of diabetes
- Carbohydrates that are not digested in the small intestine are substrates for fermentation in the colon, with probable health benefits

Introduction

The main form of dietary fat is triacyglycerol (TAG) in which three fatty acids are bound to a molecule of glycerol (Fig 4.4). It is in this form that fat is stored, predominantly in adipose tissue. Phospholipids are similar in structure, but have a phosphate group and an additional base (choline, inositol, serine) in place of one of the fatty acids. Together with cholesterol,

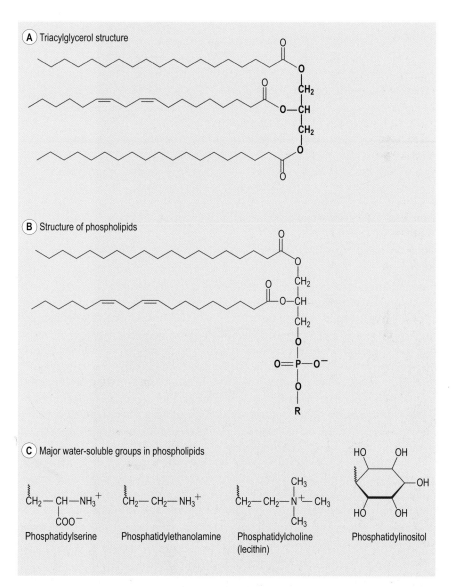

Figure 4.4 Structure of triacylglycerol (TAG) and phospholipids. Triacylglycerol (A) consists of a glycerol backbone esterified to three fatty acids. In phospholipids (B) carbon-3 glycerol is esterified to phosphate, then to one of a number of water-soluble bases shown in (C).

Structure	Class
$CH_3-(CH_2)_4-CH=CH-CH_2-CH=CH-(CH_2)_7\ COOH$	Polyunsaturated (Linoleic acid, 18:2 n-6)
$CH_3-(CH_2)_7-CH=CH-(CH_2)_7\ COOH$	Monounsaturated (Oleic acid, 18:1 n-9)
$CH_3-(CH_2)_{16}\ COOH$	Saturated (Stearic acid, 18:0)

Figure 4.5 Fatty acid structures.

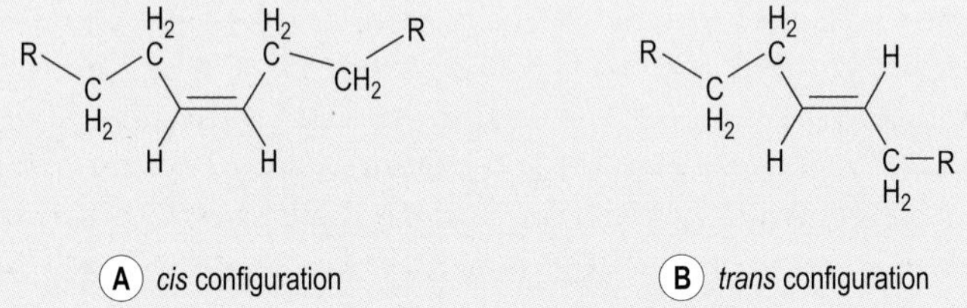

Figure 4.6 Distribution of atoms at a carbon–carbon double bond: (A) *cis* and (B) *trans* configuration.

phospholipids are important constituents of cell membranes. Fatty acids consist of hydrocarbon chains with a carboxylic acid group at the head. Typically a fatty acid has between 12 and 22 carbon atoms and may contain no double bonds (saturated fatty acid) or one (monounsaturated) or more (polyunsaturated) double bonds (Fig 4.5). The hydrogen atoms at the carbon–carbon double bond may be on the same side of the double bond (*cis*) or on opposite sides (*trans*) (Fig 4.6). *Trans* fatty acids are absent from natural plant lipids but may be found in some animal fats such as milk fat. *Trans* fatty acids may also be formed during the processing of some fats for incorporation into foods. High intakes of *trans* fatty acids have been associated with an increased risk of cardiovascular disease.

TAG molecules constitute an excellent storage form of fat because they are hydrophobic and can therefore be packed very densely. Following oxidation fat generates 9 kcal (36 kJ) energy per gram, which is considerably more than carbohydrate or protein and makes fat especially valuable as a fuel. Fat is stored in adipose tissue in the fed state and adipose tissue fat stores are mobilized in the fasted state.

Functions of dietary fat

Fat plays diverse roles in human nutrition. In addition to its importance as a source of energy, both for immediate utilization by the body and as a store for later utilization when food intake is reduced, dietary fat acts as a vehicle for the absorption of fat-soluble vitamins. Phospholipids and cholesterol are components of cell membranes and cholesterol is the precursor for synthesis of adrenocorticoid and sex hormones. Long chain (C20 and C22) polyunsaturated fatty acids in membrane phospholipids are the precursors of prostaglandins and other eicosanoids, compounds that have important local hormone effects.

Energy storage

The majority of fat is stored as TAG in the cells of adipose tissue. Following a meal, ingested fat which is not required by the body tissues for immediate use is transported to the adipose tissue in lipoproteins. The fatty acids are hydrolysed from the TAG in circulating lipoproteins by the enzyme lipoprotein lipase (LPL), taken up by the adipose tissue and re-esterified into triacylglycerol. Conversely, when dietary energy supply is limited, such as after an overnight fast, the fat in adipose tissue is mobilized and fatty acids are released into the circulation, bound to serum albumin. These fatty acids enter other tissues and are oxidized for energy production. This process is tightly regulated by the concentration of metabolites (glucose, fatty acids, TAG) in the blood and by hormones (insulin, glucagon, adrenaline). In addition to its role as an energy store, subcutaneous adipose tissue is important in the maintenance of body temperature, whereas internal fat (visceral fat) protects the vital organs such as the kidney and spleen. Accumulation of excessive visceral fat (abdominal obesity) is a risk factor for heart disease and diabetes and is linked with insulin resistance.

The structural role of fat in cell membranes

The basic structural unit of most biological membranes is phospholipid, although sphingolipids, which are based on a sphingosine rather than a glycerol backbone, are also widespread in membranes, and are particularly abundant in the brain and nervous system. The chain length and degree of unsaturation of the fatty acids within the membrane have a large impact on membrane physical properties. Dietary fatty acid composition has been shown to influence the composition of fatty acids in cell membranes. Cholesterol is also a component of cell membranes, in which its interactions with fatty acids are essential to maintain membrane structure and fluidity.

Membrane fats in cell signalling

Various lipids are involved in cell signalling and the conversion of extracellular signals into intracellular ones. Membrane phospholipids are important mediators of hormone and neurotransmitter action and as such are involved in regulation of cellular processes such as smooth muscle contraction, glycogen metabolism and cell proliferation and differentiation. Membrane sphingolipids are important modulators of cell growth and death, and of inflammatory responses.

Fat as precursors of the eicosanoids

The two dietary essential fatty acids, linoleic and α-linolenic acid, are precursors of long chain polyunsaturated fatty acids (PUFAs), including eicosapentaenoic acid (EPA) and arachidonic acid (AA). These two PUFAs (AA being the most important) are the precursors of a group of hormone-like compounds called eicosanoids, including prostaglandins, thromboxanes and leucotrienes, which are important for a wide range of processes including inflammatory responses, blood clotting and smooth muscle contraction.

Fat transport and metabolism

As TAG, cholesterol and phospholipids are not water-soluble, they cannot be transported free in the blood, but are carried in lipoproteins. Lipoproteins are particles which transport lipids between tissues. They have a hydrophobic core of TAG and cholesterol esters and a hydrophilic surface consisting of phospholipids and free cholesterol. Lipoproteins also contain specific proteins, apoproteins, which determine how the lipoprotein is metabolized. Apoproteins recognize and interact with specific receptors on the cell-surface, and the receptor–lipoprotein complex is taken into the cell. Apoproteins also determine the activities of a range of proteins, including hydrolysing enzymes (lipases), receptors and lipid transfer proteins, which are involved in all stages of lipoprotein metabolism.

Lipoprotein classes

Lipoproteins have traditionally been classified according to their density into four main subgroups: chylomicrons, very low-density lipoproteins (VLDL), low-density lipoproteins (LDL) and high density lipoproteins (HDL). Recent research has focused on a fifth category of lipoproteins, lipoprotein(a), or Lp(a), which has a strong independent association with the development of atherosclerosis. Chylomicrons formed in the gut, and VLDL formed in the liver are the least dense of the lipoproteins as they contain the lowest protein: lipid ratio. The smaller denser LDL and HDL are involved in the transport of cholesterol to and from the cells, with about 70% of total cholesterol present in LDL. LDL is derived from the metabolism of VLDL in the circulation. HDL, which is originally synthesized in the gut and the liver, is responsible for the removal of excess cholesterol from peripheral tissues and its return to the liver, a process called reverse cholesterol transport.

The exogenous and endogenous lipoprotein pathways

The exogenous lipoprotein pathway distributes fat entering the circulation from the diet whereas the endogenous fat pathway distributes fat either synthesized or stored in the liver.

Exogenous pathway

Dietary fat is packaged into chylomicrons in the enterocytes of the small intestine, which are then secreted into the lymphatic system and enter the circulation via the thoracic duct. Chylomicrons are too large to move through the capillary wall, so cells cannot take them up directly. Adipocytes, muscle and mammary cells synthesize and secrete the enzyme lipoprotein lipase (LPL), which hydrolyses the triacylglycerol in chylomicrons and releases fatty acids, which are subsequently taken up by the tissues. Once inside a cell fatty acids are rapidly converted into TAG. In adipose tissue and mammary gland the fatty acids are stored as TAG as an energy reserve and to provide milk fatty acids, whereas in the muscle the fat is used as an immediate source of fuel for muscle contraction. The lipid-depleted chylomicron remnant (CMR) is taken up by liver cells via a receptor.

Endogenous pathway

The liver synthesizes VLDL using fatty acids from a variety of sources including other lipoproteins and fatty acids synthesized in the liver. Upon secretion into the bloodstream triacylglycerols are hydrolysed by LPL and the fatty acids are taken up by tissues. VLDL remnants are either taken up by the liver or become LDL, the major carrier of cholesterol in the blood. An increased secretion or delayed clearance of triacylglycerol rich lipoproteins (VLDL and chylomicrons) is a significant risk factor for coronary heart disease. LDL transports cholesterol to the peripheral tissues and regulates *de novo* synthesis of cholesterol at these sites. On arrival at the cell surface the cell takes up the LDL–receptor complex. Once inside the cell the cholesterol can be used immediately for incorporation into cell membranes, used in the synthesis of steroid hormones or stored as cholesterol esters (cholesterol bound to a fatty acid) within the cell.

LDL that has become chemically modified, by oxidation for example, is recognized by scavenger receptors on the surface of macrophages. Macrophages take up these chemically modified LDL and in so doing accumulate lipid. This uncontrolled process of lipid accumulation leads to the formation of foam cells, which mark an early stage of atherosclerosis.

Excess cholesterol in tissues is transported in HDL back to the liver, where it can be excreted in the bile or be transported to other cells via the VLDL–LDL pathway. More than 40% of individuals who have a myocardial infarction (heart attack) have low HDL levels.

Intracellular fat metabolism

Fatty acid oxidation

Fatty acid oxidation occurs in many tissues, predominantly through a pathway of β-oxidation in the mitochondria. The substrate fatty acids are supplied to tissues either in the form of non-esterified fatty acids (NEFA), bound to serum albumin, or by the hydrolysis of the triacylglycerol component of circulating lipoproteins.

Before fatty acids can be oxidized, they have to enter the mitochondria, for which purpose they are initially converted to esters of acetyl CoA (called fatty acyl CoA). Fatty acyl CoA crosses into the mitochondria via a carnitine transport system. Mitochondrial fatty acyl CoA undergoes a repeating series of four reactions, which results in the cleavage of the fatty acid molecule to give acetyl CoA and a new fatty acyl CoA which is two carbons shorter than the initial substrate. This new, shorter, fatty acyl CoA is then a substrate for the same sequence of reactions, which is repeated until only acetyl CoA is left.

The rate of β-oxidation is high when the supply of fatty acids to tissues is high, such as in the post-absorptive state or after an overnight fast. At this time the insulin:glucagon ratio will be comparatively low and this will drive the mobilization of stored fat and its subsequent oxidation. In the fed state the insulin:glucagon ratio will be high and this will inhibit the mobilization of TAG from adipose tissue and drive the deposition of TAG instead. Skeletal muscle favours fat as a fuel over carbohydrate and active skeletal muscle will take up fatty acids from plasma and oxidize them.

Synthesis of ketone bodies

When fatty acid oxidation is occurring at a fast rate, such as following an overnight fast or during prolonged fasting, the rate of production of acetyl CoA may be too high for metabolism by the TCA cycle, and under these circumstances some of the acetyl CoA will be converted in the liver to compounds called ketone bodies. These compounds are important because they can be used as an alternative to glucose by other tissues (but not the liver). The brain cannot use fatty acids but can oxidize ketone bodies and this is extremely important as a glucose-sparing strategy. Additionally, under these conditions, with insulin:glucagon ratio low, the liver will become more likely to carry out gluconeogenesis, to make glucose available to the brain and other cells unable to oxidize fatty acids, such as red blood cells.

Fatty acid synthesis

De novo fatty acid synthesis usually signifies an excess of carbohydrate or amino acids. The acetyl CoA generated from the oxidation of these substrates leaves the mitochondria and enters the cytoplasm, the site of fatty acid synthesis. Fatty acids are synthesized by the successive addition of two-carbon units from acetyl CoA, followed by reduction. Two key multi-enzyme complexes are responsible for the synthesis of fatty acids from acetyl CoA. The first catalyses the carboxylation of acetyl CoA to malonyl CoA, which is a 3-carbon unit, and the second catalyses the successive addition of 2-carbon units to a growing fatty acid chain, using malonyl CoA as the donor of each 2-carbon unit.

Elongation and desaturation of fatty acids

Fatty acids synthesized in this way can be elongated using elongases (enzymes that add carbon atoms to preformed fatty acids) and desaturated to form fatty acids with double bonds. There are two fatty acids that the body cannot make, linoleic acid and linolenic acid, which are therefore termed essential fatty acids, and both of which are polyunsaturated. Linoleic acid belongs to the omega 6 family, so named because the first double bond starts six carbons from the methyl end of the fatty acid, whilst linolenic acid belongs to the omega 3 family. These essential fatty acids are precursors for a number of longer chain polyunsaturated fatty acids including arachidonic acid (omega 6 family), eicosapentaenoic acid (EPA, omega 3 family) and docosahexaenoic acid (DHA, omega 3 family).

Synthesis of cholesterol

Cholesterol can be obtained through the diet, but cholesterol synthesis in the liver makes a much more important contribution to body cholesterol than diet does. The process of cellular cholesterol metabolism is tightly regulated.

Synthesis and utilization of triacylglycerol

Whenever energy supply from the diet exceeds the energy expenditure of the body, TAG is deposited in adipose tissue. When a fat-containing meal is consumed, adipocytes acquire fat from circulating lipoproteins by breakdown of TAG by lipoprotein lipase. In the reverse situation, when there is a demand for fatty acids for metabolism, TAG is mobilized from adipose tissue by the enzyme hormone-sensitive lipase (HSL). These processes are integrated and controlled by the nutritional status of the individual through a number of hormones, the most important of which is insulin. Biosynthesis of triacylglycerol involves the esterification of three fatty acids to a glycerol backbone. It can occur in a number of tissues, predominantly adipose tissue, liver, enterocytes and the mammary gland during lactation. Under conditions where the demand for mobilization of fuel reserves increases, usually signalled by low concentrations of insulin, biosynthetic pathways are inhibited and hormone-sensitive lipase in adipocytes is activated. Once released, the fatty acids are bound to plasma albumin and may be taken up by tissues for oxidation.

Integration and control of fat metabolism

Following an overnight fast and during prolonged fasting hormone-sensitive lipase activity is high, mainly because of a low insulin:glucagon ratio, and fat is mobilized and fatty acids enter the plasma. The increase in concentration of fatty acids in the plasma drives uptake by tissues such as skeletal muscle and liver for subsequent oxidation. This spares glucose, which will be in short supply, for particular use by the brain. Additionally, glycerol is released from the adipose tissue when TAG is mobilized, and this is used for gluconeogenesis in the liver. Conversely, in the absorptive period, during and for a few hours after a meal, the insulin:glucagon ratio is high, which inhibits TAG mobilization from adipose tissue. The concentration of TAG in the plasma (in chylomicrons and VLDL) will be high and any excess of dietary fuel over immediate requirements will be deposited as fat. Excess carbohydrate is preferentially used to replenish liver glycogen stores, whilst amino acids will be used for protein synthesis. Any excess of carbohydrate or protein will be used for fatty acid and triacylglycerol synthesis, which can be stored in adipose tissue.

The magnitude and duration of the postprandial lipaemic response will depend on the efficiency of the regulatory mechanisms for the disposal and storage of the triacylglycerol. Lipoprotein lipase is activated by insulin and will therefore be most active following a meal; in adipose tissue its activity reaches a peak approximately 3–4 h after a meal, coinciding with the peak in postprandial plasma triacylglycerol.

KEY POINTS

- Fats perform a range of essential functions in the body – they can be stored as an energy source, used as a structural component of cell membranes, play a role in cell signalling, and act as precursors for the synthesis of hormones
- Fat is transported as triacylglycerol in lipoproteins in the plasma, or as fatty acids bound to albumin
- Fatty acids can be made from carbohydrates and amino acids, but cannot be converted to either
- Fatty acids can be converted to ketone bodies – water-soluble molecules which can be used by the brain
- The TAG in lipoproteins is hydrolysed to allow fatty acids to enter tissues. TAG stored in adipose tissue is mobilized to provide fatty acids to tissues for oxidation
- Linoleic and α-linolenic acids cannot be synthesized and are essential in the diet

4.4 PROTEIN METABOLISM AND REQUIREMENTS

Introduction

Dietary protein is a complex mixture of many different proteins, each with a distinct amino acid composition. Any individual protein may contain 50–1000 amino acids, the sequence of which is specific for that protein. The nutritional requirement is not only for total protein intake, but for specific amino acids, in the proportions that are required to maintain turnover of body proteins. There are about 30,000–50,000 different proteins in the human body, and they are broken down and replaced at different rates.

Protein structure and function

Proteins are composed of chains of amino acids in chemical linkage with one another, known as polypeptides. There are 21 amino acids involved in the synthesis of proteins, together with a number that occur in proteins as a result of chemical modification after the protein has been synthesized. In addition, a number of amino acids occur as metabolic intermediates, but are not found in proteins. Chemically amino acids all have the same basic structure – an amino group ($-NH_3^+$) and a carboxylic acid group ($-COO^-$) attached to the same carbon atom (the α-carbon). What differs between them is the nature of the other group that is attached to the α-carbon, the simplest being glycine, in which the side group is hydrogen. Polypeptide chains are formed by the condensation of the carboxyl group of one amino acid with the amino group of another, to form a peptide bond. The chain of amino acids in a polypeptide chain folds in a variety of ways to form the secondary structure, and, having formed regions of secondary structure the whole protein molecule then folds up into a compact shape, representing the tertiary structure. Some proteins have a quaternary structure, in which more than one folded polypeptide chain associate with one another.

Nitrogen balance and protein turnover

The average dietary intake of protein is about 80 g/day in Western countries but is typically much less in low- and middle-income countries. Protein is largely digested to amino acids and small peptides and these are absorbed in the small intestine. A small faecal loss of nitrogen is composed mainly of intestinal bacteria, shed mucosal cells and mucus but may include a small amount of undigested dietary protein.

A small pool of free amino acids in the body is in metabolic equilibrium with proteins that are being broken down and synthesized. Some of these amino acids are used for synthesis of a variety of specialized metabolites including hormones and neurotransmitters, purines and pyrimidines. A proportion of the amino acid pool will be oxidized, and the carbon skeletons generated will be used as metabolic fuels or for gluconeogenesis, with the nitrogen being excreted mainly as urea.

Body protein balance can be determined by measuring the dietary intake of nitrogenous compounds and the output of nitrogenous compounds from the body. Nitrogen constitutes 16% of most proteins, and the protein content of foods can therefore be calculated as: mg N $\times$ 6.25. Nitrogen is lost from the body largely in the urine and faeces, but significant amounts may also be lost in sweat and shed skin cells. The difference between intake and output of nitrogenous compounds is termed nitrogen balance. Three states can be defined:

- An adult in good health and with an adequate intake of protein excretes the same amount of nitrogen each day as is taken in from the diet. This is nitrogen balance or nitrogen equilibrium: intake = output, and there is no change in the total body content of protein.
- In a growing child, a pregnant woman or someone recovering from protein loss, the excretion of nitrogenous compounds is less than the dietary intake – there is a net retention of nitrogen in the body, and an increase in the body content of protein. This is positive nitrogen balance: intake > output, and there is a net gain in total body protein.
- In response to trauma or infection, or if the intake of protein is inadequate to meet requirements, there is net a loss of nitrogen from the body – the output is greater than the intake. This is negative nitrogen balance: intake < output, and there is a loss of body protein.

The proteins of the body are continually being broken down and replaced although the rate can vary from minutes to days, depending on the proteins. An adult catabolizes and replaces about 3–6 g of protein per kg body weight per day, with no change in total body protein content. Protein breakdown occurs at a more or less constant rate throughout the day. In contrast, replacement synthesis is greater than breakdown after a meal, and is less than breakdown in the fasting state, when amino acids are being used as substrates for gluconeogenesis. This means that there are periods of positive and negative nitrogen balance throughout the day. Even in severe undernutrition, the rate of protein breakdown remains more or less constant, while the rate of replacement synthesis falls, as a result of the low availability of metabolic fuels. It is only in cachexia (a condition of weight loss and muscle atrophy often associated with disease), that there is increased protein catabolism as well as reduced replacement synthesis.

Tissue protein catabolism

The catabolism of tissue proteins is a highly regulated process; different proteins are catabolized (and replaced) at very different rates. It is the continual catabolism of tissue proteins that creates the requirement for dietary protein. Although some of the amino acids released by breakdown of tissue proteins can be re-used, most are metabolized to intermediates that can be used as metabolic fuels and for gluconeogenesis. The nitrogen is metabolized to urea, which is excreted.

Protein synthesis

The synthesis of a particular protein is directed by the sequence of bases on a specific region of DNA in the nucleus. This information is transcribed onto a molecule of messenger RNA (mRNA), which carries the message into the cytoplasm for translation into the appropriate polypeptide chain.

DNA is a linear polymer of nucleotides. It consists of a sugar phosphate backbone in which phosphate bonds link adjacent deoxyribose molecules. Two strands of deoxyribonucleotides are held together by hydrogen bonds between bases (adenine, guanine, cytosine and thymine). The DNA double strand coils into a double helix. The order of bases in a stretch of DNA acts to code for the specific order of amino acids to be incorporated into a polypeptide chain, for protein synthesis. This code (the genetic code) is read in groups of three bases, called a codon. Most amino acids are coded for by more than one codon, which allows a degree of buffering against errors in protein synthesis.

In RNA the sugar is ribose, rather than deoxyribose, and RNA contains the base uracil instead of the thymine in DNA. There are three main types of RNA in the cell: mRNA, synthesized in the nucleus as a copy of one strand of DNA; ribosomal RNA (rRNA), that constitutes part of the ribosomes on which protein is synthesized; and transfer RNA (tRNA), that provides the link between mRNA and the amino acids for protein synthesis on the ribosome.

As a first step in the synthesis of a protein, the information on a region of DNA is transcribed onto mRNA in the nucleus of the cell; a part of the desired region of DNA is uncoiled, and the two strands of the double helix are separated. A copy of one DNA strand is synthesized using complementary bases – the copy is mRNA (see also chapter 11).

The message carried by the sequence of bases in mRNA is then translated into amino acids, and the formation of peptide bonds between amino acids generates the polypeptide chain. This process occurs on the ribosome in the cytoplasm. Each amino acid is carried to the ribosome by a specific transfer RNA molecule. The order of amino acids is directed by the mRNA base sequence.

Energy cost and control of protein synthesis

In the fasting state, when the rate of protein synthesis is relatively low, about 8% of total energy expenditure is accounted for by protein synthesis. After a meal, when the rate of protein synthesis increases, it can account for as much as 20% of total energy expenditure.

Insulin, secreted in the fed state, increases the rate of protein synthesis, both by direct actions and also by stimulating the uptake of glucose and amino acids into cells. The glucocorticoid hormone cortisol acts at a whole body level to increase the rate of muscle protein catabolism and gluconeogenesis in the liver.

Amino acid metabolism

Because different proteins contain different amounts of the various amino acids not all proteins are nutritionally equivalent. The body's requirement is not simply for protein, but for specific amino acids. Nine amino acids – lysine, histidine, leucine, isoleucine, methionine, phenylalanine, tryptophan, threonine and valine – cannot be synthesized in the body and are termed essential (or indispensable). Some amino acids, including arginine and glutamine, are termed conditionally essential (or partially dispensable) because, although they can be synthesized in the body, there are some circumstances under which requirements can overwhelm the capacity for synthesis.

Because there is continual oxidation of amino acids as a source of metabolic fuel and for gluconeogenesis in the fasting state, an adult has a daily requirement for dietary protein. Overall, for an adult in nitrogen balance, the total amount of amino acids being metabolized in a day will be equal to the total intake of amino acids ingested in dietary proteins. Amino acids are also required for the synthesis of a variety of metabolic products, including purines and pyrimidines for nucleic acid synthesis, the neurotransmitters, dopamine, noradrenaline and adrenaline, and the thyroid hormones thyroxine and tri-iodothyronine.

The initial step in the metabolism of amino acids is the removal of the amino group ($-NH_3^+$), leaving behind the carbon skeleton of the amino acid. Chemically, these carbon skeletons are keto acids, which have a $-C = O$ group in place of the $HC-NH_3^+$ group of an amino acid. Some amino acids can be directly oxidized to their corresponding keto acids, releasing ammonia, a process called deamination. Most amino acids undergo transamination, which involves the transfer of the amino group from an amino acid onto a keto acid, forming a new amino acid and a new keto acid. Thus, by deamination and transamination all of the amino acids can be converted to their keto acids and ammonia.

The carbon skeletons of amino acids may be oxidized, used for fatty acid synthesis or be used to synthesize glucose or ketone bodies (only leucine, lysine, phenylalanine and isoleucine).

The metabolism of ammonia

Ammonia is toxic and is removed from the body in the form of urea, which is synthesized in the liver and then excreted in urine. The total amount of urea synthesized each day is several-fold higher than the amount that is excreted. Urea diffuses readily from the bloodstream into the large intestine, where it is hydrolysed by bacteria to carbon dioxide and ammonium ions. Much of the ammonium is reabsorbed, and metabolized in the liver.

Protein and amino acid requirements

It has proved difficult to define protein requirements, mainly because there are no specific biochemical markers or deficiency symptoms, apart from growth failure and tissue wasting – which only mark a severe deficiency. Additionally, because the body makes adaptations to low protein intakes the relation between intake and requirements can be weak. Without biochemical indicators, protein and amino acid requirements can only be defined in terms of maintenance of body protein. Measuring the protein requirement for maintenance requires the use of balance methods, which are imprecise and difficult to carry out. Protein requirements are best discussed in terms of metabolic demand, dietary requirement and dietary allowances.

- *Metabolic demand* for protein is determined by the nature and extent of those metabolic pathways which consume amino acids, which include maintenance and special needs such as growth, rehabilitation, pregnancy and lactation. Maintenance comprises all those processes which consume amino acids and give rise to urinary, faecal and other losses (Fig 4.7). Net protein synthesis is only a very small part of maintenance.
- *Dietary requirement* is the amount of protein and/or its constituent amino acids that must be supplied in the diet in order to satisfy the metabolic demand and achieve nitrogen equilibrium. The dietary requirement will usually be greater than the metabolic demand because of factors which influence the efficiency of protein utilization. These are factors which influence the *digestibility* and consequently the amount of dietary nitrogen lost in the faeces, and the cellular bioavailability of the absorbed amino acids in relation to needs, which influences the *biological value*.

Methods of determining dietary protein requirements
Nitrogen balance and factorial models

The metabolic demand can be estimated from measurement of all losses of nitrogen in subjects adapted to a protein-free diet. This is the obligatory nitrogen loss (ONL). When losses are measured over a range of intakes, balance is

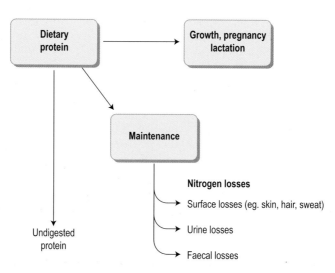

Figure 4.7   Routes of protein utilization.

calculated at each intake as intake minus losses, and the equation of the balance curve is calculated to predict the requirement. Using this approach the currently accepted maintenance requirement is 0.66 g/kg body weight/d. However, there are a number of problems with this approach:

- Nitrogen balance is the small difference between two large measurements and is associated with a high degree of imprecision.
- Nitrogen balance is usually overestimated because of an overestimation of nitrogen intake and an underestimation of output.
- Individual nitrogen balance curves are not linear and therefore curve fitting has to be used to predict nitrogen loss at zero intake.
- Nitrogen balance varies as a function of energy intake. Excess energy intake leads to weight gain, including some lean tissue, whilst insufficient energy intake will lead to oxidation of protein for energy.
- Different types of physical activity can influence nitrogen balance in ways that are currently only partly understood.
- Changes in protein intake elicit adaptive changes in metabolism. The time taken for complete adaptation is not fully understood.

Protein requirements for growth and special needs

For infants, children and pregnant and lactating women, protein requirements are derived by a semi-factorial analysis of the components of metabolic demand. The main components are maintenance requirements, dietary requirements for growth, and a factor to cover inter-individual variability. Additional requirements are associated with pregnancy and lactation.

Expression of requirements

In the past, protein requirements have been expressed as protein amounts per person or per kg body weight. Whilst this is adequate for calculating recommended intakes for an individual, it is less useful when advice is given about the types of diets and foods to be recommended and in assessing the adequacy of intakes. Energy expenditure determines overall energy and nutrient intakes, so that food-based guidelines can be more useful. Because the very high energy requirements during infancy and childhood decrease with age at a greater rate than the fall in the protein requirement, the protein:energy (P:E) ratio of the requirements for infants is low and increases with age. This means that a diet which can meet both energy and protein needs of the infant can satisfy energy needs of older children or adults while failing to meet their protein needs.

Importance of physical activity for nutrient intakes and risk of deficiency

Protein requirements are generally not considered to vary with energy expenditure and are usually provided by the increased food energy intakes. With energy requirements predicted from BMR × physical activity level, energy requirements per kg will vary markedly with age (falling), with gender (women < men), with body weight (large < small) and with physical activity.

Protein:energy ratios: key implications

- Protein dense foods are more important for adults, especially the elderly, than for infants and children.

- Energy dense foods are more important for children than adults.
- Protein deficiency is more likely in the elderly than in children.
- Protein deficiency at any age is less likely as physical activity increases.

Methods of evaluating protein quality and assessing amino acid requirements

Classic methods of evaluating protein quality were developed from rat growth studies. Protein quality can be assessed using various criteria.

Protein efficiency ratio (PER)

PER is g weight gain/g protein intake from a diet containing 9–10% of the protein. Very marked differences are apparent between proteins, with values of 3.8, 2.0 and 0.3 for whole egg, soya and wheat gluten respectively.

Digestibility

Values range from 60–80% in legumes and cereals to 97% for egg.

Biological value (BV)

BV varies mainly through the composition of the absorbed amino acid mixture in relation to the pattern of the metabolic demand for maintenance and net protein deposition. BV is low for cereals because of low levels of lysine and tryptophan and for legume proteins because of low levels of methionine and cysteine. However, BV of a diet can be increased by mixing different plant foods and mixed plant protein diets can have a BV that is similar to animal proteins.

Net protein utilization (NPU)

NPU represents a specific measure of protein utilization. It can be measured by means of N balance studies allowing separate evaluation of both digestibility and BV. Because faecal and urinary losses include ONL the measurements need to differentiate between these and exogenous losses due to poor utilization of food protein. However, it has proved difficult to differentiate protein quality of different diets in nitrogen balance studies carried out in humans partly because what is being measured is maintenance requirements and not demands for rapid growth, as in rats. Other methods have been examined, including the amino acid scoring method.

Amino acid scoring method

If the pattern of amino acid requirements is known, then in theory the measured BV of a dietary protein should be predictable from its amino acid pattern relative to that of the requirement pattern. The reference pattern is that of an ideal protein which would provide requirement levels of all amino acids when fed at the protein requirement level. So that:

reference pattern (as mg/g)
= (amino acid requirement/kg)/(protein requirement/kg)

This is the PDCAAS method: Protein Digestibility Corrected Amino Acid Score.

Stable isotope studies of protein and amino acid requirements
Stable isotopes allow tracer studies of amino acid metabolism, typically leucine, in humans.

Post-prandial protein utilization (PPU)
The efficiency of protein utilization is determined by the increases in losses in response to feeding. PPU is best measured as *change in balance/change in intake* between feeding isoenergetic low and high protein meals. The derived PPU value is a measure of biological value since the intake value is an estimate of digestible intake.

Indicator amino acid oxidation studies
A fixed amount of an amino acid mixture is fed, containing varying amounts of the amino acid under test. The oxidation of a second 'indicator' labelled amino acid is measured. When the intake of the test amino acid is too low to support net protein synthesis, the rest of the amino acid intake is oxidized, including the indicator amino acid. As the test requirement intake is approached or exceeded, all of the amino acid intake, including the indicator, will be utilized, so that indicator oxidation falls.

Definition of reference amino acid patterns

It is clear that there is much uncertainty about the actual values for amino acid requirements from which reference amino acid patterns can be constructed but there is agreement on the principles. For infants the amino acid composition of breast milk is assumed to represent an optimum pattern. Since it is quite clear that after the first year of life growth is relatively slow, there is no reason to expect amino acid requirements to vary much between the preschool child and the adult. This means that once an agreed maintenance pattern has been defined, a factorial calculation of amino acid requirements can be derived from maintenance together with the composition and amount of tissue protein gain.

Quality of animal and plant proteins

The important measure of protein quality is available protein in foods, the adjusted P:E ratio, which is determined by both protein content and quality. Animal foods generally perform well on both counts. For cereal proteins, yam and cassava, lysine is the limiting amino acid. Maize also contains less than the reference tryptophan level but lysine is the limiting amino acid and adjusting intake to supply lysine needs will supply more than enough tryptophan. Potatoes provide sufficient of all amino acids. Even after correcting for digestibility the adjusted P:E ratio of potato at 8.2% is higher than that of breast milk but the growth of a newborn could not be supported on mashed potato, because it has low energy density. The high protein level in wheat means that it provides a much higher level of utilizable protein than yam or cassava, even though wheat has the lowest lysine level of any staple.

KEY POINTS

- Proteins are large polymers of 21 different amino acids; the amino acid sequence of each protein is different, and is determined by the gene for that protein
- Folding of the protein chain produces proteins that act as receptors, transport proteins and enzymes, and structural proteins
- An adult is overall in nitrogen equilibrium, with intake of nitrogenous compounds (mainly protein) matched by excretion of nitrogenous metabolites
- In growth there is positive nitrogen balance; in response to trauma, or an inadequate intake, there is negative nitrogen balance
- In the fasting state protein catabolism exceeds synthesis, and in the fed state synthesis exceeds catabolism
- Nine amino acids cannot be synthesized in the body, but must be provided in the diet – these are the essential or indispensable amino acids
- The catabolism of amino acids leads to the formation of ammonia by transamination linked to deamination; this is transported to the liver to form urea
- The carbon skeletons of amino acids may provide substrates for energy-yielding metabolism, fatty acid synthesis or gluconeogenesis
- Protein requirements can be considered in terms of the metabolic demand for total protein and individual amino acids, and the dietary requirement, taking into account the digestibility and nutritional value of different proteins
- Protein requirements can be determined by nitrogen balance studies and factorial calculation but there are difficulties
- Protein requirements may be calculated on the basis of intake per kg body weight or on the basis of energy density

4.5 ALCOHOL METABOLISM AND HEALTH EFFECTS

In the context of this book the term alcohol refers to beverages containing ethanol, and these include beer, wine and spirits. Over most of the globe, with the exception of Africa, alcohol consumption is increasing. Whilst consumption at low levels may be associated with low risks the products of alcohol metabolism are toxic and it is well recognized that habitual over-consumption has numerous adverse effects on health.

Alcohol consumption in the United Kingdom

The alcohol content of beverages ranges from 0.5% for low alcohol beers to 40–50% for distilled spirits such as vodka or whisky. The Department of Health (UK) have recommended that alcohol consumption be limited to 2–3 Units per day for women and 3–4 Units a day for men. In the UK one

Unit of alcohol is equivalent to half a pint of beer, or one small glass of wine, or one measure of fortified wine or spirits. Taking the adult population of the UK as a whole, about 27% of males and 12% of females drink more than 21 or 14 Units per week respectively. There is evidence that alcohol consumption in children is increasing too. There are an estimated 2.8 million UK individuals classified as alcohol-dependent.

Energy content of alcoholic beverages

The energy composition of alcoholic beverages varies from about 30–220 kcal/100 ml (Table 4.1). Alcoholic beverages also contain trace amounts of compounds that impart flavour or characteristics of taste and smell such as sulphur-containing compounds, tannins, and polyphenols. Overall the current estimate is that ethanol contributes about 6.5% to energy intake in men and 3.9% in women in the UK but as this estimate includes drinkers and non-drinkers the value will in fact be much higher in those people who drink alcohol.

Alcohol metabolism

Ethanol is produced from the fermentation of carbohydrate, which generates ethanol, carbon dioxide and energy. Typically grapes, apples and grains are used, yielding wines, cider and beer respectively. Further distillation yields spirits, including whisky, vodka and rum. The immediate metabolite of ethanol oxidation, acetaldehyde (Fig 4.8), is a highly toxic and chemically reactive molecule that can bind irreversibly with proteins and nucleic acids. Acetate, the product of acetaldehyde metabolism, is either oxidized or used for synthesis of fatty acids and triglycerides. Many of the pathologies associated with drinking alcoholic beverages are due to the effects of acetaldehyde.

Ethanol requires no digestion and is rapidly absorbed, primarily in the upper gastrointestinal tract but also directly from the stomach, and appears in the blood within a few minutes of ingestion. Food in the stomach delays the absorption of alcohol and blunts the peak blood alcohol concentration. Alcohol is rapidly distributed around the body. In the post-absorption phase, the distribution of alcohol in the body will reflect body water so that for a given dose of alcohol, blood levels will reflect lean body mass.

Alcohol metabolism is initiated in the stomach but the primary site of metabolism is the liver. Alcohol is oxidized to acetaldehyde by three routes:

- alcohol dehydrogenase (ADH)
- microsomal ethanol oxidizing system (MEOS)
- catalase.

Once acetaldehyde is formed, it is further oxidized to acetate via aldehyde dehydrogenase (ALDH). Genetic or ethnic variations in ADH and ALDH may explain some of the pathologies of alcoholism, and why some individuals will develop certain diseases when others do not. Also, a lower activity of stomach ADH in women than men means that women have a higher blood alcohol concentration than men, following an equivalent load.

MAIN DIETARY COMPONENTS

Table 4.1 Composition of alcoholic beverages

(a) Per 100ml – all as g, except energy

	kcal	kJ	Alcohol	Protein	Fat	Carbohydrate
Alcohol-free lager	7	31	Trace	0.4	Trace	1.5
Low alcohol lager	10	41	0.5	0.2	0	1.5
Lager	29	131	4.0	0.3	Trace	Trace
Special strength lager	59	244	6.9	0.3	Trace	2.4
Bitter	30	124	2.9	0.3	Trace	2.2
Cider (dry)	36	152	3.8	Trace	0	2.6
Wine (red, dry)	68	283	9.6	0.1	0	0.2
Wine (white, dry)	66	275	9.1	0.1	0	0.6
Wine (white, sweet)	94	394	10.2	0.2	0	5.9
Sherry (dry)	116	481	15.7	0.2	0	1.4
Spirits (various; 40% proof)	222	919	31.7	Trace	0	Trace

(b) Per 100ml – all as mg

	Na	K	Ca	Mg	P	Fe	Cu	Zn	Cl	Mn
Alcohol-free lager	2	44	3	7	19	Trace	Trace	Trace	Trace	0.01
Low alcohol lager	12	56	8	12	10	Trace	Trace	Trace	Trace	0.01
Lager	7	39	5	7	19	Trace	Trace	Trace	20	0.01
Special strength lager	7	39	5	7	19	Trace	Trace	Trace	20	0.01
Bitter	6	32	8	7	14	0.1	0.001	0.1	24	0.03
Cider (dry)	7	72	8	3	3	0.5	0.04	Trace	6	Trace
Wine (red, dry)	7	110	7	11	13	0.9	0.06	0.1	11	0.10
Wine (white, dry)	4	61	9	8	6	0.5	0.01	Trace	10	0.10
Wine (white, sweet)	13	110	14	11	13	0.6	0.05	Trace	7	0.10
Sherry (dry)	10	57	7	13	11	0.4	0.03	N	14	Trace
Spirits (various; 40% proof)	Trace	Trace	Trace	Trace	Trace	Trace	Trace	Trace	Trace	Trace

N: significant quantities but no reliable information

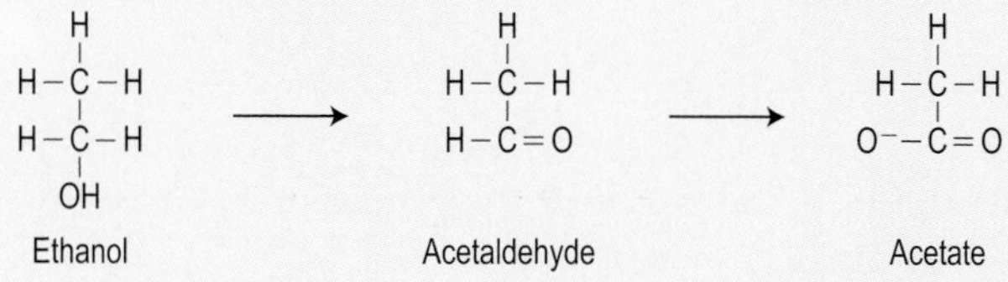

Figure 4.8 Metabolism of alcohol. Simplistic representation of conversion of alcohol to acetaldehyde and then acetate.

The MEOS is an inducible pathway of ethanol metabolism and is thus of particular significance in chronic ethanol misusers where the existing enzymes are unable to cope with the high ethanol load.

Chronic excess alcohol consumption is associated with both weight loss and obesity. Alcohol-related weight loss has been ascribed to poor dietary intake and malabsorption but there is also evidence for impaired energy production through uncoupling of metabolism from energy production.

Alcohol-related pathologies

There are at least 60–120 different alcohol-related pathologies. These include cirrhosis, gastrointestinal pathologies, fatty liver, hypertension, skeletal and bone marrow changes.

- *Fatty liver:* Traditionally, alcohol-induced liver disease has been thought to have three stages, fatty liver (steatosis), alcoholic hepatitis with fibrosis, and cirrhosis. Fatty liver occurs in about 80–90% of chronic alcohol misusers but rarely has symptoms. The excess lipid in affected liver is mainly triacyglycerol, but there is also an increase in esterified cholesterol.
- *Lactic acidosis:* Alcohol metabolism leads to an increase in the lactate: pyruvate ratio, and this may be made worse by ketoacidosis (caused by the production of large amounts of ketone bodies). In severe situations of ketoacidosis and hypoglycaemia, permanent brain damage may occur. These conditions may be exacerbated by thiamin deficiency. The high concentration of lactic acid also impairs the kidney's ability to excrete uric acid and consequently blood uric acid levels rise, causing gout.
- *Influences on hormones:* Alcohol causes increased activation of the sympathetic nervous system, with increased circulating catecholamines secreted by the adrenal medulla. Alcoholism also affects the hypothalamic–pituitary–gonadal axis, and these effects are further exacerbated by alcoholic liver disease.
- *Effects on central nervous system:* Effects are dose-dependent and begin with the so-called social modulating effects of alcohol, including increasing cheerfulness, loss of inhibitions and impaired judgement. Heavier consumption leads to agitation, slurred speech, loss of memory, with double vision and staggering.
- *Effects on cardiovascular system:* Acute effects of alcohol on the cardiovascular system involve both the heart and the peripheral vasculature. Peripheral vasodilation causes a sensation of warmth.

Cardiac effects are usually in the form of arrhythmias, such as bradycardia, tachycardia or sometimes fatal atrial fibrillation, experienced as palpitations.

- *Effects on muscle weakness:* Alcoholic myopathy is common and is a major cause of morbidity. It is characterized by muscle weakness, myalgia, muscle cramps and loss of lean tissue.
- *Effects on dehydration:* Ethanol affects hypothalamic osmoreceptors, reducing antidiuretic hormone release, so causing reduced salt and water reabsorption in the distal tubule, leading to dehydration.
- *Effects on liver function:* The pathophysiology of alcohol-induced cirrhosis is incompletely understood, but is thought to involve the production of reactive oxygen species, and associated oxidative damage. Inadequate intake of dietary antioxidants may exacerbate the effect.

Alcohol and nutritional status

Chronic ethanol misuse is often associated with impaired nutritional status either due to inadequate dietary intake or damage to the gastrointestinal system.

Alcohol consumption can displace nutrient rich foods from the diet, leading to generalized undernutrition. Inadequate intakes of micronutrients, including vitamins B_1, A, C, E and folate and zinc and selenium have often been reported in alcoholics. Effects of alcohol on the integrity of the mucosal cells of the gastrointestinal tract can impair nutrient absorption, which will exacerbate effects of nutrient displacement. The metabolism of alcohol leads to an inhibition of other metabolic pathways, principally because of depletion of NAD. This limits the oxidation of fat, carbohydrate and protein, with various metabolic consequences. Alcohol also has effects on specific nutrients, such as thiamin, and functional thiamin deficiency is a common feature of alcoholism.

Alcohol intake and chronic disease risk

Epidemiological studies suggest that a modest intake of alcohol is cardio-protective and can reduce coronary heart disease, particularly in middle-aged men and post-menopausal women. This protective effect is not seen at higher levels of intake, which increase incidence of cardiovascular disease including hypertension. Moderate to heavy drinking is associated with an increased risk of stroke. Consumption of up to 3 Units/day however, reduces ischaemic strokes but binge drinking increases the risk of all types of stroke. The reported cardioprotective effects of alcohol may be due to antioxidant properties of substances in the beverages, such as polyphenols in red wine. Protective effects may also occur via clot formation and dissolution, reducing circulating levels of fibrinogen, factor VII and plasminogen activator. Platelet aggregability may also be reduced by alcohol.

In contrast there is strong evidence that alcohol increases the risk of cancer at various sites, including breast cancer, with no evidence for a lower threshold. The public health message must therefore take into account the effects of alcohol consumption on both cardiovascular disease and cancer. A recent report of diet, physical activity and cancer (WCRF/AICR 2007) recommends that alcohol consumption be restricted to one drink per day for women and two for men.

KEY POINTS

- In the UK, the overall contribution of ethanol to total energy intake is 6.5% in men and 3.9% in women
- Alcohol absorption and metabolism is affected by a number of variables, including gastric alcohol-metabolizing enzymes, ethnicity, gender, presence of different foods and body size
- There are at least 60–120 different alcohol-related pathologies
- The immediate metabolite of ethanol oxidation, acetaldehyde, is highly toxic
- There are a number of routes of ethanol metabolism. The microsomal ethanol oxidizing system (MEOS) is particularly important in chronic alcoholism
- About 50% of alcoholics will have nutritional deficiencies; these can arise via a number of processes including poor dietary intakes, displacement of foods (empty calories theory), maldigestion and malabsorption
- Low to moderate amounts of alcohol may reduce risk of cardiovascular disease, particularly in middle-aged men

4.6 WATER BALANCE AND REQUIREMENTS

Body water balance

Water makes up about 60% of the total body weight of a healthy adult. It is a major component of extracellular and intracellular fluids. Regulation of water balance is central to survival; death occurs within a few days of water deprivation whilst humans can live from many weeks without food. The term 'water balance' simply refers to the balance between water intake and water output. Total body water is regulated to maintain an osmotic pressure in body fluids of 285 mosmol/kg. Plasma osmolality is a measure of the concentration of substances such as sodium, chloride, potassium, urea, glucose, and other ions in human blood. It is calculated as the osmoles of solute per kilogram of solvent. Body water is determined by the balance between intake and loss. Water intake is regulated by feelings of thirst or satiety whilst the extent of dilution of urine determines water loss.

Water intake

Water intake is governed by thirst and satiety. When the concentration of solutes in body fluids rises there are three routes to initiating drinking of water:

- water is drawn out of the salivary glands and the mouth becomes dry, prompting drinking
- the hypothalamus detects the increases in solute concentration and initiates a drinking stimulus
- receptors in the stomach detect hydration state and may prompt drinking.

Water loss

Water loss occurs principally in the breath, in sweat, in urine, and in exfoliated cells. Regulation of water excretion is mainly under the control of anti-diuretic hormone (ADH), which is secreted from the pituitary gland in response to stimulus from the hypothalamus. If the hypothalamus detects an increase in solute concentration in the blood it stimulates the pituitary to release ADH, which directs the kidneys to reabsorb water. Additionally, low blood pressure can result from excessive water loss, and this triggers the release of renin by the kidney. Renin activates angiotensin which has two effects; it acts as a vasoconstrictor, thereby raising blood pressure, and stimulates the adrenal glands to secrete aldosterone, which directs the kidneys to retain sodium and water. Urine osmolality can vary between 50–1200 mmol/kg depending upon the osmotic pressure of body fluids. In these ways water is recycled rather than excreted in times of water deficit.

Failure of water balance

Under some circumstances these mechanisms of regulation of water balance fail to cope. Dehydration is a feature of diarrhoea, of heavy sweat loss, and of alcohol abuse. It will also develop in untreated diabetic patients. In contrast, excessive water retention, indicated by oedema, occurs in association with congestive heart failure, which is common among elderly people, and in renal dysfunction.

Water and electrolyte balance

The movement of water across cell membranes is inextricably linked to the movement of electrolytes. The movement of water is dictated by the concentration of electrolytes, such that water will tend to cross a membrane to dilute a concentrated fluid, if the solute molecules cannot readily cross the membrane themselves. It is very important physiologically that the concentration of solutes in body fluids is regulated, and this is achieved by control over absorption and excretion. Sodium and chloride ions are present in the highest concentration in extracellular fluids and are lost most readily as a result of fluid loss such as in heavy sweating or diarrhoea. Under such circumstances drinking water will not restore sodium and chloride balance, and the person would require a source of these electrolytes, through the consumption of salty foods or the use of a special electrolyte mix. It is considered that most adults need about 1.5 g sodium and 2.3 g chloride, or 3.8 g salt daily to replace physiological losses.

Dietary sources of water

In addition to the water consumed in beverages all but the most fatty foods are a useful source of water. Fruits and vegetables commonly have high water content, some fruits and vegetable contain 95% water and even full fat cheeses and meats can be 50% or more water. Additionally the body generates water as a result of oxidative metabolism of macronutrients.

Water requirements

There are currently no evidence-based recommendations for daily water consumption in the same way as there are for energy and most nutrients. The Food and Nutrition Board of the Institute of Medicine in the USA recommend that women consume a total of about 2.7 litres of water daily and that men consume about 3.7 litres daily. Of this about 80% generally comes from water and other beverages and the remainder comes from food. People in hot climates or engaging in strenuous activity will have increased water requirements; endurance athletes can lose 1.5 litres of water with only one hour of exercise.

FURTHER READING

Bender D A 2008 Introduction to nutrition and metabolism, 4th edn. CRC Press, Boca Raton, FL

Frayn K N 2003 Metabolic regulation: a human perspective, 2nd edn. Blackwell Science, Oxford

Gurr M I, Harwood J L, Frayn K N 2002 Lipid biochemistry – an introduction, 5th edn. Blackwell Science, Oxford

Garlick P J 2006 Protein requirements of infants and children. Nestle Nutrition Workshop Series Pediatric Program 58:39–47; discussion 47–50

Lieber C S 2000 Alcohol: Its metabolism and interaction with nutrients. Annual Review of Nutrition 20:395–430

CHAPTER 5

Minor Dietary Components

OBJECTIVES

By the end of this chapter you should be able to:

- identify good food sources of water-soluble vitamins, fat-soluble vitamins, minerals and trace elements
- summarize the absorption and transport of each
- summarize the main metabolic functions of each
- describe the main effects of deficiency and excess of each
- understand the methods of assessment of status
- appreciate the metabolic interactions between different micronutrients

5.1 INTRODUCTION

The term 'minor dietary components' in this book refers to vitamins, minerals, trace elements and phytochemicals. The term reflects the fact that the amounts of these nutrients present in typical diets range from micrograms, as for vitamin B_{12}, to grams, as for calcium, in contrast to the very much higher dietary intakes of fats, carbohydrate and protein. This is a diverse group of dietary components, with wide-ranging functions. For some, such as iron, deficiency states are often encountered in human populations, even in high-income countries, whereas for other nutrients, such as sodium, dietary deficiency is uncommon. Of course, inadequate dietary intake will not be the sole determinant of poor nutritional status; many other factors, such as genotype, and lifestyle factors such as physical activity, the use of medication, alcohol consumption and smoking habits, can interact with diet to influence nutritional status. Furthermore, dietary deficiencies are not always encountered as single nutrient deficiencies, and certain dietary patterns are associated with multiple nutrient deficiencies. This chapter considers, in a brief way, the main features of metabolism, effects of deficiency and excess, dietary sources of each nutrient and daily requirements.

5.2 WATER-SOLUBLE VITAMINS

Vitamin B₁ – thiamin

Metabolic functions of thiamin

The active form of this vitamin is thiamin diphosphate (also called thiamin pyrophosphate), which acts as a coenzyme for three multi-enzyme complexes important in central energy-yielding metabolic pathways and in the metabolism of branched chain amino acids. It is also the coenzyme for transketolase in the pentose phosphate pathway of carbohydrate metabolism.

Thiamin deficiency

Deficiency can develop rapidly during depletion. In deficiency there is impaired entry of pyruvate into the tricarboxylic acid cycle, especially on a relatively high carbohydrate diet, which results in increased plasma concentrations of lactate and pyruvate, which may lead to life-threatening acidosis. Thiamin deficiency can result in three distinct syndromes: a chronic peripheral neuritis, dry beriberi, which may or may not be associated with heart failure and oedema; acute pernicious beriberi, in which heart failure and metabolic abnormalities predominate, also called wet beriberi; and Wernicke's encephalopathy, associated especially with alcoholism. Dry beriberi is associated with a more prolonged, and presumably less severe, deficiency, with a generally low food intake, while higher carbohydrate intake and physical activity predispose to oedema and hence wet beriberi.

Forms of thiamin in foods, and good food sources

In foods, most thiamin is present as the diphosphate. Thiamin is present in many foods of plant and animal origin, although pork, nuts and fish are especially rich sources.

Absorption and transport of thiamin

Thiamin is absorbed by active transport in the duodenum and proximal jejunum. There is active transport from the intestinal cells into the bloodstream; this is inhibited by alcohol, leading to thiamin deficiency in alcoholics. Much of the absorbed thiamin is phosphorylated in the liver, and both free thiamin and thiamin monophosphate circulate in plasma, bound to albumin. All tissues can take up both thiamin and thiamin monophosphate, and are able to phosphorylate them to the active di- and triphosphates.

Assessment of thiamin status and dietary requirements

The activation of apo-transketolase in erythrocyte lysate by thiamin diphosphate added in vitro is the most widely used index of thiamin nutritional status. An activation coefficient >1.25 is indicative of deficiency, and <1.15 is considered to reflect adequate thiamin nutrition.

Thiamin requirements depend largely on carbohydrate intake. In practice, requirements are calculated on the basis of total energy intake. For diets that are lower in fat, and hence higher in carbohydrate and protein, thiamin requirements will be higher. Depletion/repletion studies show that an intake of 0.3 mg/1000 kcal is required for a normal transketolase activation coefficient and this is the basis of the current recommended intakes.

Riboflavin – vitamin B$_2$

Metabolic functions of riboflavin

This vitamin is important in a wide variety of oxidation and reduction reactions central to all metabolic processes, including the mitochondrial electron transport chain. The active forms of the vitamin are flavin adenine dinucleotide (FAD) and flavin mononucleotide (FMN). Riboflavin contributes to antioxidant defences through a role in the synthesis of glutathione, an important antioxidant. Riboflavin is also important in folate and vitamin B$_6$ metabolism, and may play a role in iron utilization.

Riboflavin deficiency

Low intakes of riboflavin and associated biochemical riboflavin deficiency are common in many regions of the world including affluent Western countries. Clinically, deficiency is characterized by lesions of the margin of the lips and corners of the mouth and a painful desquamation of the tongue, so that it is red, and dry. However, the functional significance of riboflavin deficiency in humans is not completely understood. Impaired fatty acid oxidation has been reported in animals but this has not been substantiated in humans. Altered gastrointestinal development and impaired iron absorption are features of riboflavin deficiency in animals and there is some evidence to suggest that this may also be important in humans, but research is ongoing.

Forms of riboflavin in food and dietary sources

Apart from milk and eggs, which contain relatively large amounts of free riboflavin, most of the vitamin in foods is as the flavin coenzymes, FAD and FMN, bound to enzymes. Liver, milk, meat and fish are good sources of riboflavin; some green leafy vegetables also provide significant amounts. About one-third of riboflavin in Western diets comes from milk and milk products.

Absorption and transport

FAD and FMN in foods are hydrolysed to riboflavin in the gastrointestinal tract and riboflavin is taken up into the gastrointestinal mucosa. Much of the absorbed riboflavin is phosphorylated in the intestinal mucosa, and enters the bloodstream as riboflavin phosphate. Free riboflavin and FAD are the main forms in plasma. Most riboflavin in tissues is as FAD or FMN, bound to enzymes. There is no evidence of any significant storage of riboflavin, and intake in excess of tissue requirements is excreted rapidly in the urine.

Assessment of riboflavin status and dietary requirements

On the basis of depletion/repletion studies, the minimum adult requirement is 0.5–0.8 mg/day. Because of the central role of flavin coenzymes in energy yielding metabolism, reference intakes are sometimes calculated on the basis of energy intake: 0.6–0.8 mg/1000 kcal (0.14–0.19 mg/MJ).

The most commonly used method for determining riboflavin status is the activation of the erythrocyte enzyme glutathione reductase by FAD added in vitro, known as EGRAC. With decreasing intakes of riboflavin EGRAC values increase and values of about 1.40 and above are considered to indicate riboflavin deficiency.

Niacin

Niacin is the generic term for the two compounds that have the biological activity of the vitamin, nicotinic acid and nicotinamide. Niacin is the precursor of the nicotinamide part of the coenzymes nicotinamide adenine dinucleotide (NAD) and its phosphorylated form NADP, which are important as electron carriers in the metabolism of protein, carbohydrate and fat. In fact nicotinamide can be made from the amino acid tryptophan, and in developed countries, average intakes of protein provide more than enough tryptophan to meet requirements for NAD synthesis without any need for preformed niacin. It is only when tryptophan intake is inadequate that niacin becomes a dietary essential, such as in populations in which maize is the staple.

Metabolic functions of niacin

In general, NAD is involved as an electron acceptor in energy-yielding metabolism, and the resultant NADH is oxidized by the mitochondrial electron transport chain. The major coenzyme for reactions of biosynthesis is NADPH. NAD is also the precursor of messengers that act to increase the release of calcium from intracellular stores in response to hormones.

Effects of niacin deficiency and excess

Niacin deficiency can lead to the deficiency disease pellagra, which is characterized by a photosensitive dermatitis, like severe sunburn, affecting regions of the skin that are exposed to sunlight. Advanced pellagra is also accompanied by a 'dementia' or depressive psychosis, and there may be diarrhoea. Untreated pellagra is fatal.

The synthesis of NAD from tryptophan requires both riboflavin and vitamin B$_6$, and deficiency of either may lead to the development of secondary pellagra when intakes of tryptophan and preformed niacin are marginal.

High intakes of niacin through supplements cause liver damage. Sustained release preparations are associated with more severe liver damage and clinical liver failure.

Forms in foods and good food sources of niacin

Meat and fish are good sources of preformed niacin and nuts and some fruits and vegetables provide significant amounts. Most of the niacin in cereals is biologically unavailable. Because synthesis of niacin from tryptophan is more important than dietary preformed niacin, foods that are good sources of protein are also good sources of niacin. Total niacin intakes are calculated as mg niacin equivalents: the sum of preformed niacin plus 1/60 of tryptophan (the average equivalence of dietary tryptophan and niacin).

Absorption and transport of preformed niacin

Niacin is present within cells largely as the nicotinamide coenzymes. Both nicotinic acid and nicotinamide are absorbed from the small intestine by a sodium-dependent saturable process. The coenzymes NAD and NADP are synthesized from these compounds in tissues. In the liver, NAD can be synthesized from tryptophan, and then hydrolysed to release nicotinamide, which is exported to other tissues.

Assessment of niacin status and dietary requirements

There is no wholly satisfactory biochemical measurement of niacin status. The two methods in current use are measurement of blood nicotinamide nucleotides and the urinary excretion of niacin metabolites. Because of the central role of the nicotinamide nucleotides in energy-yielding metabolism, niacin requirements are conventionally expressed per unit of energy expenditure. The average niacin requirement has been estimated to be 5.5 mg/1000 kcal (1.3 mg/MJ). Allowing for individual variation, reference intakes are set at 6.6 mg niacin equivalents. The tolerable upper limit of niacin intake is 35 mg/day for adults.

Vitamin B$_6$

The term vitamin B$_6$ includes six vitamers: the alcohol pyridoxine, the aldehyde pyridoxal, the amine pyridoxamine and their phosphorylated derivatives. These vitamers are metabolically interconvertible, and have equal biological activity.

Metabolic functions of vitamin B$_6$

Pyridoxal phosphate is involved in many reactions of amino acid metabolism, is a cofactor for glycogen mobilization, and plays a role in lipid metabolism and in steroid hormone action. Vitamin B$_6$-dependent enzymes catalyse several types of reactions involving amino acids including transamination, which is central both to the utilization of amino acid carbon skeletons for gluconeogenesis or ketogenesis and also the synthesis of non-essential amino acids, and decarboxylation, to form a variety of biologically active amines such as the neurotransmitter serotonin (see chapter 4).

As pyridoxal phosphate, vitamin B$_6$ also plays a role in the control of the nuclear action of steroid hormones. In animals, vitamin B$_6$ deficiency results in increased and prolonged nuclear uptake and retention of steroid hormones in target tissues, and enhanced end-organ responsiveness to low doses of hormones.

Effects of vitamin B$_6$ deficiency and excess

Vitamin B$_6$ is widely distributed in foods and is synthesized by intestinal flora so clinical deficiency is rare, although biochemical deficiency is reported in 10–20% of the population of developed countries. Although clinical and physiological effects of vitamin B_6 deficiency in animals have been well-characterized there is relatively little documented about clinical deficiency in humans, except for neurological abnormalities in acute deficiency. Studies suggest that low vitamin B_6 status increases the risk of cardiovascular disease, probably independent of an associated elevation of plasma homocysteine.

Vitamin B_6 deficiency may result from the prolonged administration of drugs that antagonize the metabolism of the vitamin, such as penicillamine and the antitubercular drug isoniazid which reacts with pyridoxal phosphate, making it unavailable.

High dose supplements of vitamin B_6 are consumed for a variety of conditions, including premenstrual syndrome, depression, morning sickness in pregnancy, hypertension and carpal tunnel syndrome, although the evidence of efficacy is slight. High doses of the vitamin, of the order of 100 times requirements, cause peripheral sensory neuropathy.

Forms of vitamin B_6 in foods and good food sources

Meat, fish, potatoes and bananas are good sources of vitamin B_6 and milk, nuts, beans and vegetables also make a useful contribution to dietary vitamin B_6. All forms of the vitamin are found in foods but pyridoxal phosphate predominates.

Absorption and transport of vitamin B_6

Phosphorylated forms of the vitamin are hydrolysed in the intestinal mucosa and the non-phosphorylated vitamers, pyridoxal, pyridoxamine and pyridoxine, are all absorbed rapidly by carrier-mediated diffusion. Vitamin B_6 is retained in tissues by conversion to pyridoxal phosphate. Pyridoxal and pyridoxal phosphate constitute the main plasma forms of the vitamin, together with the oxidation product pyridoxic acid, which is excreted in the urine.

Assessment of vitamin B_6 status and dietary requirements

Vitamin B_6 status is usually assessed from the measurement of plasma concentrations of either total vitamin B_6 or pyridoxal phosphate, or urinary pyridoxic acid or as the activation coefficient of vitamin B_6-dependent red blood cell enzymes.

In view of the important role for vitamin B_6 in amino acid metabolism, requirements for this vitamin can be expressed relative to protein intake. On the basis of depletion/repletion studies in adults, reference intakes for the UK population range from $8\mu g/g$ protein per day in infants to $15\mu g/g$ protein per day in adults, which approximates to 0.2–1.5 mg per day.

Folates

Folic acid derivatives function in the transfer of one-carbon fragments in a variety of reactions. The term folate includes a number of compounds with a common ring structure to which one or more glutamic acid residues are attached. The compounds exist in two states of oxidation. In the reduced state the attachment of various one-carbon groups forms the biologically active coenzymes. The term *folic acid* strictly only refers to the simplest, oxidized form, carrying a single glutamic acid residue.

Metabolic functions of folate

Folate is central to reactions involving the transfer of one-carbon units, in biosynthetic and catabolic processes. It plays an important role in the synthesis of purines and pyrimidines for nucleic acid synthesis, and acts as a methyl group donor to various substrates, including DNA. There is evidence that the role for folate in DNA methylation is important for gene expression and may influence carcinogenesis. Folate plays a key role in the regulation of concentrations of the amino acid homocysteine in cells and in the plasma, through its conversion to methionine by methylation. This is important because raised plasma homocysteine is considered to be a risk factor for cardiovascular disease. Certainly increasing folate intake will reduce plasma homocysteine levels, but the role for homocysteine in determining cardiovascular disease risk is still uncertain. A commonly occurring polymorphism (see chapter 11) in the gene expressing methylenetetrahydrofolate reductase, which generates the methyl group essential for methylation of homocysteine, is associated with a reduced concentration of red blood cell and plasma folate and an increased plasma homocysteine concentration, particularly in people with low folate intake.

Effects of folate deficiency and excess

Low dietary intakes of folate are common in many countries of the world, in affluent countries as well as low-income countries. Folate status is also compromised in patients using the drug methotrexate, an anti-cancer drug also used to treat rheumatoid arthritis and psoriasis. Deficiency results in megaloblastic anaemia which involves the release into the circulation of immature red blood cells due to a failure of the normal process of maturation in the bone marrow. Deficiency is frequently accompanied by depression, insomnia, forgetfulness and irritability, and sometimes cognitive impairment and dementia. Low folate status can lead to elevated plasma homocysteine levels and there is some evidence that low folate status may alter the methylation profile of DNA.

Folate deficiency and neural tube defects

The neural tube, which runs from the brain to the lower end of the spinal cord, normally closes in embryonic development in the third and fourth weeks after fertilization. A failure of this process leads to a range of severe fetal malformations collectively known as neural tube defects. There is evidence that low folate status in women increases the risk of neural tube defects in their offspring and that supplements of 400 μg/day of folic acid, begun before conception, significantly reduce risk. Women who are planning a pregnancy are advised to take folic acid supplements.

Two groups of people are at risk of adverse effects of high folic acid intakes that might result from widespread enrichment of foods with folic acid or indiscriminate use of supplements. High intakes of folic acid may mask the development of vitamin B_{12} deficiency, which is prevalent among the elderly; this increases the risk of the deficiency progressing to irreversible neurological damage. High intakes of folic acid also antagonize the anticonvulsants used in treatment of epilepsy, leading to an increase in fit frequency.

Forms of folate in food and good food sources

All forms of folate can be present in foods, although folic acid only occurs as a food fortificant and it is in this form that folate is typically taken as a supplement. Folates are present naturally in a wide variety of foods; liver is an especially rich source, green leafy vegetables, beans, nuts and some fruits are also good sources. In some countries, including the USA, folic acid is added as a fortificant to flour and therefore many foods contain appreciable amounts of folate in this form.

Absorption and transport of folate

In the small intestine, folate polyglutamates are hydrolysed to the monoglutamate which is absorbed in the jejunum. Methyl-tetrahydrofolate (MeTHF) is the main form of the vitamin in the plasma and is taken up by tissues. Efficiency of absorption of folate from foods varies, such that folate in cereals is relatively poorly absorbed whilst that in milk appears to be well absorbed. Folic acid appears to be absorbed readily, although at single doses greater than about 200 µg it appears in the circulation in this form and there are suggestions that there may be adverse effects. Folate absorption is depressed in people who take the anti-inflammatory drug sulfasalazine, which is one reason why patients with inflammatory bowel disease often present with poor folate status.

Assessment of folate status and daily requirements

The plasma or red blood cell concentration of folate can be measured by protein-binding, radioimmunoassay, chromatography and microbiological assays but there is a lack of standardization of methodology. Folate is incorporated into red blood cells (erythrocytes) during their formation in the bone marrow, and does not enter the cells in the circulation to any significant extent. For this reason erythrocyte folate is generally considered to give an indication of folate status over 1–3 months (the lifespan of erythrocytes in the circulation is 120 days), rather than reflecting recent intake. Folate concentration can also be measured in white blood cells.

Because of the problems of determining the availability of the mixed folates in foods, reference intakes allow a wide margin of safety. Current reference daily intakes for the UK population range from 50 µg in infants to 200 µg in adults, with an increment of 100 µg during pregnancy. Dietary reference values for Europe and USA are higher, rising to 400 µg and 600 µg respectively, in pregnancy.

Vitamin B$_{12}$

Various vitamers of vitamin B$_{12}$ exist, in which different groups are attached to a central cobalt atom in the molecule; these are cyanocobalamin, hydroxocobalamin, methylcobalamin and adenosylcobalamin.

Metabolic functions of vitamin B$_{12}$

Vitamin B$_{12}$ plays a role in the metabolism of methionine, fatty acids with an odd number of carbon atoms, and the amino acid leucine. In each case vitamin B$_{12}$ acts as an enzyme cofactor. Its role in methionine metabolism is linked with the conversion of folate from the Me THF form to tetrahydrofolate and therefore vitamin B$_{12}$ deficiency is associated with the 'trapping' of folate in its methylated form in cells, which can lead to secondary folate deficiency.

Effects of deficiency and excess of vitamin B$_{12}$

The involvement of vitamin B$_{12}$ in folate metabolism is the basis of the megaloblastic anaemia that can develop during depletion, which, as we have seen, is also a feature of folate deficiency. Megaloblastic anaemia of vitamin B$_{12}$ deficiency is known as pernicious anaemia, and is associated with spinal cord degeneration and peripheral neuropathy; this is because vitamin B$_{12}$ is essential for making the fatty myelin sheath that covers nerve fibres. Vitamin B$_{12}$ deficiency is commonly due to poor absorption because of a failure to secrete intrinsic factor (IF) into the stomach, as this compound is essential for absorption. Pernicious anaemia is most common among the elderly, among whom it is typically treated with vitamin B$_{12}$ injections.

There is no evidence of adverse effects of high oral doses of vitamin B$_{12}$.

Forms of vitamin B$_{12}$ in foods and good food sources

Vitamin B$_{12}$ is found only in foods of animal origin, there are no plant sources. Rich sources include liver, fish and meat.

Absorption and transport

The major route of vitamin B$_{12}$ absorption is by way of binding to intrinsic factor, a glycoprotein secreted by cells of the gastric mucosa. There is an increased likelihood of impaired absorption in the elderly due to atrophic gastritis, which can lead to impaired secretion of intrinsic factor. The vitamin B$_{12}$–intrinsic factor complex is absorbed from the ileum into the mucosal cells. Inside the mucosal cells, the vitamin is released from IF and is bound to a protein carrier called transcobalamin, for transport into the bloodstream. The vitamin–transcobalamin complex is taken up from plasma by tissues, after which the vitamin is released as hydroxocobalamin, and converted to other vitamers. Vitamin B$_{12}$ undergoes entero-hepatic circulation, in which the vitamin is secreted in the bile and reabsorbed in the intestine.

Assessment of vitamin B$_{12}$ status and dietary requirements

Vitamin B$_{12}$ status is usually determined by measuring plasma total vitamin B$_{12}$, although there is general agreement that it does not always adequately reflect tissue depletion, especially in people with impaired renal function. Plasma holotranscobalamin (transcobalamin saturated with vitamin B_{12}), is currently under scrutiny as a marker of vitamin B_{12} status. Methylmalonic acid accumulates in cells during vitamin B_{12} depletion because of a block in a metabolic pathway, and plasma and urinary concentrations of this compound offer potential as functional markers of deficiency.

Reference nutrient intakes have been set at between 0.3–1.5 µg per day from infancy to adulthood, for the UK population, compared with an average intake of some 5 µg/day by non-vegetarians in most countries.

Vitamin C (ascorbic acid)

Vitamin C is a dietary essential for only a limited number of vertebrate species: human beings and the other primates, the guinea pig, bats, some birds and fishes.

Metabolic functions of vitamin C

Vitamin C contributes to the synthesis of collagen and the catecholamines noradrenaline and adrenaline through its role as a cofactor in enzyme-catalysed reactions. The presence of ascorbic acid in a meal containing non-haem iron can significantly affect iron absorption, through reduction from the ferric to ferrous form, and binding of the iron. This reducing effect appears also to be important in mobilizing iron from the plasma iron transport protein, transferrin. The vitamin can protect cells from damage caused by free radicals because it can react with such radicals and convert them to less damaging species. Ascorbic acid is also thought to reduce the vitamin E radical α-tocopheroxyl, formed in cell membranes and plasma lipoproteins during the oxidation of vitamin E, so sparing vitamin E. However, it can also increase the rate of production of free radicals, via a chemical reduction of transition metals like iron or copper. The normally high concentration of vitamin C in white blood cells probably contributes to an appropriate inflammatory response to stress whilst minimizing oxidant damage to surrounding tissue.

Vitamin C deficiency and excess

Various biochemical and clinical changes result from vitamin C depletion, eventually resulting in the deficiency disease scurvy. Deficiency is associated with tiredness and general malaise, and is often accompanied by anaemia. In scurvy, skin changes reflect effects on collagen synthesis, and include haemorrhage of the gum capillaries and poor wound healing. High dose supplements of vitamin C can lead to unabsorbed ascorbate in the intestinal lumen, which becomes a substrate for bacterial fermentation, and can be associated with diarrhoea.

Forms in foods and good food sources

Ascorbic acid is the physiologically important form of the vitamin. It can oxidize to dehydroascorbic acid but this retains biological activity because it can be reduced to ascorbic acid. Fruits and vegetables are rich sources of ascorbate; blackcurrants and guava provide about five times the reference intake in a single serving, and potatoes are an important source in many countries.

Absorption and transport of vitamin C

Ascorbate and dehydroascorbate are both absorbed by the duodenum and up to 90% of the vitamin can be absorbed from usual dietary intakes. The vitamin is carried in the red blood cells and plasma predominantly as ascorbic acid, in comparable concentrations, but white blood cells concentrate the vitamin and can have extremely high concentrations.

Ascorbate is excreted quantitatively with increasing intake once the renal threshold has been exceeded. Additionally, use of the antibiotic tetracycline is associated with increased urinary excretion of vitamin C and a fall in plasma concentration.

Assessment of vitamin C status and reference intakes

Vitamin C status is generally assessed by measuring plasma and white blood cell concentrations of the vitamin. At intakes above about 100 mg/day the plasma concentration of ascorbate reaches a plateau and urinary excretion increases. The reference nutrient intake for the UK population ranges from 25 mg/day in infancy to 40 mg/day in adults, with an increment of 10 mg in pregnancy. Recommended intakes are higher in the USA (up to 90 mg/day in adults).

Pantothenic acid

Pantothenic acid has a central role in energy-yielding metabolism as the functional group of a compound called coenzyme A (CoA), which is important in a wide variety of reactions. It is also essential for fatty acid synthesis through its function in acyl carrier protein. Pantothenic acid is widely distributed in all food-stuffs and it is absorbed throughout the small intestine. Intestinal bacterial synthesis contributes to intake.

There are no generally used functional tests of pantothenic acid status. From the limited studies that have been performed it is not possible to establish requirements for pantothenic acid. Average intakes in adult populations are 2–7 mg/day.

Biotin

Biotin occurs in a wide variety of foods and deficiency has only been reported in individuals consuming large amounts of uncooked egg white, which contains a biotin antagonist. Dietary deficiency of biotin sufficient to cause clinical signs is extremely rare in humans.

Metabolically, biotin is of central importance in lipogenesis (fat synthesis) and gluconeogenesis (glucose synthesis), acting as the coenzyme for enzyme-catalysed reactions. In addition, it induces the synthesis of a number of key enzymes of glycolysis and gluconeogenesis.

There is little information concerning biotin requirements, and no evidence on which to base recommendations. Average adult intakes range between 15–70 µg/day. The safe and adequate range of intakes is set at 10–200 µg/day.

KEY POINTS

- *Thiamin*
  - Thiamin functions as a coenzyme in energy-yielding metabolism
  - Thiamin deficiency, leading to central nervous system damage, is a significant problem among alcoholics
- *Riboflavin*
  - Riboflavin functions as a coenzyme in a wide variety of reactions, including key reactions in energy-yielding metabolism
  - Riboflavin deficiency can lead to impaired handling of iron
- *Niacin*
  - There are two vitamers of niacin – nicotinamide and nicotinic acid
  - Niacin is the precursor of NAD and NADP, which are central to many oxidation reduction reactions
  - Deficiency leads to skin lesions, especially where the skin is exposed to sunlight, and dementia
  - At extremely high doses niacin can cause liver damage
- *Pyridoxine*
  - Vitamin B_6 functions as a coenzyme in a wide variety of reactions of amino acids and in glycogen and lipid metabolism
  - Clinical deficiency of vitamin B_6 is more or less unknown, but marginal status is widespread
  - Very high doses of vitamin B_6 cause sensory nerve damage
- *Folates*
  - Folates function as coenzymes in one-carbon transfer reactions
  - Dietary folate deficiency is not uncommon; deficiency results in anaemia in which large red blood cells enter the circulation (called megaloblastic anaemia)
  - Low folate status is associated with neural tube defects, and periconceptual supplements reduce the incidence
  - Low folate status is associated with high levels of the amino acid homocysteine in the blood and altered methylation of DNA
- *Vitamin B_{12}*
  - Vitamin B_{12} is involved in fatty acid and amino acid metabolism
  - Dietary deficiency of vitamin B_{12} occurs primarily in vegans as there are no plant sources of the vitamin
  - Functional deficiency, due to failure of absorption, is relatively common among elderly people
  - Deficiency causes pernicious anaemia, which is megaloblastic anaemia with spinal cord degeneration
- *Vitamin C*
  - Vitamin C is important for the synthesis of collagen and catecholamines. It can act as an antioxidant but also a pro-oxidant. It enhances the absorption of non-haem iron
  - Deficiency (scurvy) results in mood and behavioural changes, skin lesions and impaired wound healing

Vitamin A

The term vitamin A includes two groups of compounds; pre-formed vitamin A, which include retinol, retinaldehyde and retinoic acid, and a variety of carotenoids which can be converted to retinal. The most important of the pro-vitamin A carotenoids in humans are α- and β-carotene, and cryptoxanthin.

Metabolic functions of vitamin A

Vitamin A has four metabolic roles: as the prosthetic group of the visual pigments, as a modulator of gene expression, as a carrier of mannosyl units in the synthesis of glycoproteins, which are important in cell-to-cell interactions, and in the post-translational modification of proteins, with effects on protein function.

Retinaldehyde in vision

Vitamin A is important for vision. In the retina retinaldehyde binds to the protein opsin, forming the light sensitive pigment rhodopsin. The absorption of light by rhodopsin results in a change in the configuration of the retinaldehyde, together with a conformational change in opsin. This results in both the release of retinaldehyde from the protein and the initiation of a nerve impulse. In vitamin A deficiency, both the time taken to adapt to darkness and the ability to see in poor light are impaired.

Genomic actions of retinoic acid

Retinoic acid has both a general role in growth and a specific role in development and tissue differentiation. These functions are the result of effects of vitamin A in the nucleus, leading to alterations in gene expression. Both deficiency and excess of retinoic acid cause severe developmental abnormalities. In the nucleus there are two groups of receptors which bind different isomers (same molecular formula but different spatial arrangement of atoms) of retinoic acid, the retinoic acid receptor (RAR) family and the retinoid X receptor (RXR) family. The receptor–retinoic acid complexes can influence gene expression through effects on protein synthesis, specifically at the level of transcription. They can act to increase or to repress gene expression. They are also known to act in association with the vitamin D receptor so there is some interaction between vitamin A and vitamin D in altering gene expression. This activity underpins the role of these vitamins in determining differentiation of monocytes into immune system cells, and both vitamins therefore are important in immune function.

Antioxidant action

Because of their extended system of conjugated double bonds, carotenoids have antioxidant activity in vitro and in lipoproteins ex vivo. This antioxidant potential may contribute to the protective effects of diets rich in fruits and vegetables against certain cancers and cardiovascular disease. However, the antioxidant properties of carotenoids depend upon a low oxygen concentration and at high oxygen concentration carotenoids may autoxidize and act as pro-oxidants. This may explain why evidence from randomized controlled trials shows that very high doses of β-carotene may increase the risk of lung cancer, especially in heavy smokers.

Effects of vitamin A deficiency and excess

Vitamin A deficiency is recognized as a public health problem in 100 countries and is widespread in the tropics. It is largely responsible for the global annual toll of 0.5 million new cases of preventable blindness. The cumulative effects of retinol deficiency on the epithelia of the surface of the eye explain the progressive signs of xerophthalmia, the term used to describe blindness of vitamin A deficiency. Night blindness, the inability to see in dim light, is an early sign of vitamin A deficiency. The action of vitamin A in promoting mucous secretion in the respiratory tract and gut explains its protective effect in acute respiratory infection, including measles, and in diarrhoeal disease. Vitamin A deficiency is also associated with a reduction in the number and cytotoxic activity of T lymphocytes. A mild infection such as measles often triggers the development of xerophthalmia in children whose vitamin A status is marginal.

Vitamin A supplements can reduce the severity of diarrhoea and several large community trials have shown a reduction in overall mortality in population groups with poor vitamin A status.

Vitamin A is both acutely and chronically toxic. Acutely, large doses of vitamin A (in excess of 300 mg in a single dose to adults) cause nausea, vomiting and headache, which disappear within a few days. After a very large dose there may also be itching and exfoliation of the skin, and extremely high doses can prove fatal. Single doses of 60 mg of retinol are given to children in developing countries as a prophylactic against vitamin A deficiency. About 1% of children so treated show transient signs of toxicity, but this is considered to be acceptable in view of the considerable benefit of preventing xerophthalmia. The chronic toxicity of vitamin A is a more general cause for concern. Prolonged and regular intake of more than about 7500–9000 μg/day by adults (and significantly less for children) causes signs and symptoms of toxicity affecting the skin, central nervous system, liver and bones. Synthetic retinoids used to treat dermatological conditions are highly teratogenic (increase the risk of birth abnormalities), and there is concern that retinol might be also, so pregnant women are advised not to take supplements containing vitamin A without medical advice. Carotenoids, in contrast, do not cause hypervitaminosis A, because of the limited conversion to retinol.

Forms and good food sources

Liver, full-fat dairy produce, fortified margarine, oily fish and kidneys are good sources of retinol. Pro-vitamin A carotenoids are found only in plant foods. Good dietary sources of carotenoids are dark green, yellow, red and orange fruits and vegetables. The total vitamin A content of foods is expressed as μg retinol equivalents, being the sum of that provided by retinoids and carotenoids – 6 μg of β-carotene is currently taken to be 1 μg retinol equivalent.

Absorption and transport of vitamin A

The important point about vitamin A absorption is that it is absorbed with fat in chylomicrons, as both retinoids and carotenoids, passes into the lymph system and from there into the plasma. Drugs that inhibit fat absorption, such as anti-hyperlipaemic drugs, can also interfere with the absorption of vitamin A. A proportion of pro-vitamin A carotenoids is converted to retinol in the intestinal mucosa before being incorporated into chylomicrons for absorption. Retinol absorption is reasonably efficient but the absorption of carotenoids less so and as little as 5% in food may be absorbed, depending upon the nature of the meal.

Vitamin A is stored in the liver in the form of retinyl esters (retinol linked with a fatty acid). Vitamin A will be released from the liver when necessary; it binds to retinol binding protein (RBP) which then forms a complex with the thyroid hormone binding protein, transthyretin. It is in this form that retinol is transported to other tissues for use.

Assessment of vitamin A status and dietary requirements

Despite certain limitations in the usefulness of plasma retinol as a measure of vitamin A status this remains the most commonly used method for assessing status. Plasma retinol concentration remains constant over a wide range of intakes because the liver-stores release retinol when necessary. It is therefore only useful as a measure of vitamin A status when liver-stores are low, so is informative only in populations with habitually low intakes or following a period of low intakes. Additionally, in response to infection plasma retinol falls, regardless of vitamin A intakes or liver-stores, further limiting the usefulness of this measurement. The relative dose response (RDR) test is more sensitive but more difficult and time-consuming. This is a test of the ability of a dose of vitamin A to raise the plasma concentration of retinol several hours later.

Reference nutrient intakes have been set at 600–700 µg retinol equivalents daily for adults in the UK, and there is reasonable consistency across countries.

Vitamin D

Vitamin D is not strictly a vitamin because it can be synthesized in the skin. Cholecalciferol is both the usual dietary form and the form of vitamin D synthesized in the skin by UV irradiation of the precursor, 7-dehydrocholesterol. Dietary sources of vitamin D are generally relatively unimportant compared with endogenous synthesis (Fig 5.1).

Metabolic functions of vitamin D

The main physiological function of vitamin D is to maintain calcium balance. Calcitriol is formed from cholecalciferol, and maintains the plasma concentration of calcium by increasing intestinal absorption of calcium, reducing excretion by increasing reabsorption in the distal renal tubule, and mobilizing the mineral from bone. Calcitriol regulates the expression of many genes, through binding to and activating nuclear receptors that modulate gene expression. This

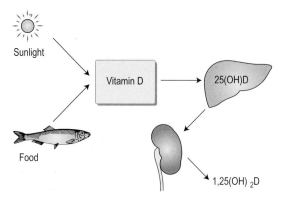

Figure 5.1 Schematic view of vitamin D metabolism.

nuclear activity may explain many of the effects of vitamin D, including effects on the secretion of insulin and the synthesis and secretion of parathyroid and thyroid hormones. Calcitriol promotes maturation and differentiation of various cell types including lymphocytes and monocytes, with associated effects on immune function. It also influences the rate of proliferation and differentiation of various cancer cell types in vitro and this may explain epidemiological data suggesting a protective effect of vitamin D against prostate cancer.

There is evidence that vitamin D suppresses development of the main cells of adipose tissue (adipocytes) and thereby helps to protect against atherosclerosis.

Effects of vitamin D deficiency and excess

Deficiency of vitamin D can lead to rickets in children and osteomalacia in adults. Rickets results from a failure of the mineralization of newly formed bone, which, as the child grows, leads to bow legs or knock knees, as well as deformity of the pelvis. Similar problems may develop during the adolescent growth spurt. Osteomalacia is the defective remineralization of bone during normal bone turnover in adults, leading to progressive demineralization and skeletal deformities. Women with inadequate vitamin D status are especially at risk of osteomalacia after repeated pregnancies and the elderly are at risk of osteomalacia because of decreased synthesis of 7-dehydrocholesterol in the skin with increasing age and low exposure to sunlight. Osteoporosis is a loss of bone mineral and matrix with age. Although it is not primarily due to a deficiency of vitamin D it is responsive to vitamin D supplements.

High intakes of vitamin D can lead to weakness, nausea, loss of appetite, headache, abdominal pains, cramp and diarrhoea and, more seriously, hypercalcaemia, which can result in hypertension. Hypervitaminosis also results in increased uptake of calcium into tissues, leading to the calcification of soft tissues, including the heart.

Forms in foods and good food sources

Vitamin D is found in foods in two forms, cholecalciferol (vitamin D_3), which is formed in the skin, and ergocalciferol (vitamin D_2), which is sometimes used as a fortificant. Good dietary sources of cholecalciferol include oily fish and eggs, and there is a modest amount in full fat milk products and liver. In many countries margarine, and sometimes also milk, is fortified with ergo-calciferol. No common plant foods contain vitamin D.

Absorption, transport and metabolism of vitamin D

Dietary vitamin D is absorbed in chylomicrons and taken up by the liver. As for vitamin A, absorption is impaired by anti-hyperlipaemic drugs. Vitamin D synthesized in the skin is bound to a plasma binding protein and is metabolized more gradually. Cholecalciferol and its active metabolites (calcidiol, calcitriol and 24-hydroxycalcidiol) are all transported bound to the same plasma binding protein. Cholecalciferol is transported in plasma lipoproteins as well. Vitamin D is converted to calcidiol (25-hydroxycholecalciferol) in the liver, which is the main circulating form of the vitamin, and this form is metabolized further, mainly to calcitriol (1,25-dihydroxycholecalciferol) in the kidney.

Vitamin D metabolism is regulated largely by the state of calcium balance. When plasma calcium levels fall parathyroid hormone secretion increases, which influences activities of the vitamin D metabolizing enzymes so as to increase circulating calcitriol. This drives an increase in plasma calcium.

Because of the low intensity radiation during the winter in temperate regions plasma concentrations of vitamin D usually show a marked fall and dietary sources become more important.

Assessment of vitamin D status and dietary requirements

The plasma concentration of calcidiol is the most sensitive index of vitamin D status. It shows a profound variation with season in temperate regions. Very low concentrations of plasma calcidiol are associated with clinical signs of rickets. Vitamin D status is determined mainly by exposure to sunlight and for this reason there are no reference intakes for adults in the UK. The reference intake for the elderly, who are more at risk of low sunlight exposure, has been set at $10\,\mu g$ per day.

Vitamin E

There are eight vitamers of vitamin E, four tocopherols which have a saturated side-chain, and four tocotrienols, which are unsaturated.

Metabolic functions of vitamin E

The best-established function of vitamin E is as a lipid-soluble antioxidant, important for preventing oxidation of lipid in membranes and lipoproteins. Vitamin E (as α-tocopherol) reacts with a lipid peroxide radical to inhibit the process of lipid peroxidation; when this happens the tocopheroxyl radical is formed. This can be reduced back to α-tocopherol by reaction with ascorbate, glutathione or other lipid-soluble antioxidants. In the absence of co-antioxidants the tocopheroxyl radical persists and causes further oxidant damage. Thus, vitamin E can also have a pro-oxidant action. Despite the known antioxidant potential of α-tocopherol there is little convincing evidence from intervention trials that supplements reduce risk of cancer, cardiovascular or neurodegenerative diseases.

α-Tocopherol, but not the other vitamers, has a role in modulation of gene expression and regulation of cell proliferation. It modulates transcription of a number of genes, including the scavenger receptor for oxidized LDL in macrophages and smooth muscle. Additionally α-tocopherol inhibits platelet aggregation and vascular smooth muscle proliferation. In animal models it has a role in immune function and there is evidence that the same may be true in humans but this has not been well established.

Vitamin E deficiency and excess

Functional effects of dietary vitamin E deficiency in humans are rare, presumably because tissue concentrations are generally adequate. Deficiency does develop in patients with severe fat malabsorption and in two groups of patients with rare genetic diseases that impair VLDL synthesis or vitamin E export from the liver. These patients develop severe neurological abnormalities.

Vitamin E deficiency may also occur in premature infants, in which case it is associated with haemolytic anaemia. Vitamin E has very low toxicity, and very high intakes are necessary before adverse effects are observed. The tolerable upper level is set at 1000 mg/day.

Forms in food and rich food sources

Tocotrienols occur in foods as both the free alcohols and as esters whilst tocopherols occur naturally as the free alcohols. Oily fish, nuts and seeds (and hence vegetable oils), beans and green leafy vegetables are rich sources of vitamin E.

Absorption and transport of vitamin E

Vitamin E is absorbed in micelles with dietary fat. Esters of vitamin E are hydrolysed in the small intestine prior to absorption. In intestinal mucosal cells, all vitamers of vitamin E are incorporated into chylomicrons, which carry the vitamin to the liver. The liver exports vitamin E as α-tocopherol incorporated into very low density lipoprotein (VLDL). The other vitamers are not incorporated into VLDL, but are metabolized in the liver and excreted. VLDL carries the vitamin E to tissues for uptake.

Assessment of vitamin E status and dietary requirements

The most commonly used index of vitamin E nutritional status is the plasma concentration of α-tocopherol, best expressed relative to plasma cholesterol or plasma total lipids. Neither the UK nor Europe has set reference intakes for vitamin E due to inadequate evidence. Vitamin E requirements are considered to increase with increasing intakes of polyunsaturated fatty acids, which oxidize readily, and therefore 0.4 mg α-tocopherol/g PUFA has been set as a safe intake.

Vitamin K

There are two naturally occurring vitamers, phylloquinone from plants (vitamin K_1) and bacterial menaquinones (vitamin K_2). The synthetic compounds menadione and menadiol are vitamin K_3.

The metabolic functions of vitamin K

The main metabolic function of vitamin K is as the coenzyme in the carboxylation of glutamate residues in proteins to yield γ-carboxyglutamate (often referred to as Gla), which is important in four proteins involved in clotting, including prothrombin. In addition, Gla is contained in proteins found in bone, the kidney cortex, atherosclerotic plaque, the inter-membrane space of mitochondria, the central nervous system, and in a number of proteins involved in cell signalling.

Vitamin K deficiency

Because vitamin K is essential for the normal synthesis of blood clotting proteins, a deficiency leads to impaired blood clotting. This can be measured as the length of time it takes for blood to form a clot, known as the prothrombin time. Osteocalcin synthesis is similarly impaired, and there is evidence that under-carboxylated osteocalcin is formed in people with marginal intakes of vitamin K despite showing no impairment of blood clotting factors. Treatment with warfarin or other anticoagulants during pregnancy can lead to bone abnormalities in the fetus, which is due to impaired synthesis of osteocalcin. Newborn infants have low plasma levels of prothrombin and the other vitamin K dependent clotting factors. It is usual to give all new-born infants prophylactic vitamin K, either orally or by intramuscular injection.

Assessment of vitamin K status and dietary requirements

The usual method of assessing vitamin K status is to measure the prothrombin time, which is a marker of clot formation. Dietary reference values have not been set for the UK or Europe but both suggest that $1\,\mu g/kg$ body weight represents a safe and adequate intake.

KEY POINTS

- *Vitamin A*
  - Vitamin A has two main functions, in the visual cycle and in gene expression and tissue differentiation
  - In addition to their role as precursors of retinol, carotenoids may act as antioxidants
  - Vitamin A deficiency is a major public health problem worldwide, and the commonest preventable cause of blindness
  - Vitamin A is both acutely and chronically toxic in excess, and is also teratogenic

- Vitamin A may be provided either as preformed retinol in animal products, or may be synthesized from dietary carotenoids, in fruit and vegetables
- *Vitamin D*
  - The main function of vitamin D is in maintenance of calcium homeostasis
  - Vitamin D also acts to regulate cell proliferation in a variety of tissues, and is involved in the secretion of a number of hormones
  - Vitamin D deficiency leads to rickets in children and adolescents, and osteomalacia in adults
  - Dietary intake is relatively unimportant compared with sunlight exposure except for infants, the elderly and ethnic groups who keep their skin covered
  - Dietary sources include oily fish, eggs and butter
- *Vitamin E*
  - Vitamin E is the major lipid-soluble antioxidant in cell membranes and plasma lipoproteins
  - α-tocopherol has actions in regulating platelet coagulability and vascular smooth muscle proliferation, and gene expression
  - Vitamin E deficiency only occurs in people with severe fat malabsorption, and some rare genetic diseases
  - Dietary sources include vegetable oils, nuts and fortified cereals
- *Vitamin K*
  - Vitamin K acts as cofactor for formation of γ-carboxyglutamate in proteins important in blood clotting and a range of other functions
  - Anticoagulants used for treatment of people at risk of thrombosis act as antimetabolites of vitamin K
  - Dietary sources include green leafy vegetables

5.4 MINERALS AND TRACE ELEMENTS

This section deals with the key minerals and trace elements essential to a number of important biochemical and physiological functions in the body. The focus is placed on dietary sources of the various minerals and their homeostatic regulation in the body. The major metabolic functions and consequences of deficiency and excess are also considered.

Calcium and phosphorus

Calcium is the most abundant mineral in the body, the majority of which is contained within the adult skeleton in the form of hydroxyapatite, a complex crystalline form of calcium phosphate, $Ca_{10}(PO_4)_6(OH)_2$.

Functions of calcium and phosphorus

The major function of both calcium and phosphorus is in the formation of the major inorganic bone component, hydroxyapatite. The rate of calcium deposition is high during skeletal development.

Both calcium and phosphorus are both important in cell signalling. Changes in the concentration of intracellular calcium play a role in a range of cellular responses including cell division, motility, contraction, and endocytosis. Phosphorus is also important in cell signalling because phosphorylation or dephosphorylation is a common mechanism for either activating or deactivating enzymes.

Calcium is an essential component of the blood clotting process and phosphorus is a component of ATP, and thereby plays a central role in energy metabolism.

Calcium and phosphorus homeostasis

Plasma calcium levels are tightly regulated by the action of parathyroid hormone (PTH) and calcitriol, which increase plasma calcium, and calcitonin, produced in the thyroid gland, which promotes calcium excretion (Fig 5.2). PTH is released in response to a decrease in plasma calcium levels and has several actions, including promoting the synthesis of calcitriol $(1,25(OH)_2 D_3)$ which in turn stimulates intestinal calcium absorption (see section 5.3). In addition, PTH (and vitamin D_3) promotes bone resorption and increases renal calcium reabsorption. Thyroid synthesis of calcitonin is promoted in

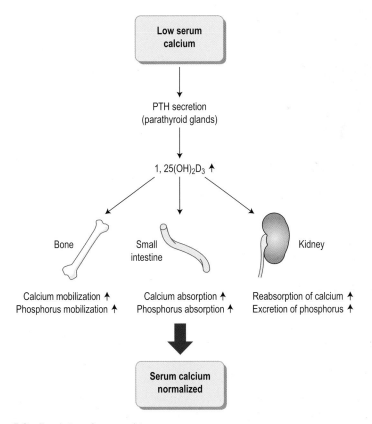

Figure 5.2 Regulation of serum calcium.

response to elevated plasma calcium levels and release of this hormone acts to antagonize the effects of PTH, to lower plasma calcium.

As a consequence of bone resorption induced by PTH and vitamin D_3, plasma phosphate levels also rise. The excess phosphate is excreted via the kidney.

Effect of deficiency and excess

Although plasma concentration of calcium is highly regulated a continual low intake of calcium will cause a severe decrease in bone mass and this, together with a number of other factors, contributes to an increased risk of osteoporosis (see chapter 9). Evidence for calcium toxicity is rare. High dose calcium supplements can interfere with iron absorption but there is little evidence for long-term effects on iron status in people taking such supplements.

Phosphorus is found in almost all foods and absorption is good so deficiency is extremely rare. Toxicity associated with high phosphorus intakes is only likely to be a problem when calcium intakes are low. Elevated phosphorus intakes manifest themselves as an increase in plasma phosphate concentration, which is thought to be a risk factor for a decrease in bone mass.

Forms in food and food sources

The most important dietary sources of calcium in the western world are milk and other dairy products including yoghurt, cheese and ice cream. Phosphorus is also abundant in these products. About one-quarter of dietary calcium and phosphorus in Western countries comes from cereals and vegetables but this value is much higher in developing countries. Carbonated soft drinks are often rich in phosphates. Meat and fish are reasonably good sources of calcium and good sources of phosphorus.

Calcium is largely present in foods as simple organic and inorganic salts; dietary phosphorus occurs in several forms including inorganic phosphate, organic phosphoproteins, phosphorylated sugars, sugar alcohols (eg phytate) and phospholipids.

Absorption and transport

Intestinal calcium absorption occurs via both active transcellular and passive paracellular pathways. Both dietary calcium and circulating calcitriol are important regulators of calcium absorption by the transcellular route. Phosphate absorption is regulated by long-term changes in dietary phosphorus content and body phosphorus status but there may also be a regulatory role for calcitriol ($1,25(OH)_2D_3$) in controlling dietary phosphate absorption.

Calcium absorption is fairly constant across the range of dietary sources. Dietary phytate, found in cereals, is the most important inhibitor of calcium absorption. Phosphorus is absorbed very efficiently, always as inorganic phosphate following the action of phosphatase on organic phosphates.

Almost all of the calcium in the body is found in mineralized tissues such as the bones and teeth, mainly as hydroxyapatite, a complex form of calcium phosphate, $Ca_{10}(PO_4)_6(OH)_2$. The remainder is found in blood and extracellular fluid. Plasma calcium concentration is tightly regulated. Similarly, the majority of phosphorus in the body is found in bone, with the remainder found in the soft tissues and blood largely as phospholipids, phosphoproteins, and nucleic acids as well as inorganic phosphate.

Status assessment and dietary requirements

Plasma calcium is highly regulated and therefore of no value as a biomarker of status. Measures of bone mass such as bone mineral content and bone mineral density have proved to be useful indicators of body calcium status. Phosphorus status is assessed by measuring plasma concentration.

Reference nutrient daily intakes for calcium for the UK and European populations range from 525 mg to 1000 mg depending upon age and gender, with an increment during breastfeeding. Except during infancy, values have been set somewhat higher for the USA. Reference nutrient intakes for phosphorus range from 400 mg to 750 mg for the UK and European populations, and again values have been set generally higher for USA.

Iron

Iron is an essential trace metal and has numerous biochemical roles in the body, including oxygen binding in haemoglobin and as an important catalytic centre in many enzymes. However, in excess, iron is extremely toxic to cells and tissues due to its ability to generate oxygen radicals. More than 2 billion people worldwide suffer from iron deficiency anaemia, making this the most common nutritional deficiency syndrome.

Functions of iron

Iron in energy metabolism

As a component of haem, iron is central to the oxygen carrying and oxygen transfer activity of red blood cells and muscle cells. Intracellular energy production from fuel molecules is also highly dependent upon iron, because it is a component of a number of key enzymes in energy metabolism. Haem-containing enzymes include the cytochromes, important in the electron transport chain. Iron is present in the non-haem form in other enzymes involved in energy metabolism such as succinate dehydrogenase, important in the tricarboxylic acid (TCA) cycle.

Iron as an antioxidant and pro-oxidant

Iron contributes to antioxidant mechanisms because it is a component of catalase and peroxidase, antioxidant enzymes that reduce hydrogen peroxide. However, there is clear evidence that iron that is not tightly bound to proteins can also contribute to the production of free radicals, and this is one of the dangers of iron overload.

Immune function

Iron seems to play a dual role in immune function. It is an important factor in a number of immune responses including lymphocyte activation and proliferation, and hence cell-mediated immunity may be compromised by iron deficiency. Several studies have shown reduced T-cell function in people with iron deficiency. However, iron is also a growth promoter for micro-organisms, and iron overload can predispose to infection.

Effects of iron deficiency and overload

The earliest signs of iron deficiency in otherwise healthy individuals is reduced iron stores, seen as low serum ferritin. Anaemia develops when there is insufficient iron available for the developing red cells, which in consequence become small and pale. Iron deficiency is treated with oral iron as a ferrous salt.

Anaemia

Iron deficiency is the most important cause of anaemia worldwide. The worst affected areas include Sub-Saharan Africa, South and South-East Asia and the West Pacific. Iron deficiency is also associated with a poor diet in affluent western countries (see also chapter 8). Work performance, particularly physical work capacity, is impaired in anaemia and this can have a serious impact on the economy of communities. Iron is also active in neurotransmitter systems in the brain and the effects of deficiency depend on the maturity of the affected individual. Children with iron deficiency in infancy demonstrate delay in developmental milestones with 'catch up' after iron repletion.

Haemochromatosis

The majority of cases of primary iron overload are accounted for by the genetic disease haemochromatosis, which leads to unregulated iron absorption. The condition leads to the deposition of iron in tissues, especially in the liver, with associated tissue damage.

Forms in food and food sources

Iron is present in food in the form of haem, found in meat and meat products, or non-haem, found in other foods. In industrialized countries about 10% of dietary iron is in the haem form, whereas in developing countries almost all dietary iron is as non-haem iron, present as iron oxides and salts as well as more complex organic chelates.

Cereals make an important contribution to iron intake throughout the world. In the UK most are fortified with iron and many breakfast cereals and infant foods are also fortified with iron.

Absorption and metabolism

Bioavailability

Dietary non-haem iron absorption is influenced by several dietary factors as well as the iron status of the individual, and the overall bioavailability is low. Some dietary factors enhance absorption, the most important being vitamin C, as ascorbic acid, although citric acid is also effective. Meat and fish consumed with non-haem iron also enhance its availability, possibly through effects of specific amino acids. Phytates, found in cereal products, and phenolic compounds (such as tannins in tea and red wine) inhibit the absorption of non-haem iron. Haem iron has a much higher bioavailability than non-haem iron, being relatively little influenced by other dietary factors.

Absorption

Both haem and non-haem iron are absorbed in the duodenum, but by different mechanisms. Haem is absorbed intact and the iron is removed once inside the enterocyte. Non-haem iron is preferentially absorbed in the reduced (ferrous) form and therefore dietary iron in the ferric form is first reduced in the lumen, mainly by dietary reducing agents such as ascorbic acid. Once in the enterocyte iron can either be stored as ferritin when the body stores are replete, or can leave the cell and be loaded onto transferrin for transport in the plasma and delivery to tissues.

Transport and homeostasis

Iron is transported in the plasma bound to the protein transferrin (Fig 5.3). The body iron content of a healthy adult is about 3–5 g and about 75% of this is found in the red blood cells, as haemoglobin, or in the site of their production, the bone marrow. Iron is also present in myoglobin in muscle cells, and a small amount is present as an essential component of some enzymes. Iron is stored in the liver, as ferritin and haemosiderin.

The body has three basic mechanisms for maintaining iron homeostasis: (1) continuous re-utilization of iron recovered from senescent red blood cells; (2) regulation of intestinal iron absorption to match body iron status; (3) storage and mobilization when appropriate. Iron losses are restricted to that stored in cells shed from the lining of the gastrointestinal and urinary tracts, skin and hair, and losses through bleeding.

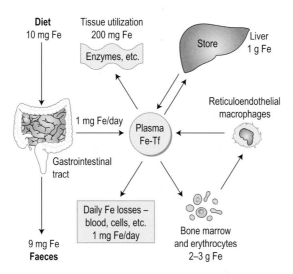

Figure 5.3 Body iron (Fe) metabolism: 75% of body iron resides at any one time in the bone marrow and circulating erythrocytes; 25% is present in body stores in the liver. Approximately 1 mg Fe/day is absorbed from the diet to replace iron lost through minor bleeding and cell shedding. Tf, transferrin.

Status assessment and dietary requirements

Iron status can be assessed using a range of biochemical measures. Some are specific to iron and these include plasma ferritin and transferrin saturation, which decrease in iron deficiency, and erythrocyte protoporphyrin and plasma transferrin receptor concentration, both of which increase in iron deficiency. As iron stores are depleted blood haemoglobin concentration falls, but a low haemoglobin concentration may reflect nutrient deficiencies other than iron.

Dietary intakes to satisfy metabolic requirements and iron losses in an individual depend largely on the bioavailability of iron in the diet. Reference daily nutrient intakes for the UK population range from 1.7 mg in infancy to 15 mg in adult females, with no increment during pregnancy as additional requirements should be met by iron stores.

Zinc

Functions of zinc

The major function of zinc in human metabolism is as a cofactor for over 100 metalloproteins and enzymes. Several key enzymes involved in the synthesis of RNA and DNA are zinc-dependent including the DNA and RNA polymerases. In addition, zinc plays a key role in gene transcription as an essential structural component of the zinc finger motifs found in several nuclear hormone receptors and transcription factors. Zinc is also an essential component of superoxide dismutase (SOD), an antioxidant enzyme.

Zinc has a range of other functions; the secretion of insulin from the pancreas is zinc-dependent, as is blood clotting. Zinc is also involved in the maturation and activity of white blood cells, as part of the immune response.

Zinc deficiency and excess

Dietary zinc deficiency is unusual in Western countries but several Middle Eastern countries in particular report severe zinc deficiency, mainly due to the inhibitory effect on absorption of dietary phytate. In these circumstances the deficiency is associated with growth retardation. Severe zinc deficiency develops mainly as a result of an inborn error of zinc metabolism leading to a decrease in the absorption of dietary zinc; it is characterized by dermatitis, diarrhoea and impaired immunity leading to greater susceptibility to infections. Mild zinc deficiency can also depress the immune response and is associated with a reduced growth rate in humans; studies have shown beneficial effects of zinc supplementation on diarrhoeal disease and improved growth in infants and children.

Acute excessive intakes of zinc can cause symptoms such as nausea, abdominal pain, vomiting diarrhoea and fever. In addition, there are some concerns that high doses of zinc over a prolonged time might inhibit iron absorption.

Food sources

Zinc is present in a very wide range of foods, but highest levels are found in protein-rich foods including shellfish and meat. Wholegrains and eggs are also good sources. In general the zinc content of green leafy vegetables and fruit is low.

Absorption and metabolism

Zinc absorption takes place mainly in the jejunum of the small intestine. The major inhibitor to absorption is phytic acid, present in large quantities in cereals, legumes and other vegetables. Animal protein is thought to act as an 'antiphytic' agent and enhances the bioavailability of zinc. Once inside the mucosal cell some of the zinc may be retained by binding with metallothionein and the rest passes into the bloodstream. It is transported to the tissues, mainly attached to albumin. Zinc taken up by the pancreas may be secreted into the small intestine along with exfoliated cells from the intestinal lining, and reabsorbed, constituting an enterohepatic circulation.

Typically an adult has about 2–3 g body zinc, predominantly in skeletal muscle and bone. The small intestine regulates both the amount of dietary zinc absorbed and the quantity of endogenous zinc that is secreted into the gastrointestinal lumen and lost in the faeces. When body zinc status is higher absorption is reduced through an increased binding by intracellular metallothionein. Zinc is excreted in the urine but unlike the intestine, zinc reabsorption in the kidney is unaffected by daily fluctuations in dietary zinc intake. Zinc is also lost from the body via skin, hair and sweat.

Status assessment and dietary requirements

There is at present no satisfactory measure of zinc status. It is usual for zinc status to be measured as concentration in plasma or white or red blood cells but these measurements are not very sensitive to changes in dietary intake. Reference daily nutrient intakes for the UK population range from 4.0 mg in infancy to 9.5 mg in adolescents. There is no increment for pregnancy.

Iodine

Functions of iodine

Iodide is taken up by the thyroid where it is used in the synthesis of mono-iodotyrosine and di-iodotyrosine which can condense to form the thyroid hormones tri-iodothyronine (T_3) and thyroxine (T_4). The major functions of the thyroid hormones are the maintenance of metabolic rate, cellular metabolism and growth. They bind to DNA and regulate the transcription of several genes in target tissues, in particular the brain, heart, liver and kidneys.

Effects of iodine deficiency and excess

Iodine deficiency causes a wide range of abnormalities collectively known as iodine deficiency disorders in which symptoms range from mild, such as goitre, to severe, including mental retardation or cretinism. The fetal brain is particularly susceptible to iodine deficiency if the mother is iodine deficient. The severe neurological damage caused by iodine deficiency in these children results in mental and physical retardation and is irreversible. Clinical deficiency is characterized by goitre which forms by enlargement of the thyroid gland in response to a fall in T_4 production. Moderate iodine deficiency leads to weight gain and tiredness. Iodine deficiency disorders are widely distributed throughout the world; Asia, Africa and the Eastern Mediterranean regions are most affected.

Exposure to high intakes of iodine may result from iodine contamination of food or water supply, in which case it may lead to an enlargement of the thyroid gland, as in deficiency.

Dietary sources

Iodine is usually found in food as inorganic iodide or iodate. The iodine content of plants and cereals varies greatly depending on the iodine content of the soil. The richest sources of iodine in the diet are generally marine fish, shellfish and sea salt but in the UK milk is a significant source of iodine because of the use of supplemented feeds to dairy cows.

Absorption and metabolism

Iodine from foods is rapidly and efficiently absorbed in the proximal small intestine as iodide. Brassicas (cabbage, broccoli etc), and the tuber cassava, a staple food in some regions of the world, contain compounds (goitrogens) that interfere with iodine absorption.

Transport and tissue distribution

Once iodide appears in the blood it is transported to the tissues where its uptake is stimulated by thyroid stimulating hormone (TSH) released from the pituitary gland. Total body iodine levels are 15–20 mg in healthy adults. Excess iodide is excreted in the urine.

Status assessment and dietary requirements

Biochemical assessment of iodine status is by the measurement of urinary iodine:creatinine ratio, which falls in deficiency. Clinical iodine deficiency is assessed by size of the thyroid, measured by palpation and ultrasound. In adults, an iodine intake of 70 µg/day appears to be the minimum necessary to avoid the appearance of goitre and has therefore been set as the lower reference nutrient intake for the UK population. The RNI has been set at 140 µg/day with a recommended upper limit of 1 mg per day.

Other important trace elements
Copper

Copper is found in high concentrations in shellfish, liver, kidney, nuts and wholegrain cereals. The major function of copper is as a catalytic centre in numerous enzymes involved in redox reactions. Dietary induced copper deficiency has not been reported in humans. Dietary copper overloading is also rare due to the body's ability to excrete excess copper in the bile, but a congenital disease, Wilson's disease, leads to copper accumulation in the body, particularly in the liver and the brain, with associated pathological damage.

Selenium

Selenium is found in a number of foods especially cereals, meat and Brazil nuts in different forms including the selenoamino acids selenocysteine and selenomethionine, and inorganic selenide, selenite and selenate. The selenium content of cereals is directly proportional to the soil Se content and there has been a considerable reduction in selenium intakes in UK over the last two decades, partly as a result of increased use of European wheat at the expense of Canadian imports.

The main function of selenium is in the active sites of about 35 selenoproteins and enzymes including iodothyronine deiodinase, responsible for the conversion of T_4 to T_3, thioredoxin reductase, which reduces nucleotides in DNA synthesis, and members of the glutathione peroxidase family of antioxidants. The best-characterized selenium deficiency syndrome is Keshan disease, a cardiomyopathy that affects children and women in rural China where soils are selenium deficient. Low selenium status may also impair immune function and thyroid function.

There is epidemiological and experimental evidence to support a role for selenium in protecting against certain cancers, including prostate, colon and lung cancers. Selenium is toxic in excess.

The current UK RNI for selenium is $75\,\mu g/day$ for men and $60\,\mu g/day$ for women.

Chromium

The main chromium-rich foods are meat, nuts, cereal grains, brewer's yeast and molasses. Chromium enhances the actions of insulin and people receiving adequate dietary chromium have better control over blood glucose than those on low intakes.

Fluoride

Fluoride is present in most foods at varying levels and also in drinking water, either naturally occurring or added deliberately. The main function of fluoride in the body is in the mineralization of bones and teeth (as calcium fluoroapatite). Adding fluoride to drinking water is a controversial issue because while low supplementary levels may be beneficial in reducing dental decay, higher intakes of fluoride are toxic leading to fluorosis but water concentrations are controlled at a low level. Symptoms of fluorosis may be mild (mottled tooth enamel) or severe (skeletal fluorosis). Skeletal changes include calcification of ligaments and tendons leading to stiffness, joint pain and spinal defects. Fluorosis is rare in the West but common in parts of southern Africa, the Indian subcontinent and China where there is a high fluoride content in the subsoil water that enters the food chain.

KEY POINTS

- Calcium and phosphorus are the major bone minerals, and in an equilibrium with the plasma that is controlled by the hormones parathyroid hormone, calcitriol and calcitonin
- Non-haem iron absorption from the diet is strongly influenced by other dietary components that may act to promote (eg ascorbic acid) or inhibit (eg phytic acid) bioavailability. Iron deficiency anaemia is the most common nutritional deficiency disease in the world
- Zinc is essential for a wide array of biochemical processes that play a central role in growth and development
- Iodine is an essential nutrient because it is a constituent of the thyroid hormones thyroxine and tri-iodothyronine. These hormones are required for normal growth and maintenance of the metabolic rate
- For these and many other key minerals and trace elements there is a need for better functional markers of body nutritional status

5.5 PHYTOCHEMICALS

This is a term used to describe a broad class of compounds found in plant foods, not essential for life (not nutrients) but with proven or probable health benefits. The term includes a diverse group of phenols and polyphenols that in turn includes flavonoids and phyto-oestrogens. Whilst they are not essential nutrients some of their properties are similar to those of micronutrients and they can be considered as non-nutritive plant components.

Phenols and polyphenols

This is a very large group of compounds, ranging in complexity from the simplest, phenol itself, to the complex tannins. The best-characterized group is the flavonoids, which include the catechins (tea, wine, fruit juices, chocolate), flavanones (orange and grapefruit juice) and anthocyanidins (blackberries and blueberries).

Beneficial effects

Epidemiological evidence suggests that certain polyphenols have protective effects against cancers at some sites, and may protect against cardiovascular disease. This evidence is supported by plausible mechanistic explanations. However, the evidence base is inconsistent and the quality of studies is sometimes poor.

Mechanisms of action

Most of the beneficial health effects of flavonoids in humans are attributed to their antioxidant properties, which have been demonstrated in many in vitro studies. Quercetin, found in plants of the allium and brassica families, also in apples and blackcurrants, has been shown to have very potent antioxidant activity in vitro, through its ability to scavenge reactive oxygen species, reactive nitrogen species, peroxyl radicals and superoxide. However, antioxidant effects of polyphenols in vivo will be influenced by the chemical nature of the parent compound, the absorption and distribution characteristics in vivo, and the nature of the active derivative, and these properties vary greatly between compounds.

Several polyphenols have chemopreventive effects in animal models and this activity has been explained by effects on cell proliferation and apoptosis as well as antioxidant activity. An additional mechanism by which polyphenols exhibit anti-carcinogenic activity is through effects on Phase II enzymes, responsible for metabolizing potential carcinogens.

Phyto-oestrogens

Some polyphenols occurring in plants have weak anti-oestrogenic activity and are known collectively as phyto-oestrogens. They can bind to oestrogen receptors and thereby antagonize the action of oestrogens. This is the explanation given for their epidemiological association with a reduced breast cancer risk, and a reduced incidence of osteoporosis. Additionally, phyto-oestrogens increase the synthesis of sex-hormone binding protein and thereby lower concentration of circulating oestrogens. Legumes, especially soya beans, are rich sources of phyto-oestrogens.

FURTHER READING

Bender D A 2003 Nutritional biochemistry of the vitamins, 2nd edn. Cambridge University Press, New York

Bender D A 2008 Introduction to nutrition and metabolism, 4th edn. CRC Press, Boca Raton, FL

Bourgeois C F 2003 Antioxidant vitamins and health: cardiovascular disease, cancer, cataracts and aging. HNB Publishing, New York

Holick F M 2007 Vitamin D deficiency. Review. New England Journal of Medicine 357: 266–281

Powers H J 2003 Riboflavin (vitamin B_2) and Health. Review. American Journal of Clinical Nutrition 77(6):1352–1360

Rayman M P 2000 The importance of selenium to human health. The Lancet 356:224–233

Sharp P A, Tandy S R, Srai S K 2003 Mechanisms involved in the regulation of intestinal iron absorption. Nutrition Abstract and Reviews Series A: Human and Experimental 73:1R–9R

Thurnham D I, Northrop-Clewes C A 2004 Effects of infection on nutritional and immune status. In: Hughes D A, Darlington L G, Bendich A (eds) Diet and human immune function. Humana Press, Totowa, NJ, p 35–64

CHAPTER 6

Diet and the Lifecycle

OBJECTIVES

By the end of this chapter you should be able to:

- outline the changing characteristics of growth and maturation from birth to adult that alter nutrient requirements
- understand the immaturity of the digestive tract and organs during infancy, and the implications for diet
- discuss the composition of maternal milk and compare with alternatives
- describe the weaning process and advantages and risks of complementary foods
- have an informed opinion about the application of 'healthy eating' beliefs
- be aware of the social and psychological factors that affect food intake and nutrition during adolescence
- describe the physiological changes during pregnancy
- describe the impact of nutrition before and during pregnancy on maternal, infant and long-term health
- outline the promotion of successful lactation
- describe problems associated with breast feeding
- describe the physiological and pathological changes of ageing relevant to nutrition
- discuss important aspects of macro- and micronutrient intakes in older people
- discuss the role of nutrition in the development, susceptibility to and outcome of common chronic disabling diseases in the elderly
- understand current important public health messages to maintain and improve nutritional status in elderly people.

6.1 INTRODUCTION TO INFANCY, CHILDHOOD AND ADOLESCENCE

Growth has specific nutritional needs but is not a steady process, proceeding rapidly in early life, slowing in middle childhood and accelerating at puberty before linear growth ceases. With increasing age also come the physical and psychomotor maturation which influence activity and body composition and, through feeding skills and food choices, dietary intakes. Percentage body weight that is fat (% BF) increases rapidly to a peak between 6 and 12 months, followed by a period of natural 'slimming' until around 5 years, then by a second phase of relatively rapid fat deposition (the adiposity rebound) which continues in girls until growth ceases. In boys the adiposity rebound ceases with the rapid lean tissue deposition of late puberty.

6.2 NUTRITIONAL ASSESSMENT IN CHILDHOOD

Body weight for age (WFA) is frequently used as an indicator of nutritional status but weight is heavily influenced by height. Childhood nutritional assessment (see also chapter 12) commonly uses either weight-for-height (WFH) independent of age, or WFA in relation to height-for-age (HFA). Reference standards for growth and development do not distinguish the abnormal from the extremes of normal. Scores of <-2 or $>+2$ SD, or <3rd and >97th centiles, are often used as cut-off points for 'normality'. Velocity of growth may be more informative than size attained.

Undernutrition

Stunting is assessed by height-for-age or length-for-age, the same cut-off points as are used for normality. Growth retardation associated with socioeconomic deprivation is a significant problem in westernized as well as in less affluent societies and usually responds better with changes in psychosocial and/or economic environments than with specifically nutritional interventions.

Overnutrition

In adults, body mass index (BMI: weight in kg/height in m^2) is used to define underweight, overweight and obesity; however in children mean BMI varies non-linearly with age and so the use of this index is less simple. The International Obesity Task Force (IOTF) defines childhood overweight and obesity as the BMI Z score (ie SD score) at any age which, if maintained throughout childhood would achieve the adult overweight and obesity BMI cut off points of 25 and $30 \, kg/m^2$ at 18 years.

6.3 DEVELOPMENT AND MATURATION

Physical maturation

Growth from the fetus through infancy and childhood is clearly one aspect of physical maturation before the onset of puberty when rapid physical maturation occurs. The age at onset of puberty and the pubertal growth spurt vary widely between individuals. Secular trends towards increased height and weight and earlier age at puberty, attributed to positive changes in health and nutrition, have slowed or ceased in recent years in much of Europe and North America, but continue elsewhere.

The typical age for onset of the secondary sexual development characteristic of puberty is considered to be between 8 and 13 years in girls and

9 and 13.5 years in boys with similar mean age (11.5 years) in both sexes. In girls the growth spurt always occurs early in the progression of puberty with most rapid growth in height on average 0.7 years after the first signs of puberty and before menarche. Growth acceleration in boys occurs later in the pubertal process, with most rapid growth occurring on average 1.5 years after the first signs of puberty, and continues longer than in girls. Peak bone mass is achieved two years after cessation of growth (mean: girls 16 years; boys 18 years). Pubertal changes in body size and composition lead to greater differences in nutrient requirements between males and females than were present in earlier childhood. In adolescent girls the nutritional needs of pregnancy and lactation may have to be added to those of growth and menstruation. In adolescent boys increased lean body mass leads to greater nutritional demands per kg body weight (see Appendix 2).

Psychomotor maturation relevant to feeding

The period of infancy (birth to 12 months) is one of almost total dependency on others for the provision of warmth, food, shelter and emotional needs. As children become more independent, they can make their wishes understood and learn to use food to manipulate those around them. Once at school, children also take their cues for food preferences from their friends and may be heavily influenced by advertising pressures. In adolescence, peer fashions can lead to haphazard eating and bizarre diets with risk of compromising the good quality diets needed to meet the demands of growth and maturation, and may be used to express independence of the family. Adolescents living away from home for the first time may lack the cooking skills required for a good diet. Lifestyles adopted in the adolescent years can continue into adult life. Adolescents (and, increasingly, younger children) may demonstrate psychiatric instability through anorexia nervosa or bulimia. These two conditions have profound, even fatal, effects (see chapter 8).

Nutrition, growth and later disease

There is increasing evidence of a relationship between fetal and early infant growth and nutrition with health and disease in adulthood (fetal origins hypothesis). Low birth weight (LBW), particularly when there is rapid catch-up growth postnatally, is associated with increased prevalence of coronary heart disease and Type 2 diabetes mellitus in adult life.

Immunological development

Food allergy and intolerance and the maturation of the immune system in relation to dietary components are discussed in chapter 10. Infants are born with unchallenged and immature immune systems. Gastrointestinal resistance to invasion by foreign proteins relies in part on protective substances such as immunoglobulins (eg IgA and IgM) and enzymes which destroy histamine and active substances in the gut. Low levels of secretory IgA (sIgA) and lack of specifically sensitized immunoglobulins make young infants more at risk of sensitization to foreign proteins which cross the mucosal barrier.

Infant eczema has been attributed to foreign proteins either in maternal milk, infant formula, or early weaning foods. Maternal allergen exclusion diets during lactation may reduce the prevalence of eczema in breast fed infants, at high risk of atopy (allergic hypersensitivity), in the early months of life. The nature and pattern, rather than simply the timing, of solid feeding are important for subsequent development of food allergy.

Development of gastrointestinal function

Digestion and absorption in breast fed infants are promoted by many specific components in breast milk, such as lactose, lipase and lactoferrin. Immaturity of gastrointestinal enzymatic function makes digestion and absorption less efficient with infant formula than with breast milk in the first months of life. Fat absorption is less in formula fed infants than in breast fed infants. Pancreatic lipase, amylase and bile salt pool size are low in the newborn compared with older infants. Lactase levels in the newborn are quite low, increase as milk feeding begins and may decline later as milk ceases to be the predominant feed. Low lactase levels and lactose intolerance are common in older African and Asian children and adults but less common in Caucasian children and adults.

Development of renal function

Young infants cannot dilute or concentrate their urine as much as older children and adults. This makes them particularly susceptible to fluid overload and to overload from other substances which have to be excreted via the kidneys. The unmodified cow milk formulas used before 1972 gave young infants difficulty excreting sufficiently concentrated urine to expel the necessary solutes. The ensuing intracellular hyperosmolality, especially in the brain, had disastrous, often fatal, consequences.

The high phosphate content of unmodified cow milk based formulas precipitated falls in plasma calcium, hypocalcaemic tetany and convulsions in otherwise healthy infants around 7–10 days old. UK legislation in the early 1970s lowered the acceptable levels of sodium, phosphate and protein in infant formulas and this was followed by similar EC directives. Changes to low phosphate infant formula have virtually eliminated the problem of tetany.

6.4 NUTRITION IN INFANCY

Breast milk

There is now almost universal consensus that breast milk is the best food for normal infants with healthy mothers, because of its composition, digestibility, and anti-infective properties. Despite this consensus, most one-month-old infants in UK have received some infant formula and by 10 weeks 64% of infants are wholly formula fed. It is proving difficult to improve 'breast feeding statistics' in UK despite widespread education and publicity promoting breast feeding.

The composition of human milk is variable. The first milk, colostrum, is low in volume and high in proteins, especially immunoglobulin A, as well as vitamin A and zinc. As the volumes of milk secreted increase, milk

Table 6.1 Energy and selected nutrients/100 ml of colostrum, mature human milk, infant formula, and cow milk

Nutrient	Colostrum	Mature human milk	Infant formula (whey dominated)	Cow's milk
Energy (kcal) (kJ)	69 (290)	70 (295)	67 (280)	67 (280)
Protein (g)	10.0*	1.3	1.5	3.3
Fat (g)	2.6	4.2	3.6	3.8
Carbohydrate (g)	6.6	7.0	7.2	4.8
Calcium (mg)	28	35	46	115
Sodium (mg)	47	15	16	55
Zinc (mg)	0.6	0.3	0.6	0.4
Iron (mg)	0.1	0.1	0.8	0.05
Retinol (μg)	115	60	75	52
Vitamin D (μg)	N	0.04	1.0	0.03
Vitamin C (mg)	7	4	9	1

*Since much of this protein is s IgA it is not clear how much is digested and absorbed and how much remains in the gastrointestinal tract.

N: significant quantities but no reliable information.

Information derived from various sources.

composition modifies to 'transitional' and then 'mature' milk. Table 6.1 outlines the biochemical composition of colostrum, human milk, modern infant formula and cow's milk. Volumes of milk produced and precise composition of breast milk vary between women, over time and by time of day. Human milk contains cells (macrophages, lymphocytes, neutrophils) and humoral components, eg sIgA, which protect infants against infection in the first months of life. *Lactobacillus* and *Bifidobacterium* spp promote lactic and acetic acid production from lactose, which discourages growth in the large bowel of potential pathogens such as *E. coli* and *Shigella* spp.

Lactose, the main carbohydrate in milk, accounts for approximately 40% of total milk energy and facilitates calcium absorption. Human milk protein is 30–40% casein and 60–70% whey. Whey proteins include lactalbumin, sIgA, lactoferrin and lysozymes, whereas casein is a mixture of proteins bound with calcium. Human milk casein forms smaller micelles with looser structure than the casein of cow's milk, which facilitates digestion. Nutrient binding proteins in milk such as lactoferrin (which binds iron) facilitate absorption of some specific nutrients. The quantities of fat in human and cow's milk are similar, but human milk fat is higher in unsaturated fat, particularly the essential fatty acids linoleic and α-linolenic acids, and also contains the long chain polyunsaturated fatty acids arachidonic, eicosapentaenoic and docosahexaenoic acids (22:6ω3), which are important for neurological development (see chapter 4).

The fats in human milk are more readily digested and absorbed than those of cow's milk. Most infant formulas now contain mainly vegetable oils with rather different proportions of fatty acids than those found in human milk fat, which partly depends on maternal dietary fatty acid content. Human milk has a high level of cholesterol and of carnitine, which is involved in mitochondrial oxidation of fatty acids. Premature infants and those undergoing very rapid (catch-up) growth may be unable to synthesize carnitine at a sufficiently rapid rate to meet demand.

Vitamin supplementation

In 1994 the Department of Health for the UK stated that 'Breast fed infants under six months do not need vitamin supplementation provided the mother has an adequate vitamin status during pregnancy. From the age of six months infants receiving breast milk as their main drink should be given supplements of vitamins A and D'. Plasma vitamin K levels are low in the newborn because they lack colonic flora synthesizing vitamin K. Vitamin K deficiency can cause minor bruising, blood loss, or major haemorrhage in the brain. All term newborn infants in UK should receive prophylactic oral vitamin K (1 mg) at least once. Breast fed infants should be offered four further oral doses at two-weekly intervals.

Formula feeding

All infant formulas are now highly modified from their base of cow's milk or soya protein (Table 6.1). Many formulas are available and differ according to content, eg long chain polyunsaturated fatty acids, taurine, carnitine. Since the 1970s a series of government reports have made recommendations on the composition and promotion of infant formula. In 1991 an EC directive on the composition, labelling and marketing of infant and follow-on formulas was incorporated into the UK *Infant Formula and Follow-on Formula Regulations*. New EU regulations came into force in January 2008 but in the UK the labelling legislation will not be in force until 2010.

Specialized infant formulas

Most infant formulas are for non (exclusively) breast fed infants from birth until the age at which neat cow's milk is introduced (not before 12 months). Other more specialized formulas fulfil various purposes, eg

- *Follow-on formulas*, intended for infants over six months who are receiving complementary foods.
- *Formulas for LBW infants* which aim to meet the enhanced nutrient needs of very LBW and pre term (PT) infants.
- *Hypoallergenic formulas* for infants with strong family history of atopy and/or already diagnosed atopic disorders.
- *Vegan formulas* which are usually soya protein based formulas with vegetable fats.
- *Other formulas* – there are many very specific formulas developed to meet the needs of infants with inborn errors of metabolism and other specific illnesses.

6.5 THE TRANSITION TO MIXED FEEDING: WEANING OR COMPLEMENTARY FEEDING

Definitions

Weaning, also known as complementary feeding, has been defined as 'The process of expanding the diet to include foods and drinks other than breast milk or infant formula'. Since the term 'weaning' is also used to indicate complete cessation of breastfeeding, WHO recommends that the terms 'weaning' and 'weaning foods' are avoided. The term complementary feeding is used here to embrace the use of all foods and liquids other than breast milk or infant formula.

Maternal milk output averages 650 ml/day at one month of lactation, 750 ml/day at 3–4 months' lactation and peaks at about 900–1000 ml/day at 4–5 months' lactation. Average infants would need 850 ml and 1450 ml of breast milk to meet energy requirements at 6 and 12 months respectively on exclusive breast feeding. From six months, and probably before this for some infants, additional sources of energy and nutrition are needed to complement breast milk. The World Health Organization and the UK Department of Health have formally adopted the policy:

> Breast milk is the best form of nutrition for infants. Exclusive breastfeeding is recommended for the first 6 months (26 weeks) of an infant's life, as it provides all the nutrients a baby needs. Breastfeeding (and/or breast milk substitutes, if used) should continue beyond the first 6 months along with appropriate types and amounts of solid foods. Mothers who are unable to, or choose not to, follow these recommendations should be supported to optimize their infants' nutrition.

However, a survey in 2000 found that 90% of infants are introduced to some non-milk, non-formula, food *before 4 months*, despite education about the age of introduction of complementary foods.

Maternal choice in complementary feeding

Depending on the choice of food, complementary feeding can provide necessary extra energy and micronutrients. It encourages development of feeding techniques and ability to eat with the family, but is less likely to be sterile and early introduction can lead to allergic reactions to foods.

Complementary foods may be home prepared or commercially produced. Initially one small feed is introduced per day but feed frequency can increase quite quickly. Whilst breast milk (or formula) remains the main source of energy early in complementary feeding, cereal based complementary foods, with energy density enhanced by additional fat source, should be introduced early. Rice preparations are usually recommended since rice is gluten free. With wheat based foods there is slight risk of malabsorption from either temporary gluten intolerance following gastrointestinal infection, or permanent gluten intolerance in coeliac syndrome. Fats increase the energy density of foods, thus facilitating energy sufficiency and optimum infant growth with the relatively small volumes of food tolerated by infants' small gastric capacities. Fats are also sources of fat-soluble vitamins, essential fatty acids and exogenous cholesterol and enhance taste and food texture and therefore palatability. Provided breast milk, formula, or (later) cow's milk intakes are around 500 ml/day, protein intakes are likely to be adequate even if complementary feeds are low in protein and amino acid variety (eg in diets with a single plant staple).

Home-prepared versus commercial complementary foods

About 40% of home prepared complementary foods have an energy content lower than breast milk and are lower in fat, iron and vitamin D and higher in sodium than commercially prepared infant foods. UK legislation specifies a range of nutritional contents for commercially produced infant foods. Thus infants receiving commercial complementary foods may have more balanced nutrient intakes than those fed home prepared foods. If only commercial fruit, vegetable and pudding products are offered as complementary foods, energy needs are unlikely to be met as the foods displace breast milk and formula in the diet but are usually less energy dense.

Early foods offered are semisolid. Infants quickly learn to cope with solid and lumpy foods and ultimately foods which require chewing prior to swallowing. This progression is important. Prolonged bottle feeding (beyond one year) can lead to failure to thrive due to the 'comfort' aspect of sucking and the low energy density of fluids proffered. Infants should be moved from fluids fed by bottle to predominantly fluids fed by cup over the second six months of life. Current UK recommendations are that cow's milk should not be given as a drink to infants under one year, but when it forms part of family recipes, small amounts may be safe before this age.

Vegan infants and other at-risk groups

Vegan mothers have higher levels of unsaturated fatty acids in their milk than omnivore mothers. This may be advantageous to the infants. Soya-based infant formulas (supplemented with micronutrients and appropriately balanced energy and protein) can be used as alternatives to breast milk as breast milk output declines, and continued beyond infancy. Vitamin deficiencies in infants born to deficient mothers (particularly for B_1 and B_{12}) may be exacerbated by low breast milk vitamin content.

6.6 NUTRITION IN CHILDHOOD AND ADOLESCENCE

Digestion and absorption in preschool children enable them to consume the same foods as adults but nutrient needs and feeding skills are different. Children's small stomachs limit the amounts of food taken at any one meal. They should therefore be fed three meals a day and perhaps two between-meal snacks, with one snack or meal close to bedtime. Recommendations for adults to consume <35% dietary energy from fat do not apply to young children. The transition from >50% dietary energy derived from fat provided by exclusive breast feeding to <35% energy derived from fat should spread over the first five years of life. Similarly adult recommendations for fibre intake should not apply in early childhood since high fibre content lowers food energy density and phytates reduce absorption of micronutrients. Diets with <30% energy derived from fat are quite common amongst preschool children who consume large quantities of 'juice' and sweets instead of meals of varied content. They are likely to lead to failure to thrive if prolonged. Persuading children to eat family meals is not always easy. Children are often reluctant to eat green leafy vegetables, partly due to inexperience with chewing.

Nutritional problems in children and adolescents
Failure to thrive

Failure to thrive (FTT) is failure to gain in weight and height at the expected rate. Resolution through catch-up growth can be very rapid if the cause is treatable and extra nutrients are provided. Where the precipitating cause cannot be resolved, increasing the energy and nutrient density of the diet can lead to improved growth rates. Psychosocial deprivation may be the commonest cause of FTT in the UK today although often unrecognized. Overt cases come from homes where the nurturing environment is in some way deficient in the love, warmth, enjoyment and stimulus which enable normal growth. Changing the adverse environments so as to provide more positive nurture rapidly normalizes hormone levels and results in catch-up growth.

Obesity

Childhood obesity (see also chapter 8) is of major public health concern. Psychological distress and the physical handicap of being obese contribute to underachievement at school. Type II diabetes mellitus (previously considered only an adult disease) shows an increased prevalence in children and adolescents in Western Europe (including the UK) and North America. The vast majority of obese children have no recognizable underlying medical cause for their obesity. Around 80% of obese children have one obese parent and 20–40% have both parents obese.

Explanations for the rise in childhood obesity must be multifactorial. Total energy intakes for 10–11-year-old UK children have decreased by an average of 1.6 MJ/day between 1983 and 1997, while the percentage of energy derived from fat decreased from a mean of 37.4% to 35.7%. Energy expenditures must have declined more than energy intakes to explain the increased prevalence of obesity. Obesity in teenage boys increases in proportion to time spent watching television, a pastime associated with very low energy expenditure. Increased sedentary behaviour could be the most significant societal change leading to increased prevalence of childhood overweight/obesity. An environment of deprivation which includes, for example, lack of shops selling fresh fruit, vegetables, and wholemeal breads and lack of places to play or walk, and which leads to parental depression, may have a role in driving the obesity epidemic.

Programmes to treat already existent obesity have not been impressive in their results even when treatments have been very invasive. Drastic energy intake reduction can lead to impaired linear growth although modest 'slimming' programmes usually allow continuation of normal linear growth. There are sustainable dietary and lifestyle practices which should balance energy intakes and expenditures in the obese quite successfully. Fat loss through such practices may be slow and may do no more than keep weight static; 'growing into' their weight is a practical possibility. Grossly obese children and obese adolescents already at more than their expected adult weight and close to the end of linear growth must aim for some weight reduction through developing significant negative energy balance by increasing activity (not easy for the very obese) and modifying energy intakes. Quite small losses of body fat can improve morale, make physical activity easier, and decrease the prevalence of problems such as high blood pressure and insulin resistance so children who 'slim' but do not achieve normal BMI may nevertheless benefit.

Anorexia nervosa

See chapter 8.

Anaemia

The definition of anaemia (see also chapter 8) in childhood is not straightforward because of physiological variations in haemoglobin levels with age. In utero haemoglobin levels are high in order to maximize oxygen uptake from the low oxygen tension of the environment. At birth a high haemoglobin concentration is no longer necessary and haemoglobin concentration falls. After 4–8 weeks haemoglobin levels remain low because red blood cell production only just keeps up with the increasing body size and blood volume. Anaemia is not uncommon in UK children; in 2000 anaemia affected 9% of boys and girls aged 4–6 years and 9% of teenagers. Deficiencies of other micronutrients, such as folic acid, vitamins A, B_{12}, C, E, riboflavin and copper can contribute to anaemia.

Iron deficiency

The level of consumption of breakfast cereals (mostly fortified with iron in UK) is positively associated with dietary iron intakes in children over 11 years. Non-meat eaters and non-Caucasian adolescent girls have the greatest risk of poor iron status. Most iron is transferred across the placenta in the last trimester so premature infants have less iron/kg body weight than term infants. By six months, and often earlier in infants born prematurely, iron stores are minimal. Complementary foods providing good sources of iron are necessary. Iron stores build up only after growth has slowed considerably around five years of age. Iron requirements increase in adolescence with increase in body size and the needs for growth and, in girls, the onset of menstruation. Depletion of iron stores even in the absence of anaemia may lead to psychological changes. Depression, irritability, loss of appetite, apathy, and evidence of impaired learning and cognition and slowed growth rates have all been associated with iron deficiency anaemia (IDA). Oral iron, provided it is taken, is an effective treatment. Additional vitamin C can enhance absorption of non-haem iron.

Bone mineralization: calcium and vitamin D (see also chapters 5 and 9)

Although the total daily calcium increment is highest in adolescence, the proportion of calcium taken up compared with total body, or total bone mineral, is highest immediately after birth. At term, 300 mg of calcium are transferred across the placenta to the fetus each day. Children at most risk of deficiency are those growing most rapidly – infants, especially LBW, and adolescents. Most children with adequate summer sunshine exposure should have no need for dietary vitamin D but those with heavily pigmented skin and/or little exposure to summer sunlight in Britain are at risk. The clinical signs of vitamin D deficiency in childhood are those of rickets. Vitamin D has effects on many tissues other than bone. Muscle tone is reduced leading to hypotonia and weakness with distended abdomen due to lax abdominal musculature. Weak respiratory muscles lead to ineffective coughing and thus a tendency for lower respiratory tract infections.

Bone health and later life (see chapter 9)

The loss of bone mineral in middle and old age leading to clinical osteoporosis is partly determined by Peak Bone Mass (PBM). In childhood weight-bearing activity contributes positively to developing PBM. Normal bone mineralization can take place on diets which are very low in calcium compared with recommended requirements.

6.7 MEALS AND SNACKS IN CHILDHOOD

Growth, dependency and development make infants and children susceptible to nutritional imbalance and deficiencies. It is wise to promote meals varied in content, texture and taste for children. Variety leads to nutritionally adequate combinations of macro- and micronutrients. Meals should be made enjoyable social affairs offered without excessive pressure to eat. Snacks should be planned rather than opportunistic (or continuous). Wholemeal cereals, fruits and vegetables should be seen as enjoyable components of the diet. In this way children can eat to requirement whilst allowing opportunity to develop and recognize satiety and hunger. Linking family nutrition with a caring stimulating environment encourages both normal growth and development, and the prospect of sustainable healthy lifestyles continuing into adulthood.

KEY POINTS FOR INFANCY, CHILDHOOD AND ADOLESCENCE

- There are sound and varied physiological reasons why breast milk is most suitable for the young infant
- The adaptations in modified formula milks accommodate the needs of young infants, even for those such as very low birth weight or with inborn errors of metabolism, or for whom breast milk may have limitations
- The transition from breast milk/formula milk to a solid diet is a time when young children are vulnerable to nutritional problems
- Vitamin and mineral deficiencies present problems in child nutrition even in affluent developed countries
- Overnutrition as overweight and obesity is a problem of increasing concern in public health and child nutrition
- Adolescence is an age of both nutritional vulnerability and opportunity for nutritional education for a healthy adult lifestyle
- Healthy nutrition encompasses not only what is eaten but when and how it is consumed and includes many aspects of lifestyle such as activity

6.8 INTRODUCTION TO PRE-PREGNANCY, PREGNANCY AND LACTATION

Of couples across the globe attempting to achieve a pregnancy 90% will have been successful after approximately 18 months of regular sexual intercourse. The remaining 10% are sub-fertile but many of these couples can now be helped to have a successful pregnancy as a result of medical management. In developed countries and in the absence of any medical interference the maternal death rate is approximately 1 in 200 pregnancies and 1 in 20 babies will die before or around birth. Intervention by health professionals, including nutritional advice, reduces these figures to 1/10,000 and 1 in 200 respectively. Both these figures are higher than this in the developing world.

6.9 PRE-PREGNANCY

Nutritional requirements for healthy conception

Healthy fertile women who are ovulating on a monthly basis have an average body fat proportion of 28%; a body fat of less than 22% of bodyweight is associated with the absence of ovulation. Menarche and the onset of fertility can be delayed by athletic training or eating disorders and accelerated by excess nutrient consumption. Early menarche may be a particular problem in girls exposed to famine in childhood who are then re-fed with a high energy diet. The basic mechanism involved in body fat as a determinant of a healthy conception appears to be a requirement for a certain energy store to permit reproduction to take place. However, obesity doubles the rate of ovulatory infertility. Weight reduction returns ovulation, menstruation and fertility in many cases.

Periconceptional nutrition and fetal malformations

In human populations major handicapping or lethal malformations complicate 1 in 80 pregnancies. The major nutritional influence on malformation which has been scientifically tested is the benefit of folic acid supplementation in the prevention of neural tube defects (NTD). The neural tube which runs from the brain to the lower end of the spinal cord normally closes in embryonic development in the third and fourth post-fertilization weeks. Periconceptional supplementation with 400 µg of folic acid per day or a diet rich in folates can reduce the incidence from 3–4/1000 pregnancies to less than 1/1000 pregnancies. Countries where folic acid fortification has been made universal through addition to flour are reporting reductions in the rate of NTD of up to 40% for their populations. It is recommended that for the small group of women who have had a previous pregnancy affected by NTD the periconceptional supplement should be 5 mg of folic acid not 400 µg. In the UK major efforts to disseminate the public health message have resulted in take-up of voluntary supplementation by 35–50% of eligible women.

Nutrition in planned and unplanned pregnancies

A large proportion of pregnancies are unplanned and in these circumstances the majority of women are not taking periconceptional supplements. The groups who are either planning a pregnancy but not taking supplements or who are more likely to have unplanned pregnancies include teenagers, women who smoke and those on low incomes. These groups are particularly at risk of low intakes of folates and other micronutrients, which may partly explain the social class gradient in the incidence of NTD which are more common in low income women.

6.10 PREGNANCY

Physiological changes in pregnancy

The physiological changes which the mother experiences precede fetal demands, are in excess of possible fetal requirements, and favour placental exchange of nutrient substrates and fetal metabolic processes.

The genital organs

The uterine weight rises from 46 g to 1000 g during pregnancy. There is hyperplasia of the mammary tissue and an increase in breast volume of about 50% by the end of pregnancy.

Blood volume and haemodynamics

There is an increase in the circulating blood volume of approximately 1600 ml by the end of the pregnancy. Thus although the red cell mass is increasing and oxygen carrying capacity is enhanced there is a dilution of the red cells because of the relatively greater increase in plasma volume. This leads to a fall in the haemoglobin concentration from a non-pregnant average of 13–14 g/dl to levels of 10–11 g/dl in late pregnancy. This reduces blood viscosity to improve placental perfusion, and therefore oxygen and nutrient exchange at the placental bed. The heart rate increases from an average non-pregnant rate of 70 beats per minute to a rate of 80–85 beats per minute at full term.

Respiratory system

The pregnant woman has an increasing metabolizing mass and an increasing requirement for oxygen as the pregnancy develops. The amount of air inspired per breath increases and oxygen consumption is increased by about 15%.

The renal system

Renal plasma flow increases by about 30% with the corresponding increase in glomerular filtration rate. There is a fall in serum albumin. An unwanted effect of the increased glomerular filtration is that significant amounts of glucose and amino acids in the urine are common in normal pregnancy.

Gastrointestinal system

There is a generalized relaxation of smooth muscle in the GI tract from about 10 weeks of gestation which persists through to term. Women commonly report altered appetite often with dulled sensation leading to craving particularly for highly flavoured or spiced foods or for sweets, chocolate, milk and dairy foods. They may also develop aversions to common dietary items such as tea, coffee and meat and some women thereby experience a major alteration in their pattern of nutrient intake from early pregnancy onwards. Pica is a rare condition where non-food items are eaten, such as coal, clay, toothpaste or chalk. This habit is potentially harmful and requires medical referral.

Endocrine changes are probably responsible for the symptoms of anorexia, nausea, and vomiting, which are particularly common problems from about 10–16 weeks of gestation. Relaxation of the cardiac sphincter in the stomach causes the common symptom of acid reflux which results in heartburn, and delayed gastric emptying can lead to a feeling of fullness after meals. Transit time from stomach to caecum is increased and nutrient absorption may be increased. The reduced peristalsis in the large bowel leads to increased water reabsorption and production of hard stools, leading to the common symptom of constipation.

Placental transfer

The placenta is responsible for maternal–fetal exchange and grows with the fetus. Barriers to adequate placental perfusion and therefore normal late fetal growth include the effect of maternal cigarette smoking.

Maternal homeostasis of fetal nutrients

Plasma levels of water-soluble and fat-soluble nutrients change in the maternal plasma in pregnancy. A fall in concentration of the water-soluble nutrients and a relative rise in the lipid-soluble nutrients occur at two stages in pregnancy. By the end of the first trimester most changes have taken place. A second wave of changes occurs at the end of the mid trimester, approximately 24–28 weeks into the pregnancy, when women in the developed world almost universally show a picture of relative insulin resistance associated with an increased availability of substrates for the fetus, particularly in the post-prandial period when plasma glucose, amino acid and lipid levels are raised, as well as during overnight fasting in pregnancy.

Macronutrients

Glucose provides at least 75% of fetal energy requirements. There is increased glucose flux across the placenta during the post-prandial period particularly in the second half of pregnancy. The human feto-placental unit appears to have no mechanism to prevent excess glucose transfer across the placenta below the saturatable maximum and in maternal diabetes the excess glucose transfer has serious harmful effects on fetal growth and development. Although small IgG class immunoglobulins may cross the placenta, the placenta is effectively a barrier to the transport of larger protein molecules. Amino acids are actively transported across the placenta and appear in higher concentrations in the fetal than maternal circulation. Fat accumulates in the fetus at a rapid rate in the last third of pregnancy when fetal synthesis makes a significant contribution. Selective transport mechanisms for essential fatty acids required for fetal central nervous system (CNS) development are present during the second half of pregnancy.

Micronutrients

Some micronutrients, such as Cu and Se, are transferred across the placenta by passive diffusion, others by active transport mechanisms, some resulting in higher concentrations in the fetal circulation than in the mother (eg vitamin C, Ca, riboflavin, Zn). Other mechanisms protect the fetus from the risks of excess of some nutrients, and fetal levels are lower than maternal (eg vitamin A, E)

Growth and development of the conceptus

Following fertilization human gestation goes through three phases, blastocyst formation, embryogenesis and fetal growth. The first stage, blastocyst formation, lasts for 2 weeks after fertilization, followed by embryogenesis which lasts for 6 weeks. During embryogenesis all the tissues and organs are defined anatomically, and any teratogens are likely to have their greatest impact. Therefore at the stage when a pregnant woman is 10 weeks post her last menstrual period the structure and anatomical relationships of her infant's tissues and organs have been established. During the remaining 30 weeks the fetus grows from a weight of about 10–30 g to its birth weight, which is on average 3.3 kg in Caucasian women. The average total weight of the products of conception including placenta and amniotic fluid at full term is about 4.8 kg.

Energy costs of pregnancy

The nutritional costs of pregnancy comprise the energetic value of new tissue laid down both by the mother and in the products of conception, and the additional energetic costs associated with the increasing metabolizing mass of the pregnant woman. This gives a total average maternal weight gain from uterus, breasts, blood, extracellular fluid, and fat of 7.2 kg which combined with the weight of the products of conception produces an average weight gain for human pregnancy of 13 kg. The theoretical energy requirements for pregnancy based on weight gain are 80,000–85,000 kcal (356 MJ), or a daily calorie increase of approximately 320 kcal (1.3 MJ), giving rise to the widespread advice that in order to have a successful pregnancy women must increase their energy intakes by 250–300 cals/day (1–1.5 MJ). However dietary surveys do not match the theoretical calculations. The calculated total extra energy intake in pregnancy is less than 20,000 kcal (84 MJ) as basal metabolic rate (BMR) falls in early pregnancy followed by a rise during the last 10 weeks. There is no excess requirement for energy in the first 30 weeks of pregnancy and the increase in the last trimester could be met by either a small increase in energy intake or a reduction in physical activity.

Effects of activity on pregnancy

Women who maintain a high level of recreational exercise throughout pregnancy gain less weight, deliver their children earlier, and produce infants of lower birth weight. In the developing world women who are involved in hard physical work show lower birth weights.

Nutrition and adverse pregnancy outcomes

Food-borne disease in pregnancy

Pregnancy represents a state of relative immune compromise and in the rare case of primary infection with *Listeria* during pregnancy transplacental infection of the fetus has been responsible for fetal death. Because *Listeria* proliferates in common foodstuffs such as mould ripened cheese, liver pâté and cook–chill foods sensible advice is that women should avoid mould ripened cheese whilst pregnant and only eat pâté from manufacturing processes where pasteurization has taken place. As far as cook–chill food is concerned food should be consumed within the recommended shelf life and properly heated through before serving.

Toxoplasma gondii is a parasitic protozoal infection which non-immune women may be at increased risk of during pregnancy. It is caught from the ingestion of parasites from undercooked meat or from contact with cat faeces as a result of gardening or cleaning cat litter trays. In the fetus it can be responsible for brain infection and defects of vision. Sensible advice to women in pregnancy who may be at risk is to cook all meat thoroughly before consumption and to either avoid gardening or cat litter trays or only to undertake these tasks with strong rubber gloves.

Maternal mortality

Maternal mortality rates are extremely low in the developed world, in the order of 1 in 10,000 births, but in the developing world rates may be as high as 6 per 1000 pregnancies. Protein–energy malnutrition in the mother may contribute to this increased mortality, as might rickets in childhood, leading to short stature and inadequate pelvic dimensions and obstructed labour in adulthood. Obstructed labour is a major cause of maternal death where facilities for safe Caesarean section are not available. Severe anaemia is also a contributor to maternal death, often in association with intercurrent illness such as malaria and the absence of safe blood transfusion to deal with antepartum or postpartum haemorrhage. Moderate anaemia is not a major risk factor but severe anaemia (Hb $< 8.0\,g/dl$) doubles death rates in urban women and quadruples death rates in rural women.

Low birth weight

The two principal causes of low birth weight are preterm delivery, in which the infant may be normally grown but born in an immature state, and intrauterine growth retardation (IUGR), where inefficient placental transfer of oxygen and/or nutrients has led to a reduced rate of growth. The WHO definition is a birth weight of less than 2.5 kg. Low calorie intakes do not significantly contribute to low birth weight above a threshold value of an average energy intake somewhere between 1400 and 1700 kcals (5.8–7.0 MJ). Below this threshold supplementation can significantly reduce the number of low birth weight babies. Above the threshold supplementation has negligible effects on birth weight and indeed experiments with protein dense supplements have been associated with a relative *reduction* in birth weight. Calcium supplements appear effective both in the reduction of preterm birth and the incidence of low birth weight, possibly due to a role in the prevention of pregnancy-induced hypertension, allowing prolongation of pregnancy.

Obesity and pregnancy outcome

A BMI above 30 is associated with a doubling of the rate of ovulatory infertility and an even greater increase when the obesity is associated with the polycystic ovarian syndrome. During pregnancy obese women are at increased risk of developing gestational diabetes, venous thromboembolism and pregnancy-induced hypertension. Labour in obese women is more likely to be prolonged and unsuccessful and should delivery be necessary by Caesarean section, there are difficulties with surgical access to the uterus through the obese abdomen. Offspring of obese mothers are heavier than offspring of non-obese women.

Nutrition and the hypertensive disorders of pregnancy

Pregnancy is complicated by the development of hypertension in about 8% of cases worldwide with a predominance of first pregnancies. When accompanied by proteinuria the condition is referred to as pre-eclampsia and is associated with increased maternal and perinatal mortality and morbidity. There have been many attempts to identify the causes of pre-eclampsia and several nutritional hypotheses have been tested. More recently attempts to prevent the condition have been made by dietary interventions. A recent large study investigated the effects of supplementation with large doses of the antioxidant vitamins C and E. These had no effect on pre-eclampsia, but increased the prevalence of low birth weight. Calcium supplements have been shown to reduce mean blood pressure compared to placebo.

6.11 LACTATION

In many societies 99% of women lactate and produce enough milk to satisfy their infant's nutritional requirement for at least the first 6 months of its life and a significant component for up to two years. In other societies, particularly in the developed world, lactation rates may be as low as 30% or 40% and artificial formula feeding is more common.

Promoting successful lactation

Volumes of milk increase over the first months of lactation as infants develop appetite and grow. Successful lactation is promoted by early onset, frequent and night-time suckling, especially in the first days of lactation. Breast feeding for 6 months may be ideal but most women in developed societies stop breast feeding either exclusively or altogether long before that time. Their choices, once made, should be supported. Many need, or want, to work outside their homes. Some formula feeding, whilst continuing to breast feed, may enable mothers to avoid abandoning breast feeding altogether, although the introduction of other formula almost invariably leads to reduction in the volume of breast milk secreted.

Nutrient requirements of lactation

During lactation the mother has increased requirements for energy, protein and the micronutrients, especially calcium, to match losses in the milk. In prolonged lactation bone mineral density reduces in relation to the volume of breast milk produced. The bone mineral density is restored rapidly on cessation of lactation and there is no evidence that lactation contributes to an increased risk of osteoporosis in post-menopausal life.

Problems associated with breast feeding

Breast feeding is not without problems, for example:

Transmission of infection via breast milk

Breast milk may transfer viral infection, most notably Hepatitis B, cytomegalovirus, and human immunodeficiency virus, from mothers to infants. Infants of mothers positive for Hepatitis B surface antigen are at risk irrespective of the feeding method and should be actively immunized at birth. HIV risk of infection increases with duration of breast feeding and is greatest when breast feeding is not exclusive. Current UK advice for HIV positive and high-risk women is to avoid breast feeding. Where the risks of infection and undernutrition make formula feeding undesirable, breast feeding should be exclusive for 6 months and then infants should be moved on to complementary feeding and breast feeding stopped as quickly as practical.

Unwanted components of maternal diet which pass into milk

General concerns about the effect of components of the maternal diet on infants' tolerance of breast milk are probably overstated. Essential oils in foods such as garlic and some spices produce characteristic odours in milk which the infant may object to. Foods which can produce problems of tolerance for the infant are cabbage, turnips, broccoli and beans which seem capable of producing colic in some infants. The same effect has been ascribed to rhubarb, apricots and prunes. It might be sensible to exclude such food items when a breast fed infant appears to be distressed by colic after feeds.

Undernutrition in lactation

There are significant adaptive mechanisms to protect the newborn despite acute or chronic maternal undernutrition. Most mothers maintain an appropriate energy balance, compromising neither their own health status nor that of their developing infants. Mothers on low energy intakes in lactation maintain their weight well and lactate successfully, suggesting that important adaptive mechanisms are operating.

Lactational amenorrhoea, birth spacing and effects of maternal nutritional status

Fertile couples reproducing in the developing world without access to contraception typically show birth intervals of 3–4 years. This includes the duration of the pregnancy and approximately 18–24 months of lactational amenorrhoea during which there is no ovulation. In the developed world lactational amenorrhoea may be as short as 6–8 weeks after the delivery. Thus paradoxically a high nutritional plane may be associated with a shorter inter-pregnancy interval, compared with the developing world. There may be a trigger related to body mass index for the resumption of ovulation and menstruation.

KEY POINTS

- Nutritional status throughout the human reproductive cycle can affect outcome
- Anovulatory infertility is seen in under- and over-nourished women
- Periconceptual nutritional deficiencies may be associated with congenital malformations
- Energy costs of pregnancy are variable and unpredictable
- Food-borne diseases such as listeriosis may be fatal for the fetus
- Maternal nutrient deficiencies such as iron predict increased mortality in the developing world
- Reduced diet-induced thermogenesis is an energy sparing mechanism in lactation

6.12 INTRODUCTION TO AGEING AND OLDER PEOPLE

The number of older people is growing rapidly worldwide, creating a need for a more complete understanding of the role of nutrition in the prevention and treatment of chronic disabling diseases in the elderly. Undernutrition is a potential problem among the elderly, especially in the oldest age groups, but there are difficulties in diagnosis because of physical and biochemical changes which may take place as part of normal ageing, and nutritional assessment in acute clinical medicine is neglected. In Britain, undernutrition is prevalent but largely unrecognized in elderly patients on admission to hospital and tends to deteriorate further during their hospital stay, although good nutrition contributes to the health and wellbeing of elderly people and to their ability to recover from illness.

Since the early 1930s the number of people aged over 65 in England has more than doubled and today a fifth of the population is over 60. Between

1995 and 2025 the number of people over the age of 80 is set to increase by almost a half and the number of people over 90 will double. The National Health Service (NHS) spends around 40% of its budget on people over the age of 65 and social services spend nearly 50%.

6.13 AGE-RELATED PHYSIOLOGICAL AND PATHOLOGICAL CHANGES RELEVANT TO NUTRITION

Anorexia and weight loss are common and important clinical problems in the oldest age groups. The causes are multifactorial, predisposing to protein–energy undernutrition, particularly in the presence of other 'pathological' factors associated with ageing, such as social, psychological, physical, and medical factors, some of which are responsive to treatment.

Physiological changes

Hormonal

The mechanisms of physiological anorexia of ageing include an increase in the satiating effects of cholecystokinin (CCK) (see chapter 2), and an increase in the time taken for the emptying of the stomach after large volumes of food. This may explain why older adults feel a greater satiating effect of an average meal compared to younger adults. Other hormones (eg leptin), neurotransmitters (eg opioids & nitric oxide) and cell signalling molecules (eg cytokines) may also have a role to play in anorexia and weight loss of ageing.

Gastrointestinal

Changes in smell and taste are common and may decrease food intake or alter the type of foods which are selected. The use of drugs, particularly antihypertensive medication, is a contributing factor. Some 45% of the free-living elderly in the UK are edentulous and there is a link between dentition and nutritional status. Absorption of some nutrients, in particular vitamin B_{12}, may be impaired because of mild ageing-related achlorhydria.

Body composition

Changes in body composition seen with ageing include a decrease in lean body mass, which occurs faster after the eighth decade, and an increase in body fat. The decline in lean body mass is predominantly that of muscle, which contributes to a loss of mobility and an increased frequency of falls in elderly people. This is associated with a reduction in energy expenditure which will lead to a reduction in energy intake. Exercise can halt the decline in lean body mass with ageing, and limit the usual fall in energy intake with increasing age.

Bone mass and composition (see chapter 9)

Peak bone mass, which is higher in men than women, is achieved at around 30 years of age and is a determinant of bone mass in old age. Osteoporosis is particularly common in post-menopausal females. Severe osteoporosis may cause the bones in the legs to bow under the weight of the body and to changes of the spine.

Pathological changes
Medical and social factors

Physical changes such as decreased visual acuity, joint problems, hand tremors and hearing problems, often occurring in combination, may make the task of food preparation and eating more difficult for the elderly. Other factors which may affect nutritional status in the elderly include isolation and reluctance to go out shopping, loss of spouse, depression and bereavement, decreased mobility, dementia, anorexia due to disease (especially cancer), medications, poor dentition, alcoholism and most important of all, acute illness. In institutions, lack of supervision and assistance at mealtimes may be an important determinant of poor food intake. Because old people are disproportionately isolated, on low income or disabled, socioeconomic factors and disease are likely to have more influence on their nutritional status than age alone.

Immune function

Aspects of the immune response are known to deteriorate with ageing and to be influenced by poor nutritional status. However, studies in healthy elderly people have shown that many modifications in immune responses previously reported to be due to ageing *per se* may in fact be associated with pathological conditions. While ageing may induce dysregulation of the immune system, undernutrition seems to be one of the main factors leading to poor immune responses, particularly in cell-mediated immunity. Protein–energy undernutrition and micronutrient deficiencies, such as zinc, selenium, iron, copper, vitamins A, C, E and vitamin B_6, and folic acid, may all influence immune response.

Cognitive function

Cognitive decline and dementia are common in old age. Dementia affects one in 20 people over the age of 65 and one in five over the age of 80. The central nervous system requires a constant supply of glucose, and adequate brain function and maintenance depend on almost all essential nutrients. Although the nutritional determinants of cognitive decline are not well understood, there is some evidence that inadequacies of vitamins C, E and the B group may be important.

Obesity

Obesity now affects large numbers of people worldwide. Ageing is associated with a high incidence of diseases such as hypertension, diabetes, atherosclerosis, arthritis and disability, most of which are associated with obesity.

6.14 AGE-RELATED CHANGES IN ENERGY AND PROTEIN REQUIREMENTS

Energy requirements

The average energy intake of elderly men and women in the UK and other countries has been falling over several decades and the most recent National Diet and Nutrition Survey of British people aged 65 years and over in 1998 reported an overall intake of 1909 kcal in free living men and 1422 kcal for women. Changes in requirements with age depend on changes in the components of energy expenditure (see chapter 2).

Basal metabolic rate (BMR)

BMR increases with body size, particularly with lean body mass, and this explains why it is higher in men than women, and 10–20% lower in old people compared with younger adults because of reduced muscle mass and increased fat mass with ageing.

Physical activity

In most working populations physical activity accounts for 10–35% of total energy expenditure. The energy expenditure of different activities depends on the amount of work being carried out, the weight of the individual and the efficiency with which that work is carried out. In general, ageing is associated with a reduction in efficiency, which may make everyday tasks up to 20% more energy-expensive in older people. A variety of degenerative and chronic diseases such as chronic obstructive airway disease, angina and arthritis are likely to limit physical activity in the elderly.

Thermogenesis

A fall in the capacity for thermogenesis with age may explain the increased risk of hypothermia in the elderly.

Protein requirements

Lean body mass protein falls with age and protein synthesis, turnover, and breakdown all decrease with advancing age. The progressive loss of protein appears to be a major feature of ageing throughout adult life, affecting some tissues, notably skeletal muscle, more than others but this erosion of tissue protein does not appear to be due to lack of adequate amounts of protein in the average diet. Ill health, trauma, sepsis, and immobilization may upset the equilibrium between protein synthesis and degradation.

6.15 AGE-RELATED CHANGES IN MICRONUTRIENT INTAKES AND REQUIREMENTS

Vitamins

Because of a reduced energy requirement and the associated lower food intake and the increased incidence of physical diseases, which may interfere with absorption, metabolism and utilization, deficiency of certain vitamins is more likely in the elderly than in younger adults. In the United Kingdom average vitamin intakes of most vitamins are above current RNIs but there are subgroups in which deficiencies are more likely. For example, vitamin D status is more likely to be poor among institutionalized elderly, particularly during the winter months, and intakes of folate and vitamin C are lower in low socioeconomic groups.

B group vitamins

Low intake of riboflavin in institutionalized elderly has been a consistent feature of surveys of the elderly in the United Kingdom, with some evidence of biochemical deficiency in a modest proportion of elderly people. Numerous studies have suggested an association between neurocognitive function and B vitamin status in the elderly.

Homocysteine

Elevated plasma homocysteine is a risk factor for cardiovascular disease. Plasma homocysteine levels increase in the elderly, partly because of impaired renal function but low vitamin B_{12}, vitamin B_6, and riboflavin intakes contribute to elevated plasma levels of homocysteine in the elderly. Some medications may impair B vitamin status such as folate antagonists including methotrexate, phenytoin, carbamazepine, and vitamin B_6 antagonists such as theophylline and azarabine. Subjects with an elevated plasma homocysteine compared with the lowest quintile have a significantly increased risk of death from vascular and non-vascular causes. Also, cognitive function is inversely related to plasma homocysteine concentrations.

Antioxidant vitamins

Low intakes of vitamin C and associated biochemical deficiency has been reported in many studies of the elderly, with those living in institutions most at risk. There is a strong inverse association between mortality from stroke and plasma ascorbic acid. Low plasma concentrations of ascorbic acid and α-tocopherol are associated with an increase in oxidative damage after acute ischaemic stroke. Poor vitamin C status in the elderly may also be relevant to other diseases with a clear age-profile, such as senile macular degeneration and cataract.

Minerals

Sodium and potassium

Hypertension and stroke are both more common in older people. Excess salt intake causes hypertension and enhances thrombosis by the acceleration of platelet aggregation. On the other hand, dietary potassium may protect against these effects.

Calcium and vitamin D

Many institutionalized and free-living elderly (up to 50% in some studies) have poor vitamin D status, and the possible causes for this include sunlight deprivation, decreased intake of dairy products, lactose intolerance and malabsorption of fat-soluble vitamins. Bone mass declines with age, especially in white females; this is associated with osteoporosis and an increased fracture risk. Calcium supplements of 1000 mg daily with exercise slows postmenopausal bone loss. Dietary supplementation with calcium and vitamin D significantly reduces bone loss and reduces the incidence of non-vertebral fractures.

Magnesium

Magnesium deficiency in the elderly can occur due to low dietary intake and the use of diuretic therapy. Acute magnesium or potassium deficiency can produce cerebrovascular spasm, and the lower the extracellular concentration of either magnesium or potassium the greater the magnitude of cerebral arterial contraction.

Iron

Because of a higher prevalence in elderly people of disorders which interfere with efficient iron absorption, such as atrophic gastritis and post-gastrectomy syndromes, a proportion of elderly people have reduced dietary availability of iron. Blood loss due to peptic ulcer, haemorrhoids, cancer and non-steroidal anti-inflammatory drug use is more likely in elderly people.

Zinc

Studies suggest that, in the UK, institutionalized elderly subjects are at increased risk of zinc deficiency. Both zinc deficiency and pharmacological doses of zinc may adversely affect cell-mediated immunity.

6.16 ASSESSMENT OF NUTRITIONAL STATUS IN OLDER PEOPLE (SEE CHAPTER 12)

The combination of advanced age, multiple chronic diseases and use of drugs leads to an increased risk of protein–energy undernutrition. Problems in diagnosing undernutrition in the elderly are common because of physical and biochemical changes which may take place as part of normal ageing processes. In addition, overt clinical signs of undernutrition may be late to appear and much subclinical damage may have gone uncorrected. Of particular importance are involuntary body weight changes or values below an established population standard, arm muscle circumference, skinfold measurement and depressed secretory proteins.

6.17 NUTRITIONAL STATUS IN OLDER PEOPLE

In the community

Provided individual elderly people are in good health, their dietary patterns and the foods eaten are no different from those of younger people. However, risk factors for undernutrition in elderly people in the community include those described above under 6.13.

In acute and non-acute care settings

In hospitals and residential/nursing homes food intakes are less than those reported for free-living elderly people. Undernutrition is prevalent and often unrecognized in patients admitted to hospitals and institutions. The effect of ill health on the nutritional status of hospitalized patients can be limited to the time of acute illness, but elderly people are particularly at risk because of decreased nutritional reserves and the effects of repeated ill health. There is a strong correlation between undernutrition and an increased risk for subsequent in-hospital morbid events.

6.18 NUTRITIONAL SUPPORT OF OLDER PEOPLE

Prior to coming into hospital elderly people in the community are likely to have decreased energy or calorie intake, low lean body mass and impaired immune response, all of which may be associated with poor nutritional status. Their nutritional status is likely to deteriorate further as the result of the catabolism associated with an acute illness. This is compounded by the demands of the sometimes prolonged period of rehabilitation. Nutritional depletion during rehabilitation, however, may be more serious than during acute illness, since rehabilitation periods may extend over weeks and months, and weight loss, although less marked than in the early catabolic phase, may be greater overall. Most stroke patients who remain in hospital show marked and significant deterioration in all measures of nutritional status during the hospital stay. Nutritional status is a strong and independent predictor of morbidity and mortality at three months following acute stroke.

A systematic Cochrane Library review on protein and energy supplementation in elderly people at risk from malnutrition concluded that supplementation produces a small but consistent weight gain with statistically significant beneficial effect on mortality and a shorter length of hospital stay. The poor outcome in elderly patients following acute illness may at least be partly due to undernutrition, and aggressive nutritional support during the convalescent period is more likely to improve nutritional status and lead to better rehabilitation outcome, decreased readmission rate, improved quality of life and contribute to reducing NHS cost.

KEY POINTS

- Healthy elderly people's dietary patterns and the foods eaten are unlikely to be very different from those of younger people
- The majority of 'pathological' factors associated with ageing, which may predispose to malnutrition, are responsive to treatment
- Older people should be advised to eat a balanced diet containing a variety of nutrient-dense foods
- Elderly people should be encouraged to lead an active life, especially after episodes of inter-current illness

FURTHER READING

Department of Health and Social Security 1992 Nutrition in the elderly (Report on health and social subjects 43). HMSO, London

Mittlemark R A, Wiswell R A, Drinkwater B L 1991 Exercise in pregnancy, 2nd edn. Williams and Wilkins, Baltimore

Morgan J B, Dickerson J W T (eds) 2003 Nutrition in early life. John Wiley and Sons, Chichester, p 291–323

World Health Organization 2002 Programming of chronic disease by impaired fetal nutrition. Evidence and implications for policy and intervention strategies. WHO, Geneva

World Health Organization 2003 Promoting optimal fetal development: report of a technical consultation. WHO, Geneva

World Health Organization 2002 Keep fit for life. Meeting the nutritional needs of older people. WHO, Geneva

CHAPTER 7

Diet for Sport and Exercise

OBJECTIVES

By the end of this chapter you should:

- understand the basic physiology of muscle contraction
- appreciate how fuels are used for different types of exercise
- understand feeding strategies for optimum physical performance for different situations
- know of the ergogenic aids in current usage

7.1 INTRODUCTION

Much of the daily energy and nutrient requirements for a healthy adult is for the maintenance of basal metabolism, which accounts for an average of 60–75% of daily energy expenditure (see chapter 2). Requirements increase incrementally with increased energy expenditure, however modest, and whether incorporated into a normal working day or as part of a fitness regimen. However, although the principles of energy and nutrient requirements do not change, people engaged in recreational or competitive sports may find that a particular dietary regimen improves performance. Some individuals strive to enhance their performance through the use of foods and supplements targeted for the competitive sportsperson, with a variable evidence-base for their efficacy.

Physical fitness need not be the exclusive domain of the sportsperson and there is now a wealth of evidence that exercise makes an important contribution to good health and helps to reduce the risk of chronic disease such as cardiovascular disease and cancer.

This chapter considers the relationships between diet, exercise and fuel metabolism.

7.2 MUSCLE STRUCTURE AND FUNCTION

To perform physical exercise our bone structure needs to be moved by muscle force, which is generated when chemical energy is transformed to

135

mechanical energy within the muscle. Skeletal muscle consists of an outer layer of connective tissue covering small bundles of muscle fibres. A muscle fibre represents the individual muscle cell and usually extends the entire length of a muscle. At both ends the muscle fibre fuses with a tendon, which is attached to the bone. The muscle fibre contains numerous myofibrils, which represent the contractile elements of the muscle. There are two types of muscle fibres, slow twitch fibres (also called type I), which are particularly important for aerobic exercise and are well suited for prolonged endurance exercise like marathon running and cycling, and fast twitch fibres (also called type II), which are more important for anaerobic work such as in short-term high intensity activities like weight-lifting or sprinting (see chapter 2). Interestingly, fibre composition differs considerably between individuals, which is largely determined by genetic background. Individuals seem therefore to have a genetic disposition towards high performance in some sports.

A single motor nerve innervates several muscle fibres, and together they are referred to as a single motor unit. Muscle contraction is preceded by a series of events. First, a motor nerve impulse is generated and conducted through the motor neuron towards its nerve endings. There, an electrical charge can be generated and conducted throughout the entire muscle fibre. Muscle contraction is dependent upon the presence of calcium ions in the muscle fibre and requires energy, which is provided by adenosine triphosphate (ATP), the universal energy donor in the living cell. An extremely complex, well-orchestrated series of muscle contractions within numerous muscle fibres from various muscle groups are needed to enable even the simplest of movements.

7.3 SKELETAL MUSCLE SUBSTRATE UTILIZATION

The immediate source of chemical energy required for skeletal muscle to contract is provided by the hydrolysis of ATP. Because intracellular ATP stores are small, metabolic pathways for ATP synthesis need to be activated directly in response to an increase in ATP demand. The transition from rest to exercise is associated with an increased demand for ATP, which, at the muscular level, can increase more than 100-fold. ATP can be generated during anaerobic metabolism in all cells, through the glycolytic pathway (chapter 4), but muscle cells can also rely on creatine phosphate. Creatine phosphate is a high-energy compound stored in the muscle, the hydrolysis of which generates energy for ATP synthesis. A high rate of synthesis of ATP can be achieved through these routes but substrates are rapidly depleted. The majority of ATP required for muscle contraction is generated through oxidative phosphorylation, primarily from the oxidation of fat and carbohydrate.

Fuel storage

Muscle contraction occurs continuously and therefore the body needs to ensure a continuous supply of ATP. It does this through the use of fuels made available through diet and from stores (Table 7.1). Carbohydrate is stored as glycogen in skeletal muscle and in the liver. A normal healthy adult stores about 100 g glycogen in the liver and about three times this in skeletal muscle. Fat is stored in adipose tissue; stores are generally between 9 and 15 kg in

Table 7.1 Available fuel in an average person

Fuel source	in weight (g)	in energy (kJ)
Fat		
plasma free fatty acids	0.4	16
plasma TAG	4.0	156
TAG stores	12,000	468,000
Carbohydrate		
plasma glucose	20	360
liver glycogen	100	1800
muscle glycogen	350	6300

Based on estimates for a normal, non-obese person with a body mass of $\pm70\,kg$; fat provides 39 kJ/g and carbohydrate 18 kJ/g.

the non-obese adult male weighing about 70 kg but can be a great deal more. Additionally, the energy provision from fat is 39 kJ/g, more than twice that from carbohydrate.

Exercise intensity and duration

Fat and carbohydrate are the main substrates that fuel aerobic ATP synthesis during prolonged exercise. Though both substrates will always contribute to total energy provision, their relative utilization has been shown to vary with the intensity and duration of exercise.

During low intensity exercise (less than 30% of maximum oxygen consumption, VO_2max), most of the energy requirement comes from the oxidation of fat, principally from fatty acids in the circulation. During moderate intensity exercise fat and carbohydrate each contribute about half of the energy requirement. At high exercise intensity muscle glycogen becomes the most important source of energy. However, muscle glycogen stores are limited, and cannot sustain exercise of long duration; this is a reason behind the onset of fatigue during prolonged endurance exercise. This means that pre-exercise muscle glycogen concentration is a determinant of the time of onset of exercise fatigue.

Effects of training on fuel use

The relative contribution of fat and carbohydrate oxidation to total energy expenditure during exercise is also determined by training status. Endurance training leads to an increased capacity to utilize fat as a substrate source and reduces the reliance on the limited endogenous carbohydrate stores during exercise. Evidence suggests that the increase in fat oxidation is accounted for by an increase in the concentration of intramuscular triacylglycerol and an increased rate of utilization.

7.4 NUTRITIONAL STRATEGIES FOR OPTIMUM PERFORMANCE

Increased physical activity, however modest and through whatever means, will increase the requirement for energy. Exercise training or competition can increase the daily energy expenditure by 2–4 MJ/hour (500–1000 kcal) of exercise, depending on physical fitness, duration, type and intensity of sport. For this reason, athletes must increase food consumption to meet their energy needs, according to the level of daily energy expenditure. This increased food intake should be well balanced with respect to macronutrient and micronutrient composition.

It can be difficult to maintain the required increment in energy intake associated with high intensity exercise, especially during competition events. A professional cycling race, such as the Tour de France, can cost an athlete up to 40 MJ/day (9,550 kcal). And there is a practical limit to ingesting this amount of energy through solid meals. Some athletes resolve the problem by consuming specially-formulated fluids.

In contrast, some athletes with high profiles, such as gymnasts and ballet dancers, are known to reduce their energy intake, despite their high rate of energy expenditure. This leads inevitably to low BMI and fat mass with associated effects on performance.

Carbohydrate

Endurance performance capacity is often limited by the availability of endogenous carbohydrate. For this reason athletes involved in moderate to high intensity exercise lasting more than 45–60 min may adopt strategies to increase muscle glycogen concentration prior to competitive events. Increases in muscle glycogen can be achieved through carefully-regulated exercise and carbohydrate-feeding regimens (carbohydrate loading) and it seems that this practice is commonly employed by endurance athletes throughout the world.

Endurance exercise performance has also been shown to benefit from the consumption of carbohydrate during exercise itself. In this case carbohydrates are best provided in combination with water. Studies indicate that although monosaccharides and disaccharides are absorbed and oxidized at similar rates, exercise inhibits oxidation of carbohydrate, so no more than ~60–70 g of carbohydrate should be ingested per hour. Additionally, sports drinks should not have a high osmolality as this would result in impaired gastric emptying. Following prolonged endurance exercise the restoration of muscle glycogen is slow. Muscle glycogen synthesis rates are highest during the first two hours after exercise and this offers an opportunity for the use of carbohydrate-rich sports drinks immediately post-exercise, to aid in recovery. Thereafter, moderate-to-high glycaemic index foods (cakes, biscuits, white bread) should be consumed rather than low glycaemic index foods (brown bread, fruit, pasta).

Fat

Far less information is available on the role of fat compared with the role of carbohydrate as a fuel during exercise. However, as endurance training increases fat oxidative capacity, there is interest in the potential for nutritional interventions to increase fat oxidative capacity. Interest has focused on the use of medium chain triacylglycerols, as these are relatively water soluble and less likely to inhibit gastric emptying than long chain triglycerides.

Furthermore, medium chain fatty acid oxidation is not as limited by transport into the mitochondria as long chain fatty acids are. However, performance studies have failed to show effects greater than carbohydrate feeding.

As well as the use of fat supplements during exercise, research has also focused on the effect on performance of using high fat diets over a long term. The use of such diets provokes adaptive responses, leading to an increase in the capacity to oxidize fat as a fuel and the sparing of endogenous carbohydrate stores during exercise. However there is little evidence that such diets improve exercise performance, and from a general health perspective such diets cannot be encouraged.

Protein

Evidence shows that according to the type and duration of exercise there is an associated increase in protein requirement. This has been explained by the need to repair exercise-induced muscle damage, as an additional substrate source during prolonged exercise, and to support training-induced muscle reconditioning with an associated increase in lean tissue mass. However, there is a strong relationship between energy and protein intake in athletes and increased protein needs are likely to be covered by the increase in overall food intake that is usual in athletes. Nevertheless, protein requirements may not be met by normal dietary intake in athletes who are trying to lose weight, as is reported in some gymnasts, and female long distance runners. Resistance training is thought to increase protein requirements more than endurance exercise, and it is recommended that experienced male body-builders and strength athletes consume up to 1.6 g/kg body weight per day.

The use of protein and/or free amino acid supplements is currently popular in both strength and endurance athletes, as a means of supporting post-exercise recovery. The combined ingestion of carbohydrate with protein and/or specific free amino acids in the post-exercise phase has been shown to increase post-exercise insulin production, accelerate muscle glycogen synthesis, decrease muscle proteolysis and stimulate protein synthesis, leading to net protein anabolism. Besides providing ample substrate for protein synthesis and increasing insulin and/or growth hormone levels the ingestion of protein and/or free amino acids may also directly stimulate muscle protein synthesis. Research is currently underway to investigate the properties of individual amino acids to directly stimulate muscle protein synthesis.

Fluids and electrolytes

Most of the energy required for intensive endurance exercise is produced by oxidative metabolism, with an associated heat production. Much of this heat will be lost in sweat and at maximal sweat rates a 70 kg male athlete may lose >30 ml/min or >1800 ml sweat/hour. Dehydration substantially impairs exercise performance, with a ~10–15% decrease in performance capacity with each degree increase in body temperature. With sweat loss, electrolytes are also excreted but because sweat has a lower mineral content than plasma and water intake is inadequate to fully compensate the losses, the electrolyte concentration in blood normally increases as a result of intense endurance exercise.

Restoration of fluid balance after exercise is an important part of recovery. Rehydration after exercise can be achieved effectively only if both electrolyte as well as water losses are replaced. An ideal post-exercise rehydration drink should contain around 1100 mg/L sodium to optimize water retention. In comparison, ordinary soft drinks contain virtually no sodium and are therefore less suitable as a rapid rehydration solution.

Micronutrients

Vitamin supplements are widely used by both professional as well as recreational athletes but there is little evidence that this is either necessary or beneficial. Athletes who achieve an increased energy intake to address their increased requirements will generally do so with an associated increase in micronutrients. An exception may be athletes who have extremely high energy requirements and who choose to consume very high energy dense foods, which can be of low nutrient density, such as cakes and carbohydrate-rich fluids. Those sports men and women consuming diets of low energy content may also be prone to a marginal vitamin intake. However, vitamin supplements in individuals showing no biochemical evidence of inadequacy have not been shown to improve performance.

A specific role for antioxidant micronutrients might be argued for people who exercise regularly. Exercise has been associated with increases in free radical production in skeletal muscle, with potential for tissue damage. However, there is also evidence that athletes may compensate by increasing the intracellular activities of antioxidant enzymes and the benefit to be gained from antioxidant supplements is doubtful.

There may be a stronger case for the use of iron supplements by some athletes. Iron loss is increased in athletes, partly due to loss in sweat, increased gastrointestinal and/or urinary blood loss and foot strike haemolysis, but is usually well compensated for by the increased dietary intake associated with the higher energy expenditure. Female athletes are more likely to be iron depleted than their male counterparts, but iron deficiency anaemia is seldom reported. A lower than average haemoglobin concentration sometimes seen in athletes can be a training-induced physiological condition, caused by an increase in plasma volume, so-called 'athletes' anaemia'. This physiological condition does not respond to iron supplementation. Iron supplements have only been shown to enhance performance capacity in situations in which iron deficiency anaemia exists.

7.5 ERGOGENIC AIDS

Sports men and women the world over, seeking to enhance their performance, have turned to the wide range of heavily-marketed sports supplements now available. These products range from sports drinks, high-energy bars and protein-shakes to a multitude of nutrient supplements containing vitamins, minerals and free amino acids. Additionally, some products, marketed as ergogenic aids, contain active ingredients other than nutrients, or nutrients to be consumed in pharmacological amounts and may be marketed as functional foods. Evidence for their efficacy is generally lacking.

Caffeine

Caffeine has been used as an ergogenic aid but is currently included on the banned substances list used by the IOC (International Olympic Committee). Several studies have provided evidence for the ergogenic properties of caffeine ingestion during prolonged endurance exercise tasks. An effective ingestion dose lies between 2–5 mg/kg body weight, equivalent to about 2–6 cups of coffee. Its efficacy has been ascribed to a stimulating effect on the central nervous system, through the release and/or activity of adrenaline. Side-effects associated with caffeine use include gastrointestinal distress, decreased motor-control, shivering, headache, dizziness, and minor elevations in blood pressure and resting heart rate.

Creatine

In healthy individuals, the total endogenous creatine pool is approximately 120 g, most of which is located in skeletal muscle. It is replenished by endogenous synthesis and dietary intake (meat and fish). Studies have shown that oral creatine supplementation increases total creatine and creatine phosphate concentrations in human skeletal muscle and can enhance performance in repeated high-intensity, short-term exercise tasks, during which energy transfer is primarily derived by the ATP-creatine phosphate system. Consequently, creatine supplementation has become a common practice in both professional and amateur athletes.

Carnitine

Carnitine plays an important role in the transport of long chain fatty acids across the mitochondrial membrane, for oxidation. It has been suggested that increasing the intramuscular carnitine pool by using carnitine supplements could improve fatty acid import into the mitochondria and increase fat oxidative capacity. Carnitine is present in the diet (red meat and dairy products) and can be synthesized endogenously. Studies have generally failed to show that supplements can raise the concentration of carnitine in muscle or improve exercise performance.

Sodium bicarbonate

Sodium bicarbonate ($NaHCO_3$) better known as 'baking soda' has also been used as an ergogenic aid, on the basis that it will correct a fall in intracellular pH associated with anaerobic glycolysis. The accumulation of lactate in the anaerobic muscle leads to muscular pain and fatigue and the inability to maintain exercise intensity for a more prolonged period. Bicarbonate loading in athletes can improve performance in exercise tasks lasting between 0.5–6.0 min of near-maximal performance. Gastrointestinal distress and hyperosmotic diarrhoea have often been reported following bicarbonate loading.

KEY POINTS

- Quantitatively, muscle glycogen stores are the most important energy source during moderate to high intensity exercise
- Endogenous carbohydrate stores are relatively small and usually limit endurance performance capacity
- Carbohydrate loading in the days preceding endurance competition represents an effective means to optimize pre-exercise glycogen content
- During prolonged endurance exercise carbohydrate ingestion can significantly improve performance capacity
- Depending upon intensity and duration of exercise, people who exercise regularly may need to increase their energy and nutrient intakes
- Under most circumstances, increased protein requirements in athletes are provided by a general increase in energy intake
- Studies have failed to show that supplements of medium chain triacyglycerols enhance physical performance over carbohydrate feeding
- Fluids and electrolytes need to be supplied during prolonged exercise to compensate for sweat loss
- Vitamin and/or mineral supplementation does not improve performance capacity when no deficiencies are present

FURTHER READING

Frayn K 2003 Metabolic regulation: a human perspective, 2nd edn. Portland Press, London

Burke L M, Deakin V 2006 Clinical sports nutrition, 3rd ed. McGraw Hill, London

Maughan R J, Burke L M, Coyle E F 2004 Foods, nutrition and sports performance II. Routledge, London

McArdle W D, Katch F I, Katch V L 1999 Sports and exercise nutrition. Lippincott, Philadelphia

CHAPTER 8

Diet and Disease

OBJECTIVES

At the end of this chapter you should be able to

- describe the prevalence of important chronic diseases in different parts of the world and be aware of the changing mortality rates in different countries
- use appropriate terminology to define and describe the disease or condition
- describe the process of development of the disease or condition
- describe the risk factors for the diseases and their nutritional and other determinants
- discuss the short- and long-term risks
- discuss the main approaches to prevention and treatment

8.1 INTRODUCTION

Much of our early understanding of the nature of the relationship between diet and disease arose from observational or experimental studies of effects of nutrient deprivation. In other words, diseases of deficiencies were the focus of interest. Thus, the 1930s, 40s and 50s saw great advances in our understanding of the effects of undernutrition. In some areas of the world, in low- and middle-income countries, effects of undernutrition, in terms of energy and micronutrients, are still evident, but for a great number of the world population malnutrition is largely a problem of over-consumption rather than deficiency. This chapter examines the prevalence and causes of some diseases of public health importance worldwide, and discusses the role of diet as a preventative and therapeutic agent.

8.2 CARDIOVASCULAR DISEASE

Introduction

Cardiovascular diseases account for a significant proportion of total morbidity and mortality in adults throughout the world. An understanding of the following terms should be useful in interpreting the literature.

143

Atherosclerosis is the basic pathological lesion which tends to occlude the arteries to a varying extent. A *thrombus*, or clot, may further narrow the artery to the extent that it becomes totally blocked. When atherosclerosis affects the arteries supplying the heart muscle (coronary arteries) the person may experience *angina pectoris* or *myocardial infarction*. Angina pectoris is characterized by pain in the chest which is brought on by exertion or stress, whilst a *myocardial infarction* results from death of some of the heart muscle and is experienced as very acute and prolonged chest and often arm pain. Together these two conditions are referred to as *coronary heart disease* (CHD) or *ischaemic heart disease*. When a similar disease process influences the blood supply to the brain a *stroke* occurs which typically results in weakness or paralysis of one side of the body.

Prevalence of cardiovascular disease

In most industrialized countries CHD is the commonest single cause of death. Overall rates are higher in men than women, though as women age CHD contributes a greater proportion of total mortality. There is a wide variation in rates between countries; at the extremes, states comprising the former Soviet Union have a rate of 500 per 100,000, ten times the rate of Japan. Even across Europe there are notable differences; rates are much higher in Scotland, Finland and Poland (all more than 300 per 100,000) than in France (about 100 per 100,000) for example. These differences are attributed mainly to differences in lifestyle and this is borne out by the fact that migrant populations usually adopt the risk profile of their host country. Migrants from Japan to USA, for example, have a much higher CHD risk than in Japan. In the last 30 years rates of CHD have declined in Western European countries, North America and Oceana whilst in Eastern European countries rates are rising. In some countries, said to be in a state of nutritional transition, such as India and South Africa, affluence and poverty tend to coexist and rates of CHD are rising rapidly.

Box 8.1 shows accepted risk factors for CHD. These include non-modifiable factors such as age or gender, and lifestyle factors including smoking, physical activity and diet, or their biomarkers. Risk factors for CHD have principally been identified in prospective cohort studies. Many of these modifiable factors are associated with a graded increase in risk and in the case of cholesterol and blood pressure there is convincing evidence from randomized controlled intervention trials that lowering the risk factor reduces risk.

Epidemiological and experimental evidence linking diet with cardiovascular disease

The link with saturated and n-6 polyunsaturated fatty acids

The Seven Countries Study of Ancel & Keys and co-workers was absolutely central to our early understanding of a link between dietary intake and CHD risk. This study examined the associations between dietary intakes and 10-year CHD mortality rates of 16 population groups in seven countries.

Box 8.1 Risk factors for coronary heart disease

- *Irreversible*
  - Masculine gender
  - Increasing age
  - Genetic traits, including monogenic and polygenic disorders of lipid metabolism
  - Body build
- *Potentially reversible*
  - Cigarette smoking
  - Dyslipidaemia: increased levels of cholesterol, triglyceride, low-density and very-low-density lipoprotein; low levels of high-density lipoprotein
  - Oxidizability of low-density lipoprotein
  - Obesity, especially when associated with large waist circumference or waist:hip ratio
  - Hypertension
  - Physical inactivity
  - Hyperglycaemia and diabetes
  - Increased thrombosis: increased haemostatic factors and enhanced platelet aggregation
  - High levels of homocysteine
  - High levels of C-reactive protein
- *Psychosocial*
  - Low socioeconomic class
  - Stressful situations
  - Coronary-prone behaviour patterns: type A behaviour
- *Geographic*
  - Climate and season: cold weather
  - Soft drinking water

A strong correlation was noted between CHD and the percentage of energy derived from saturated fat and weaker inverse associations were found between CHD and percentages of energy derived from monounsaturated and polyunsaturated fat. Saturated fat was believed to increase coronary heart disease risk because of its ability to elevate blood cholesterol levels, and polyunsaturated fat (chiefly n-6 fatty acids) provided its modest protective effect via cholesterol-lowering. These observations led to many more studies and it is now clear that dietary saturated and n-6 polyunsaturated fatty acids act predominantly through effects on low-density lipoprotein (LDL) cholesterol, for which total cholesterol is a surrogate measure. In fact the effect of altering dietary cholesterol on LDL is much smaller than the effects of altering the intakes of various fatty acids. Experimental studies have shown large inter-individual variation in the lipoprotein responses to altering lipid intakes. It is thought that this can be explained by polymorphisms in key genes, but what these gene polymorphisms are is not yet clear. Saturated fatty acids can also increase CHD risk through mechanisms other than effects on lipoproteins, including a lowering of insulin sensitivity and an increase in platelet aggregation.

Nutritional and dietary determinants of cardiovascular risk

Understanding the relationships between diet and cardiovascular disease risk depends upon reliable methods for estimating dietary intake as well as accurate incidence or mortality statistics. Early studies used national food consumption data, the food balance sheets of the Food and Agriculture

Organization, or household food surveys. Positive associations with saturated fat, sucrose, animal protein and coffee, and negative correlations with flour (and other complex carbohydrates) and vegetables are some of the associations described. However, these early studies were important principally as hypothesis-generating and could not prove cause and effect.

The following sections consider some of the dietary components for which more recent evidence suggests an association with CHD risk.

Fish and n-3 polyunsaturated fatty acids

Evidence has accumulated to suggest that the regular consumption of oily fish is protective against cardiovascular disease. The effect is ascribed to the high content of the n-3 polyunsaturated fatty acids eicosapentaenoic acid (EPA; C20:5) and docosahexaenoic acid (DHA; 22.6), which reduce platelet aggregation. The n-3 fatty acids may also reduce cardiovascular risk via effects on cardiac electrophysiology, arterial compliance, endothelial function, blood pressure, vascular reactivity and inflammation.

n-6 Unsaturated fatty acids

In addition to their potential to reduce LDL, polyunsaturated fatty acids of the n-6 series may also reduce CHD risk by reducing platelet aggregation. Oleic acid may also act as an inhibitor of platelet aggregation, though the effect is less than for polyunsaturated fatty acids.

Trans unsaturated fatty acids

Partial hydrogenation of polyunsaturated fatty acids generates trans fatty acids. Metabolic studies have shown that trans fatty acids elevate LDL cholesterol, decrease high-density lipoprotein (HDL) cholesterol and increase lipoprotein(a), which constitutes a particularly atherogenic profile. Several large cohort studies have found an increased risk of CHD associated with an increased intake of trans fatty acids. Even though trans fatty acids have been reduced in retail fats and spreads in many parts of the world, deep-fried fast foods and baked products are a major and increasing source.

Antioxidant nutrients, flavonoids

LDLs are atherogenic when the constituent lipid is oxidized. Several dietary antioxidants, notably β-carotene, vitamin E and vitamin C, have been shown to reduce LDL oxidation in vitro and some prospective epidemiological studies confirm these observations, especially for vitamin E and flavonoids. A high intake of nutrients and other substances with antioxidant activity may partially explain the 'French Paradox', the term used to describe the observation that the French have a low rate of CHD despite blood cholesterol levels which do not differ markedly from those in other European countries with much higher rates of CHD. However interventions using dietary antioxidants have not generally been effective at reducing CHD risk.

B vitamins

Folate and vitamins B_2, B_6 and B_{12} may help to protect against cardiovascular disease through effects on the metabolism of the amino acid homocysteine.

Many (mainly case-control) studies have shown that an elevated plasma homocysteine concentration is associated with an increased risk of cardiovascular disease. Diets rich in folate tend to be associated with low plasma homocysteine, and supplements of folic acid, or vitamins B_2, B_6 or B_{12} all have homocysteine-lowering potential. However, there is little convincing evidence that lowering plasma homocysteine reduces risk of cardiovascular disease.

Wholegrain cereals and dietary fibre (non-starch polysaccharides)

High intakes of wholegrain cereals reduce the risk of cardiovascular disease. The protective effects may be due to the presence of non-starch polysaccharides, which have cholesterol-lowering properties, or mediated by associated low intakes of total and saturated fat.

Sodium and potassium

High sodium intake is directly associated with high blood pressure, a major risk factor for CHD and stroke. Studies suggest that a reduction in sodium intake of about 2 g per day (about 5 g NaCl), has the potential to significantly lower blood pressure in both hypertensive and normotensive individuals. Similar effects are seen with potassium supplements and many studies have reported an inverse association between dietary potassium intake and blood pressure. The DASH (Dietary Approaches to Stop Hypertension) trials, which examined dietary approaches to reducing blood pressure, found the maximum effect to be achieved by a high intake of vegetables, fruit and low fat dairy products in conjunction with a low sodium intake.

Nuts

Several large epidemiological studies have demonstrated that frequent consumption of nuts is associated with decreased risk of CHD, probably because of their high polyunsaturated fatty acid content.

Alcohol

There is evidence that low to moderate alcohol consumption (equivalent to 1–6 Units per day) lowers the risk of CHD, particularly in middle-aged men, possibly by raising HDL or through antioxidant effects. However, other cardiovascular and health risks associated with alcohol do not favour a general recommendation for its use as a preventive measure against cardiovascular disease.

Cardioprotective dietary patterns

A number of dietary patterns across the globe have been shown to be protective against CHD (Box 8.2). These include the Mediterranean diet, which traditionally has high intakes of fruit and vegetables and unsaturated vegetable oils; and certain traditional Asian diets. Unfortunately, health benefits associated with such traditional diets are being lost with the transition to more contemporary lifestyles.

Clinical trials of dietary modification

While prospective epidemiological studies provide strong evidence of risk or protection associated with individual nutrients or foods, proof of causality

> **Box 8.2** Attributes of cardioprotective diets
>
> - Low intakes of saturated fatty acids
> - High intake of raw or appropriately prepared fruit and vegetables
> - Lightly processed cereal foods and wholegrains are preferred
> - Fat intakes are derived predominantly from unmodified vegetable oils[*]
> - Fish, nuts, seeds and vegetable protein sources are important dietary components
> - Meat, when consumed, is lean and eaten in small quantities
> - Energy balance reduces rates of obesity
>
> ---
>
> [*]*Coconut oil and palm oil are not encouraged because they tend to elevate LDL*

and the ultimate level of evidence for dietary recommendations requires randomized controlled trials. The early trials all focused on lowering cholesterol levels, usually by increasing the dietary polyunsaturated:saturated (P:S) ratio. More recent trials have involved multifactorial interventions, including dietary change intended to improve all nutrition-related risk indicators as well as attempts to modify risk factors which are not diet-related, such as cigarette smoking. Dietary intervention trials have been undertaken in people with and without evidence of CHD at the time the study was started – called secondary and primary prevention trials respectively. This section describes briefly a few landmark trials (Table 8.1) and presents an overview of the important investigations of this kind.

The Los Angeles Veterans Administration Study examined the cholesterol-lowering effect of an intervention to reduce cholesterol and saturated fat intake in male volunteers between 55 and 89 years of age. The intervention was successful in lowering cholesterol and this was associated with a decrease in mortality from cardiovascular disease. The beneficial effect of the cholesterol-lowering diet was most evident in those with high cholesterol levels at the start of the study.

The Oslo Trial was a programme of dietary advice and support to stop smoking among Norwegian men. All those who participated in the study were either smokers or had elevated serum cholesterol at the outset. The intervention elicited a decrease in serum cholesterol and a reduction in the incidence of coronary events.

The Diet and Reinfarction Trial (Dart trial) was carried out among men who had already experienced a myocardial infarction, thus it was a secondary prevention trial. Men were randomized to one of three interventions – (1) a reduction of fat intake and an increase in the ratio of polyunsaturated to saturated fat, (2) an increase in fatty fish intake (or fish oil supplement), and (3) an increase in cereal fibre. The consumption of fatty fish elicited a decrease in all-cause mortality but the other interventions had no effect over the two years of the study.

The Lyons Heart Study was a secondary prevention trial among men with ischaemic heart disease. Patients either received conventional dietary advice or advice to follow a traditional Mediterranean diet which included more bread, legumes, vegetables and fruit and less meat and dairy products. This diet was lower in saturated fat and richer in n-3 fatty acids than the control diet. The group consuming the Mediterranean diet experienced a reduction in cardiovascular events as well as total mortality.

Table 8.1 Results of selected intervention trials (confidence intervals are given in parentheses)

Trial	No. of subjects	% reduction in cholesterol	Odds ratios (experimental vs control)	
			Total mortality	**Fatal and non-fatal CHD**
Veterans Administration	846	13	0.98 (0.83–1.15)	0.77
Oslo	1232	13	0.64 (0.37–1.12)	0.56
DART				
Fat advice	2033	3.5	0.98 (0.77–1.26)	0.92
Fish advice	2033	Negligible	0.74 (0.57–0.93)	0.85
Lyons Heart	605	Negligible	0.30 (0.11–0.82)	0.24
CHAOS	2002	NA	1.3	0.60
GISSI-Prevenzione				
n-3 fatty acids	2836	NA	0.80 (0.67–0.94)	0.80
vitamin E	2830	NA	0.86 (0.72–1.02)	0.88
HOPE	1511	NA	1.00 (0.89–1.13)	1.05

The Cambridge Heart Antioxidant Study (CHAOS) was a secondary prevention trial in which 2000 men and women were randomized to receive α-tocopherol (at two doses), or placebo. After 1.4 years non-fatal myocardial infarction was substantially reduced in those receiving α-tocopherol at either dose compared with the control group but there were marginally more total deaths in the α-tocopherol than the control group.

The GISSI-Prevenzione Study was also a secondary prevention trial, in this case using long chain n-3 fatty acids (eicosapentaenoic and docosahexaenoic acids), vitamin E (300 mg), or both, in subjects who had had a myocardial infarction. The group who received the n-3 fatty acids showed a decrease in cardiovascular events, including non-fatal myocardial infarction. A smaller, non-significant reduction in event rate was seen with vitamin E supplementation.

No cardioprotective effect of vitamin E was seen in the *Heart Outcomes Prevention Evaluation (HOPE) Study* in which patients at high risk of cardiovascular events were randomized to receive placebo, 400iu vitamin E (268 mg) or drug treatment (an angiotensin-converting-enzyme inhibitor) and followed for 4.5 years.

Conclusions

Cholesterol lowering by dietary means reduces coronary events in the context of both primary and secondary prevention. An increase in polyunsaturated fatty acids, a reduction in saturated fatty acids, and an increase in non-starch polysaccharide (dietary fibre) and starch, may all help to reduce cardiovascular risk. Monounsaturated fatty acids have a neutral effect. Antioxidant nutrient supplementation is less likely to be effective.

Dietary advice to reduce risk of occurrence or recurrence of cardiovascular events includes a reduction in saturated fatty acids and an increase in fruit, vegetables and low fat dairy products. Foods to be eaten regularly include pulses, fresh fruit, vegetables (starchy and non-starchy, salad vegetables), breads and cereals, brown rice and wholemeal pasta, fish, lean meat or poultry, nuts. Foods to eat only occasionally include cakes, crisps, chips, white bread, full fat cheeses, butter. Foods to avoid include chips cooked in dripping, lard or hardened margarine, sugar-coated cereals, meat fat, processed meat, cream.

KEY POINTS

- The nature of dietary fat is an important determinant of CHD in populations
- Saturated and trans unsaturated fatty acids increase CHD risk; n-6 and n-3 polyunsaturated fatty acids are protective
- Antioxidant nutrients, flavonoids, folate and other B vitamins, non-starch polysaccharides, whole grain cereals, nuts, soy protein and alcohol may protect against CHD
- Randomized controlled clinical trials demonstrate the potential for dietary change to reduce CHD rates

8.3 DIABETES

Introduction

Diabetes mellitus is a metabolic disorder of multiple aetiology characterized by chronic hyperglycaemia associated with impaired carbohydrate, fat and protein metabolism. These abnormalities are the consequence of either inadequate insulin secretion or impaired insulin action, or both. A diagnosis of *diabetes mellitus* is made on the basis of elevated plasma glucose concentration, either in a fasted or non-fasted blood sample or following a glucose load. The three most common forms are type 1, type 2 and gestational diabetes, which is defined as any degree of glucose intolerance with onset or first recognition during pregnancy. Type 2 diabetes is often associated with other metabolic disturbances and cardiovascular risk factors, collectively referred to as the *metabolic syndrome* (see section 8.5).

Aetiology and pathophysiology of diabetes mellitus
Type 1 diabetes mellitus

Type 1 diabetes is considered to be an autoimmune disease characterized by a cell-mediated autoimmune destruction of pancreatic β-cells that results in a partial or total inability to secrete insulin, and life-long need for insulin administration. Genetic factors make an important contribution to this condition but do not fully explain its aetiology. Environmental factors could contribute to the pathogenesis of type 1 diabetes mellitus through a direct toxic effect on the β-cells, triggering an autoimmune reaction against the β-cells, or damaging β-cells so as to increase their susceptibility to autoimmune destruction. Environmental factors include drugs or chemicals, viruses and dietary factors. There is, for example, evidence for a close relationship between cow's milk consumption and incidence of type 1 diabetes in childhood.

Type 1 diabetes develops over many years, and can be considered as a multistage process starting with a genetic susceptibility, requiring a triggering event, progressing to active autoimmunity, gradual loss of glucose-induced insulin secretion and finally to overt diabetes. In metabolic terms, a failure to secrete insulin leads to hyperglycaemia because of increased glucose production by the liver and reduced glucose utilization by peripheral tissue (Fig 8.1). The liver increases the rate of gluconeogenesis from extra-hepatic fuels including alanine, lactate and glycerol. Glucose utilization decreases as a result of the failure of insulin to adequately facilitate glucose entry into cells, resulting in an increased availability of free fatty acids. An increased rate of fatty acid oxidation leads to an increase in the production of ketone bodies by the liver. Ketone bodies are an important fuel for the brain in times of reduced glucose availability. All these metabolic abnormalities account for the classic symptoms and signs of the disease, such as glycosuria, polyuria, polydipsia (thirst), and weight loss.

Type 2 diabetes mellitus

Type 2 diabetes mellitus accounts for the great majority of all cases of diabetes. Type 2 diabetes, until recently referred to as non-insulin-dependent diabetes, is characterized by disorders of insulin action and secretion. These individuals may not require insulin treatment. Most of these patients are obese or have increased body fat predominantly in the abdominal region. The incidence and prevalence is increasing in the adult population but reports also indicate an emerging problem among children and adolescents.

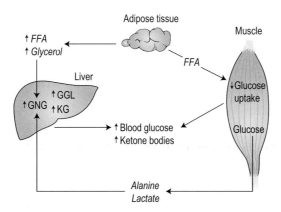

Figure 8.1 Consequences of high insulin deficiency in type 1 diabetes mellitus. FFA, free fatty acids; GNG, gluconeogenesis; GGL, glycogenolysis; KG, ketogenesis.

Patients with type 2 diabetes have two major metabolic defects: (1) impaired insulin secretion, and (2) resistance to insulin action at the liver, skeletal muscle and adipose tissue. Although genetic factors may play a role in the development of this disease, diet, including a high intake of saturated fats, obesity and a sedentary lifestyle are considered to be the main risk factors predisposing to the disease. Macrovascular complications such as myocardial infarction, heart failure and acute stroke account for much of the morbidity and associated mortality. Type 2 diabetes is often associated with other factors including raised arterial blood pressure, raised plasma triacylglycerols and central obesity together comprising the condition known as 'metabolic syndrome'.

Although type 2 diabetes is understood to be a disease primarily of insulin resistance at peripheral tissues, the secretion of insulin by the β-cells of the pancreas is inappropriately low for a given plasma glucose concentration. The main feature of the defect in insulin secretion seems to be a loss of sensitivity to glucose by the β-cell and a resulting impaired insulin secretion. The exact mechanisms for this defect are not understood but people with type 2 diabetes do have a smaller number of β-cells in their pancreas, and the β-cells themselves have certain abnormalities.

The main pathological feature of type 2 diabetes is insulin resistance, in which a given concentration of insulin produces a less than normal biological response. Insulin has a range of metabolic effects in the body, predominantly leading to the storage of nutrients (as glycogen, fat and protein). In addition, insulin regulates water and electrolyte balance and stimulates cell growth and differentiation. The underlying mechanisms for insulin insensitivity are not completely understood but evidence suggests that defects in insulin signalling, glucose transport and metabolic pathways of intracellular glucose utilization may all be involved.

Central to the altered biochemistry of type 2 diabetics is the fact that the uptake of glucose by skeletal muscle and adipose tissue is impaired with a net rise in blood glucose in both the fasted and the post-prandial state. It has been demonstrated that the ability of insulin to stimulate glucose uptake by the skeletal muscle is reduced by 40–50% in diabetic patients compared with normal subjects. Additionally, in type 2 diabetes, particularly when associated with obesity, the ability of insulin to suppress lipolysis is markedly impaired and there is an increased flux of free fatty acids (FFA) from adipose tissue into the plasma. The result is a chronic elevation of plasma FFA and triglyceride levels together with excessive deposition of fat in various tissues. In addition, type 2 diabetic patients tend to have abnormally increased glucose production in the post-absorptive state, which contributes to fasting hyperglycaemia. Although lifestyle factors are considered to be the most important determinants of type 2 diabetes there may be a contribution by mutations in some genes important to insulin secretion and effectiveness. Evidence suggests that defects in individual genes are unlikely to be important unless they occur in a large number at the same time.

Vascular complications

Microvasculature

Patients with diabetes can develop a number of complications, including those of the vasculature. Retinopathy can result from abnormalities in the microvasculature, is a feature of longstanding type 1 diabetes and can occur in type 2 diabetes. In some patients this leads to blindness. Nephropathy (damage to the kidney) occurs in about one-quarter of patients with type 1 diabetes, but is much rarer in type 2 diabetes.

The degree and duration of hyperglycaemia seems to be a key factor in the development of these vascular complications. Additionally, hypertension, smoking and hyperlipidaemia are contributory factors. Intervention trials in type 2 diabetic patients have clearly shown that improving blood pressure control significantly reduces the onset and progression of both nephropathy and retinopathy.

Macrovasculature

Diabetic patients have an increased risk of cardiovascular disease, primarily because several important risk factors are raised in diabetes, such as plasma cholesterol and triacylglycerol. Atherosclerotic arterial disease may manifest clinically as coronary heart disease, cerebrovascular disease or peripheral vascular disease. Improved blood lipid profile and a reduction in blood pressure significantly reduces cardiovascular risk in these patients. Multi-targeted interventions that include a better control over blood glucose seem to be particularly effective.

The increased risk of cardiovascular disease in diabetic patients may be mediated by endothelial damage. Endothelial damage may lead to atherosclerotic plaque formation, and an associated increased likelihood of thrombus formation and acute ischaemia.

Strategies to reduce risk of cardiovascular disease in diabetic patients should pay attention to blood glucose control, but should also address plasma lipid profile, blood pressure, platelet aggregation, obesity, physical activity, and smoking habits.

Management of diabetes mellitus
Diet

The overall objective in the management of patients with diabetes mellitus is to reduce the risk of cardiovascular disease. Nutritional management is the cornerstone of treatment, both for types 1 and 2, and complements the use of hypoglycaemic drugs or insulin. Dietary recommendations for people with diabetes are very similar to those given to the general population for the promotion of good health. Dietary strategies for patients with diabetes have to be considered as lifelong strategies.

The majority of patients with type 2 diabetes are overweight or obese, and this is becoming more common in patients with type 1 diabetes, especially in those following intensive insulin therapy. Reduction in body weight improves outcomes in patients with both type 1 and 2 diabetes. Blood glucose control, insulin resistance, blood pressure and lipid abnormalities have all been shown to improve in association with weight reduction.

Dietary intervention can also be effective in preventing the onset of type 2 diabetes in high risk individuals. Intervention trials have shown that weight loss achieved in high risk individuals consuming diets with reduced saturated fat and increased dietary fibre, in conjunction with increased physical activity, can reduce risk of type 2 diabetes.

Experts agree that patients with diabetes should consume diets in which the energy from saturated fat is less than 10% of total energy intake and cholesterol intake less than 300 mg per day. Foods rich in dietary fibre and/or with a low glycaemic index make an important contribution to glucose control and can improve blood lipid profile, therefore legumes, fruits, cereals and other vegetables are recommended. The effectiveness of a meal in modulating blood glucose is related to the glycaemic index of the constituent foods. The glycaemic index is a measure of the extent to which a food raises blood glucose concentration compared with an equivalent amount of a reference carbohydrate (glucose or white bread). A diet containing mainly low glycaemic index foods improves the metabolic control in diabetic patients and may have favourable effects on other cardiovascular risk factors. Therefore foods with a low glycaemic index (eg legumes, oats, pasta, parboiled rice, and certain raw fruits) should replace, whenever possible, those with a high glycaemic index. Additionally, in accordance with general guidelines for the promotion of good health, diabetic patients should consume less than 6 g salt per day to control blood pressure and restrict their daily alcohol intake to one or two units alcohol (women and men respectively).

Physical activity

Aerobic physical activity of moderate intensity but performed on a regular basis (daily or at least 4 times/week) has been shown to improve blood glucose control, reduce insulin resistance, induce favourable effects on other cardiovascular risk factors, prevent the incidence of type 2 diabetes and reduce cardiovascular and total mortality. In type 1 diabetic patients, glycaemic changes during exercise depend largely on blood insulin levels and, therefore, on insulin administration. Hyperinsulinaemia may cause hypoglycaemia, while hypoinsulinaemia may lead to hyperglycaemia. The risk of hypoglycaemia during exercise can be reduced by consuming 20–40 g extra carbohydrate before and hourly during exercise and/or by reducing pre-exercise insulin dosages. In type 2 diabetic patients, exercise reduces insulin resistance and therefore increases peripheral glucose uptake but an associated decrease in insulin secretion means that hypoglycaemia is rare and extra carbohydrate is generally not required.

Hypoglycaemic oral agents and insulin therapy

Patients with type 2 diabetes who do not respond adequately to a diet and exercise regimen will be given oral hypoglycaemic medication. Metformin induces weight loss and contributes to the normalization of blood glucose and for these reasons is considered the first choice drug in the treatment of overweight diabetic patients. Sulphonylureas are generally employed for normal weight patients. If adequate glucose control is not achieved with the use of either or both of these drugs or other drugs in current use, insulin therapy can be included in the treatment.

Insulin is central to the management of type 1 diabetes, and, when diet and oral hypoglycaemic drugs prove inadequate, may also be useful for type 2 diabetic patients. Insulin therapy is tailored to each patient but is commonly administered by injection three times a day, the goal of the treatment being maintenance of blood glucose within defined limits, both under fasting and post-prandial conditions.

KEY POINTS

- Diabetes mellitus is a major cause of morbidity and mortality. Its prevalence is increasing globally, both in adults and children, due to increased prevalence of obesity and low levels of physical exercise
- Type 1 diabetes is characterized by impaired insulin secretion and requires insulin therapy to prevent ketoacidosis and death
- Type 2 diabetes is frequently associated with obesity and is caused by a defect in β-cell function and insulin resistance
- Lifestyle modification including dietary change and increased physical activity can improve prognosis

---

8.4 CANCERS

Introduction

Cancer is defined as a disease in which the normal control of cell division is lost, so that an individual cell multiplies inappropriately to form a tumour. Cancer can arise from different tissues and organs in the body, thus there are many different types of cancer. The commonest sites of origin of cancer among people in Western, industrialized countries are the lung, breast, large bowel and prostate. In developing countries, the commonest sites are cancers of the lung, stomach, breast and liver.

Various factors can cause cancer, such as tobacco, alcohol, ionizing radiations, ultraviolet light, certain infections and hormones. The causes of cancer in different parts of the body vary – for example tobacco causes cancer of the lungs and many other tissues, but has almost no effect on the risk for developing cancers of the breast and prostate. Dietary factors are thought to be very important in determining the risk for developing cancer, but establishing the exact effects of diet on cancer risk has proved difficult, and currently few dietary factors have been clearly shown to be important.

Distribution of cancers throughout the world

Figure 8.2 shows age-standardized incidence rates for the common cancers in developed and developing countries. Lung cancer is the commonest cancer in men in both developed and developing countries. Cancers of the prostate and colorectum are the next most common in developed countries whilst in developing countries cancers of the stomach and liver are the most common after

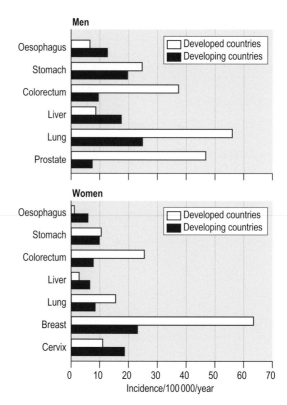

Figure 8.2 Age-standardized incidence rates of the most common cancers in men (top) and women (bottom) in developed and developing countries.

lung cancer. Breast cancer is by far the most common cancer among women in both developed and developing countries. Cancers of the colorectum and lung are the next most important in developed countries, whilst in developing countries cancer of the cervix has a similar incidence to breast cancer.

Cancer rates in the UK

The four commonest cancers in the UK are cancers of the lung, breast, colorectum and prostate – together these account for over half of all new cancer cases. In men, lung cancer rates have shown a steady fall since the 1970s due to reductions in cigarette smoking (Fig 8.3). In contrast, prostate cancer rates have increased markedly over the last 40 years, due partly to increased and earlier detection. In women, breast cancer incidence rates have increased over the last 40 years, with a steep increase around 1990 largely due to increased and earlier detection. Lung cancer rates have increased substantially in women due to increases in cigarette smoking.

Pathophysiology of cancer

Most cancers develop from a single cell that grows and divides more than it should, resulting in the formation of a tumour or cancer. Cancers growing in most tissues take the form of a lump that grows, invades local non-cancerous tissues, and may spread to other parts of the body through the bloodstream.

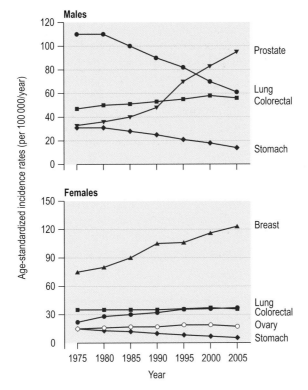

Figures 8.3 Trends in incidence for the four commonest cancers among men (top) and woman (bottom) in England and Wales 1971–1998.

Cancers arising in the cells of the blood, such as leukaemia, do not form a lump because the cells are floating freely throughout the bloodstream. Most deaths due to cancer are caused by the spread of the cancer from its site of origin into adjacent areas and to other parts of the body. The transfer of the cancer from one site to another site not directly connected with it is called metastasis.

The change from a normal cell into a cancer, termed carcinogenesis, is a multi-stage process and can take several decades; consequently incidence of most cancers is highest among the elderly. Carcinogenesis is fundamentally a process of alterations (mutations) in DNA. Typically the change from a normal cell to cancer requires mutations in a few different genes. Mutations in genes involved in the control of cell division and cell death (apoptosis) are especially important. Some mutations are inherited, while others are caused by factors such as ionizing radiation, chemical carcinogens and viruses.

The key genes in carcinogenesis can be considered in two classes: oncogenes, genes that when over-activated lead to over-stimulation of cell growth and cell division; and tumour suppressor genes, which normally limit the rate of cell division.

Inherited genetic factors in carcinogenesis

For the common types of cancer, current estimates are that inherited genetic factors contribute no more than 5% to the cases of cancer arising in a population. Inherited genetic factors (as opposed to mutations in genes that can occur during a person's lifetime) can be considered in two classes: high risk mutations and low risk genetic polymorphisms.

Inherited *high risk mutations* increase the risk of cancer by up to 50 times, but such mutations are quite rare. These types of mutations cause clusters of cancers within families; well known examples are HNPCC (hereditary non-polyposis colon cancer gene) that gives a high risk for colon cancer, and BRCA1 and BRCA2 (breast cancer 1 and 2 genes) that give high risks for both breast and ovarian cancer. At present, there is no strong evidence that dietary factors can modulate the effects of genes such as these on cancer risk.

Low risk polymorphisms: Mutations that occur with a frequency of more than 1% in a population are termed polymorphisms and they typically confer only a small increase in risk for cancer and do not cause clusters of cancers in families. There is currently great interest in the impact that gene polymorphisms can have on the cancer burden of a population, and the interaction of diet with gene polymorphisms is an area of active current research (see chapter 11).

Non-dietary causes of cancer

The proportions of cancer due to avoidable causes have been estimated by Doll & Peto and are shown in Table 8.2. These estimates apply to Western countries such as the USA or the UK; in developing countries the proportion of cancer due to infective factors would be higher. Worldwide, the most important preventable cause of cancer is tobacco, which causes cancers of the mouth, pharynx, oesophagus, larynx, lung, pancreas, kidney (pelvis) and bladder. Infectious agents are responsible for about 9% of cancers worldwide, with the proportion being higher in developing countries. For example, hepatitis B and C viruses cause liver cancer, human papillomavirus causes cervical cancer and the trematode worm, *Schistosoma haematobium*, is a major cause of bladder cancer in Egypt and Tanzania. Hormonal and reproductive factors are important determinants of cancers of the breast, ovary and endometrium

Table 8.2 Proportions of cancer deaths attributable to different lifestyle and environmental and behavioural factors in countries such as the United Kingdom

Factor	Best estimate of proportion (%)
Tobacco	30
Diet	25
Hormonal factors	15
Alcohol	6
Infections	5
Ionizing radiation	5
Occupation	2
Pollutants	2
Ultraviolet light	1
Medical drugs	<1

Adapted from Doll & Peto 2003

and childbirth reduces the risk for all three. Ionizing radiation makes a modest contribution to cancer causation; in the UK, for example, approximately 5% of lung cancers are due to naturally occurring radon gas inside buildings. Finally, a small proportion of cancers is caused by factors such as ultraviolet light, medical drugs, occupational exposures and pollution.

Diet and cancer

Dietary factors can both increase or reduce the risk for developing cancer, and the size of the effect on risk may be small or moderate (usually less than two-fold), compared to the very large effects of some other agents.

For all the common cancers, rates vary widely between populations in different parts of the world and when people migrate from one country to another they typically adopt the cancer rates of their new host country, indicating the importance of environment in determining cancer risk. Comparisons of dietary patterns and cancer rates in different countries have generated useful hypotheses linking diet with cancer risk. For example, this type of study led to the hypothesis that high intakes of meat may increase the risk for colorectal cancer, and that high intakes of fat may increase the risk for breast cancer. Hypotheses generated by these sorts of studies can be tested in case control and prospective cohort studies and randomized controlled trials (refer to chapter 12 for an explanation of study design).

Case control studies compare dietary intake, or biomarkers of dietary intake, in people with cancer with people who do not have cancer. However, case control studies suffer from bias in dietary recall in cancer patients and results need to be interpreted cautiously. Prospective cohort studies collect dietary intake data, or collect blood for biomarkers measurements, in a healthy cohort and make comparisons between those people who develop cancer with those who do not, at a later date. Randomized trials eliminate bias, and positive results from such trials provide clear evidence that the intervention has caused the change in cancer risk. Generally however, such trials test the efficacy of a nutrient supplement and intervention trials of foods or dietary patterns are uncommon even though they would be much more informative.

Mechanisms for effects of dietary factors on cancer risk

Dietary mutagens
Dietary factors may affect the chances of developing cancer in various ways. Diet may increase risk by supplying mutagens that directly damage the host DNA. Two important examples are aflatoxin and Chinese-style salted fish. Aflatoxin is a food contaminant produced by the fungus *Aspergillus*; high levels of aflatoxin can occur in foods such as grains, oilseeds, nuts and dried fruit stored in hot and humid conditions, and, together with active hepatitis due to hepatitis B virus, can cause liver cancer. Chinese-style salted fish, which can contain high levels of nitrosamines, increases the risk for nasopharyngeal cancer.

Other food components that may increase cancer risk due to their mutagenic effects include nitrites and their related compounds found in smoked, salted and some processed meat products. Cooked meat and fish can contain moderately high levels of heterocyclic amines and polycyclic aromatic hydrocarbons, which might increase risk in particular for colorectal cancer.

Alcohol

High alcohol consumption causes cancers of the mouth, pharynx, larynx, oesophagus and liver, and even moderate alcohol intakes causes a small increase in the risk for breast cancer. This effect of alcohol may act through enhancing the action of carcinogens or via the effects of acetaldehyde which is produced when ethanol is metabolized (see chapter 4). The increase in breast cancer risk due to alcohol intake may be from effects on oestrogen metabolism.

Energy balance

Obesity in humans increases the risk for several types of cancer (oesophagus, colorectum, breast, endometrium, kidney). Although the underlying mechanisms are not well understood, effects of obesity on breast and endometrial cancer are likely to be mediated by the actions of oestrogen, which is present in higher levels in the blood of obese women than non-obese women and which enhances cell proliferation in vitro.

Dietary fibre and bowel function

Diets high in fibre have generally been associated with a reduction in the risk of colorectal cancer in both animal and human studies, although it is not clear whether the fibre itself or other substances found in high fibre foods such as vegetables, fruits, cereals and pulses are associated with the beneficial effect. High intakes of fibre reduce transit time through the colon and may thus minimize the absorption of carcinogens by the colonic mucosa. Dietary fibre may also reduce exposure to carcinogens through dilution of the gut contents and/or by binding the carcinogens for faecal excretion. Finally, fermentation of fibre in the large bowel produces short chain fatty acids, such as butyrate, which may protect against colorectal cancer through the ability to promote differentiation and induce apoptosis.

Vitamins and minerals

Some prospective cohort studies suggested that some vitamins and minerals with antioxidant activity might protect against certain cancers. However, results of randomized controlled trials have generally been unsupportive. There continues to be an interest in folate because of its role in DNA synthesis and stability, and some prospective cohort studies support a role for folate in protecting against colorectal cancer.

Plant anti-carcinogens

In addition to vitamins and minerals, many compounds in plants that are not nutrients are under investigation for possible anti-carcinogenic properties. Examples include: flavonoids such as quercetin found at high levels in apples, onions and tea; carotenoids such as lycopene and lutein found in tomato products and green vegetables, respectively; isothiocyanates, predominantly found in cruciferous vegetables; sulphur-containing compounds found predominantly in the *Allium* species, garlic, onions and leeks; and phytosterols, found in a wide variety of fruit and vegetables. Some of these compounds are cholesterol-lowering agents and may also exhibit anti-cancer properties via several pathways such as regulation of signal transduction pathways that regulate tumour growth and apoptosis. Phyto-oestrogens such as isoflavones derived from soyabeans, and lignans derived from whole grain products, have received particular attention because of their possible anti-oestrogenic effects that might reduce breast cancer risk.

Recommendations for reducing cancer risk

Various bodies have made recommendations for reducing cancer risk. The most recent set of recommendations comes from the recent WCRF/AICR Report on Diet, Physical activity and Cancer. The personal recommendations are summarized in Box 8.3.

Box 8.3 WCRF/AICR Recommendations for cancer prevention

1. Ensure that body weight through childhood and adolescent growth projects towards the lower end of the normal BMI range at age 21. Maintain body weight within the normal range from age 21. Avoid weight gain and increases in waist circumference through adulthood.
2. Be moderately physically active, equivalent to brisk walking, for at least 30 minutes every day. As fitness improves, aim for 60 minutes or more of moderate, or 30 minutes or more of vigorous physical activity every day.
3. Consume energy-dense foods sparingly. Avoid sugary drinks. Consume 'fast foods' sparingly, if at all.
4. Eat at least 5 portions/servings of a variety of non-starchy vegetables and of fruits every day. Eat relatively unprocessed cereals (grains) and/or (legumes) with every meal.
5. People who eat red meat to consume less than 500 g (18oz) per week – very little, if any, to be processed.
6. If alcoholic drinks are consumed, limit consumption to no more than two drinks a day for men and one drink a day for women.
7. Avoid salt-preserved, salted or salty foods; preserve foods without using salt.
8. Dietary supplements are not recommended for cancer prevention.
9. Aim to breastfeed infants exclusively up to six months and continue with complementary feeding thereafter.
10. All cancer survivors to receive nutritional care from an appropriately trained professional. If able to do so, and unless otherwise advised, aim to follow the recommendations for diet, healthy weight and physical activity.

KEY POINTS

- The change from a normal cell to cancer requires mutations in a few genes
- The accumulation of enough mutations in a single cell to cause cancer depends on endogenous processes, exogenous mutagens, and chance
- Diet-related factors may account for about 30% of cancers in developed countries
- Evidence-based recommendations exist for dietary intake and physical activity, for the prevention of cancer

8.5 OBESITY

Introduction

Obesity has become the major nutrition related disease of this decade, and is defined as a condition of excessive body fat accumulation to an extent that increases the risk of complicating diseases. Obesity is largely preventable through changes in lifestyle, especially diet.

Epidemiology of obesity
Definition of obesity

Obesity is not a single entity, but it is most commonly classified by a single measure, the body mass index (BMI), which is weight as a function of height:

$$BMI = weight\ (kg)/height^2\ (m^2)$$

The World Health Organization (WHO) classifies underweight, normal weight, overweight and obesity according to categories of BMI (Table 8.3). BMI does not, however, distinguish fat from lean tissue or water nor identify whether the fat is accumulated in particular sites such as the abdomen where it has more serious metabolic consequences. Techniques such as bioelectric impedance to estimate body fat and DEXA-scans to separate body mass into fat-free mass (FFM) and fat mass are increasingly used, although simple waist circumference is increasingly recognized as an easy and valid measure of abdominal obesity and risk of the metabolic syndrome (see below) and associated diseases. Waist:hip ratio and skinfold thickness may also be used to verify fatness in individuals. The cut off points for waist circumference and waist:hip ratio are shown in Table 8.4.

Prevalence and time-trends of overweight and obesity

The prevalence of obesity is increasing worldwide in almost every country and in all age groups. In 2001 in the UK 21% of men and 24% of women were

Table 8.3 The classification of underweight, normal weight and classes of overweight Caucasians according to WHO

Classification	BMI (kg/m²)	Risk of co-morbidities
Underweight	<18.5	Low (but risk of other clinical problems increased)
Normal range	18.5–24.9	Average
Overweight*	>25	
Pre-obese	25.0–29.9	Mildly increased
Obese	>30.0	
Class I	30.0–34.9	Moderate
Class II	35.0–39.9	Severe
Class III	>40.0	Very severe

*The term overweight refers to a BMI > 25, but is frequently adapted to refer to the BMI 25–29.9, differentiating the pre-obese from the obese categories

obese and a further 47% of men and 33% of women were overweight (BMI 25–30 kg/m²). In the United States of America the situation is even worse. In the USA in 2000 the prevalence of obesity was 31% compared to 23% in 1988–94. Europe is following the track of the USA, but is about 10 years behind. Obesity is now apparent in even some of the poorest countries of the world. The proportion of obese people increases with age until around the age of retirement.

Attention is increasingly focused on young people, in whom the problem of overweight and obesity has become more pronounced. In the UK in 1997, 4% of 14–18-year-olds were obese and a further 15% were overweight. There is a higher than expected level of obesity among certain ethnic groups living in Europe, probably due to increased genetic susceptibility to the European lifestyle. Obesity rates are highest among people of Indian, Pakistani and black Caribbean origin, and the prevalence of obesity in young people of Asian origin is 3–4 times higher than among whites.

Risks of obesity

Obesity is a risk for health and social and psychological reasons. The increase in obesity rates has an important impact on the global incidence of cardio-vascular disease, type 2 diabetes mellitus, cancer, osteoarthritis, infertility, birth complications, work disability and sleep apnoea. Obesity has a more pronounced impact on morbidity than on mortality, but a BMI of 40 kg/m² is associated with a decreased life expectancy of around 10 years.

Psychological and social

Most overweight subjects suffer from low self-esteem. They are discrimi-nated against and can experience heat intolerance, difficulties with physical activity, and sexual problems of a psychological and physical nature.

Type 2 diabetes

Overweight and obesity are the major causes of the development of type 2 diabetes in individuals with a high genetic susceptibility to the disease. Type 2 diabetes (see section 8.3) occurs 50–100-fold more frequently in obese subjects than in lean subjects. Diabetes is the most important medical consequence of obesity because it is common, has serious complications, is difficult to treat,

Table 8.4 Cut-off points for increased risk of disease for waist circumference and waist:hip ratio

	Increased risk		Substantially increased risk	
	Male	**Female**	**Male**	**Female**
Waist circumference (cm)	≥94	≥80	≥102	≥88
Waist:hip ratio	>0.9	>0.85	>1	>1

reduces life expectancy by 8–10 years and is expensive to manage. Some of the metabolic defects accompanying impaired glucose tolerance (IGT) and type 2 diabetes are reversible with weight loss, unless the diabetes has persisted for too long. Even a modest weight loss of 3–5% achieved by diet and slightly increased daily physical activity is sufficient to prevent nearly 60% of all new cases over a 4–5-year period. It is the weight loss per se, not a specific diet or the physical activity that is important.

Cardiovascular disease

See section 8.2.

Increased blood pressure (hypertension)

The risk of developing hypertension is 5–6 times greater with obesity. Blood pressure is positively correlated with both abdominal circumference and with the degree of obesity. Insulin resistance and hyperinsulinaemia appear to be responsible for the hypertension. Even a small weight loss can result in a marked drop in blood pressure, and weight loss is a much more effective treatment than salt restriction.

Atherosclerosis, ischaemic heart disease and stroke

The risk of developing ischaemic heart disease or stroke is 2.5 and 6 times greater, respectively, in people with a pronounced abdominal fat distribution.

Arthritis urica (gout)

Gout is a frequent complication of obesity. Plasma urate is increased in the majority of patients, but clinical symptoms are observed in only a minority.

Metabolic syndrome

The metabolic syndrome encompasses insulin resistance, hypertension, increased plasma VLDL and reduced HDL cholesterol and abdominal obesity. Hormones and substrates secreted by the adipose tissue are thought to be the main cause. This syndrome is also known as insulin resistance syndrome, since the main consequence is reduced sensitivity to the action of insulin. A variety of risk factors for the development of cardiovascular disease appear to be associated with this syndrome, which links obesity with the most significant health complications (type 2 diabetes, hypertension and atherosclerosis). Factors other than obesity are significantly associated with the metabolic syndrome, including fat distribution, level of physical activity and genetic disposition. Treatment of the metabolic syndrome is weight loss and physical activity. A suggested definition of the syndrome by WHO is:

Insulin resistance (hyperinsulinaemia), and at least two of the following components:

- abdominal obesity
- glucose intolerance
- high blood pressure
- dyslipidaemia: high triglyceride and/or low HDL cholesterol.

Other complications

Obesity is a risk factor for osteoarthritis in the weight bearing joints, infertility and numerous endocrinological conditions, hypoventilation syndrome and sleep apnoea, liver and gallstone diseases, osteoarthritis and numerous cancers, especially colorectal cancers in men, and endometrial, gall bladder, cervix, breast and ovary cancer in women. Surgery has an increased risk of complications and hospital admission time is generally prolonged.

Causes
Genetics

In only a minority of cases is obesity caused by a chromosome abnormality, a mutation in a single gene or classic endocrine disorder. Most cases of obesity are due to an inadequately functioning appetite regulation and energy metabolism, where the energy density and fat content of food and drink are too high, mealtimes are irregular, daily physical activity is limited and inactivity has become a characteristic of everyday life. An unlimited supply of cheap, tasty foodstuffs and larger food portions also help to promote overweight and risk of obesity. Single-gene mutations that cause obesity in humans are extremely rare. One example is the Prader–Willi syndrome caused by absence of a paternally-derived region on chromosome 15.

It is commonly observed that obesity 'runs' in families, but could be genuine genetic inheritance or inheritance of environmental/lifestyle factors. The genetic component is rather perceived as a predisposition, which is expressed only when certain environmental factors are favourable. The most important environmental factors that are generally acknowledged to trigger obesity are a high dietary fat content, energy-rich drinks, a low level of physical activity and irregular mealtimes, though stopping smoking and pregnancy also play a role. The genetic component may be expressed in a number of ways such as abnormal lipid metabolism, poorly regulated appetite at a low level of physical activity, increased preference for fatty tastes, and a reduced ability to spontaneously increase energy expenditure during periods of overeating.

Changes in environment and lifestyle
Physical activity

In high- and middle-income countries the level of physical activity has fallen dramatically in the last 50 years, with the replacement of manual labour with machines and the increased use of physical aids for housework, transport and leisure pursuits. Low daily physical activity is a risk factor for weight gain and one or two short weekly walks are not sufficient to compensate for this. Only by regular physical activity is the capacity for fat oxidation increased and appetite regulation improved, depending on the intensity, length and frequency of the bouts of activity. The 30-minute daily physical exercise currently recommended by the American Heart Foundation and WHO, for example, is not enough to prevent weight gain and obesity in individuals predisposed to obesity – 45–60 minutes of daily activity is required.

Energy metabolism

A low relative basal metabolic rate (BMR in kJ/kg FFM) is known to increase the risk of weight gain, but this is likely in only a minority of obese people. Physical activity is often reduced, but as a result of the increased body mass the energy expenditure in carrying out a given activity increases, so energy expenditure is not reduced with obesity. Overweight patients often claim that they eat next to nothing and their dietary records apparently verify that the patient ingests only 4–6 MJ/d, despite weight stability. Measuring energy metabolism in these patients using double-labelled water (see chapter 2) shows the phenomenon to be due to a systematic under reporting, presumably not acknowledged by the patients themselves.

Diet composition and drinks

The prevalence of obesity in high income countries has risen slowly from about 1920, with a dramatic increase in the years after the Second World War. During this period the diet has changed from consisting mainly of carbohydrate-rich foods (potatoes and other root vegetables, legumes, vegetables, grains, wholemeal bread) with a modest amount of fat, to the recent diet, where the consumption of meat, cheese, butter and other rich milk products and alcohol has increased at the cost of more energy-poor, carbohydrate-rich foods. The fat content of the diet has risen considerably. Obesity is seldom seen among people who traditionally live from a diet with moderate fat content and a high content of energy-poor vegetables and wholemeal products.

The weak satiating effect of a fat-rich diet is linked to the high energy density. Typical carbohydrate rich foods with a low content of fibre are less satisfying than similar products with a high fibre content. Sugar in drinks satiates less than sugar in solid form and studies have suggested that a high consumption of sugary drinks leads to a marked weight increase.

It is normally assumed that the energy content of alcohol is added to the energy from the diet, such that alcohol increases the total energy intake. However the Health Survey of England indicated that non-drinkers are more likely to be obese than those who consume alcohol.

Macronutrient balance

A low relative energy expenditure (kJ/kg FFM) can contribute to the development of obesity, but the positive energy balance is mainly caused by excessive energy intake, so-called hyperphagia. Hyperphagia is produced in individuals with a genetic predisposition to obesity by a failure in appetite regulation, which in particular can be brought about by a fat-rich diet and low level of physical activity.

Carbohydrate and protein are not converted to fat under normal circumstances in humans as de novo lipogenesis is an energetically expensive process, which is suppressed when the fat intake of the diet is greater than about 20% energy intake. This means that the fat in adipose tissue almost completely originates from the fat in the diet; the balance of each macro component of the diet (alcohol, fat, carbohydrate and protein) is regulated separately.

The alcohol balance has the highest priority in the combustion hierarchy, since alcohol cannot be stored in the body and is oxidized at the expense of the other macronutrients in the diet. The balance of protein and of carbohydrate have the next highest priority, because of the limited size of both the glycogen depots in the liver and muscle and the protein stores compared with the much larger fat depots. Excess food intake is mainly stored as fat. It is the total energy balance that determines whether a person will gain or lose weight.

Triggering factors

Several factors can potentially disturb the energy balance to such an extent that a large weight increase is involved. These include:

- *Pregnancy*, with the average gain from conception to a year after birth being 2 kg
- *Immobility*, with acute weight gain often seen following sudden cessation of a habitually high level of physical activity due to a specific occupation or sport, and in sedentary occupations such as taxi and bus drivers, and in chronically immobilized patients
- *Stress*, as glucocorticoid excess has a powerful stimulating effect on appetite and fat deposition which is typically of the male, abdominal pattern
- *Psychological trauma* is often accompanied by over eating and weight increase in some individuals, whilst others react with anorexia and weight loss, and weight increase may follow the use of psychotropic drugs
- *Stopping smoking,* as tobacco smoking suppresses appetite and nicotine stimulates the sympathetic nervous system, so that 15–20 cigarettes a day can increase the daily energy metabolism by 10% and this weight increase is the most frequent reason for taking up smoking again
- *Endocrine obesity* can be due for example to hypothyroidism or excess cortisol production, but this represents a minority of causes
- *Drug-induced obesity* caused by a number of prescription drugs including psychotropic drugs, lithium, cyclic antidepressants, and some epilepsy drugs, as well as oestrogen, glucocorticoids and insulin and some anticancer drugs such as tamoxifen, while treatment of AIDS patients with anti-viral agents can induce lipodystrophy.

Prevention and treatment
Principles for weight loss

In almost every overweight and obese patient the diet must be adjusted to reduce energy intake. Dietary therapy consists of instructing patients as to how to modify their dietary intake to achieve a decrease in energy intake while maintaining a nutritionally adequate diet. For patients with class I obesity this requires an energy deficit of 300–500 kcal/day, and with class III obesity 500–1000 kcal/day. The desirable rate of weight loss for most people is 0.5–1 kg/week after the first month of dieting, with younger, taller and more overweight subjects aiming for the upper limit and older, shorter and less overweight for the lower rate. With higher rates of loss there may be excessive loss of lean tissue. During the first month weight loss will be more rapid because of the loss of water associated with glycogen. Differences in diet composition have less clinical importance compared with the major goal to reduce total energy intake. However advantage can be taken of the differences in the satiating power of the various dietary components in order to cause a spontaneous reduction in energy intake. This is the principle of the ad libitum low-fat diet.

Calculating energy deficit

The initial target of a weight loss programme should be to decrease body weight by 5–10%, when a new target can be set. Even a 5% weight reduction improves risk factors and risk of co-morbidities. To calculate a defined energy deficit it is necessary to estimate the actual energy requirements of the subject, by measuring resting metabolic rate (RMR) or estimating using equations based on body weight, gender and age (see chapter 2) and multiplying by an activity factor (PAL; physical activity level) to give the energy requirement (Table 8.5). The energy level of the prescribed diet is then the energy requirement minus the defined daily energy deficit.

Weight loss diets

Low-energy diets (LED) usually provide 800–1500 kcal/day and use fat-reduced foods, and normally consist of natural foods. LED are also called 'traditional diets' and 'calorie counting diets'. They are low-fat, carbohydrate-rich diets with a fixed energy allowance and should be supplemented with a daily vitamin and mineral tablet. LED introduces healthy eating habits early in the weight reduction programme to familiarize the patient with the dietary changes that are a central element in a weight maintenance programme.

Very-low-energy diets (VLED) are modified fasts providing 200–800 kcal/day that replace normal foods. Starvation (less than 200 kcal/day) is the ultimate dietary treatment of obesity, but it is no longer used because of the numerous and serious medical complications. VLED aim to supply very little energy but all essential nutrients. However, use without medical supervision has generally been abandoned and they should not be recommended due

Table 8.5 Estimating energy needs

Revised WHO equations for estimating basal metabolic rate (BMR)		
Men	18–30 years	$(0.0630 \times$ actual weight in kg $+ 2.8957) \times 240$ kcal/day
	31–60 years	$(0.0484 \times$ actual weight in kg $+ 3.6534) \times 240$ kcal/day
Women	18–30 years	$(0.0621 \times$ actual weight in kg $+ 2.0357) \times 240$ kcal/day
	31–60 years	$(0.0342 \times$ actual weight in kg $+ 3.5377) \times 240$ kcal/day

Estimated total energy expenditure = BMR × activity factor:

Activity level	Activity factor
Low (sedentary)	1.3
Intermediate (some regular exercise)	1.5
High (regular activity or demanding job)	1.7

to their questionable cardiac safety and the fact that they do not facilitate the gradual modification of the patient's eating behaviour, nutritional knowledge and skills, which seems to be required for long-term weight maintenance.

Ad libitum low-fat diets (<30% energy from fat) do not restrict energy intake directly, but restrict fat intake to 20–30% of total energy intake so that energy intake is spontaneously reduced because of the higher satiating effect of this diet, and a modest weight loss occurs.

Ad libitum low-carbohydrate diets (<25 g/day carbohydrate) have become very popular as part of a popular physiological concept which link surges in blood glucose and insulin to weight gain and obesity. The Atkins diet is the most popular and recommends a daily intake of <25 g carbohydrate. However low carbohydrate generally means high fat, and when the weight loss has slowed it is likely that the low-carbohydrate (high-fat) diet will have very negative effects on most cardiovascular risk factors, and despite the weight loss, may increase insulin resistance and risk of type 2 diabetes. Low-carbohydrate diets cannot therefore be recommended.

LED that are low-fat are more effective in inducing weight loss than ad libitum low-fat diets, and they allow a better adjustment of the reduction in energy intake. LED are therefore the preferred dietary treatment for obesity.

Weight maintenance

Most people can lose weight. The real challenge is to maintain the reduced body weight and prevent a subsequent relapse. Diet combined with group therapy leads to better long-term success rates (27%) than diet alone (15%), or diet combined with behaviour modification and active follow-up, though active follow-up produces better weight maintenance than passive follow-up (19% vs 10%).

Diet

Whereas the principle of energy restriction (LED) is successful for weight loss induction independent of dietary composition, the low-fat, high-protein/carbohydrate diet seems to be more effective for long-term weight maintenance and preventing weight regain. Numerous popular diet books promote changing diet composition in accordance with principles that are claimed to have a particularly favourable impact on weight loss and maintenance. Generally these claims are unsubstantiated and scientifically improbable, and some may even promote nutritionally insufficient diets. Some principles of diet composition follow:

Carbohydrate types

The high carbohydrate content of low-fat diets stems mainly from the complex carbohydrates of different vegetables, fruits and whole grains, which are more satiating for fewer calories than fatty foods and are a good source of vitamins, minerals, trace elements and fibre. High fibre content may further improve the satiating effect of the diet and a diet rich in soluble fibre, including oat bran, legumes, barley, and most fruits and vegetables, may be effective in reducing blood cholesterol and blood pressure levels. The recommended intake is 20–30 g of fibre daily. Low-fat diets, high in either complex or simple carbohydrates, induce similar fat loss in overweight and obese subjects, and a diet high in simple carbohydrates has no detrimental effects on blood lipids. However, recent evidence suggests that a high intake of sugar from soft drinks may be particularly obesogenic.

Glycaemic index (GI)

High-GI foods such as potatoes, white bread, and white rice produce rapid and transient surges in blood glucose and insulin which may in turn be followed by rapidly returning hunger sensations and excessive caloric intake, and so some scientists advise people to eat more whole grain products, and other foods characterized by a low GI. It is likely that this dietary change will have beneficial effects on risk factors of cardiovascular disease and diabetes but their effect on body weight regulation lacks robust evidence (see chapter 4). The GI concept is complicated and the GI of meals cannot accurately be calculated by the carbohydrate source alone, but also requires information about the energy, fat and protein content.

Protein content

Protein has a higher satiating power per calorie than carbohydrate and fat. More freedom to choose between protein-rich and complex carbohydrate-rich foods may encourage obese subjects to choose more lean meat and dairy products and hence improve adherence to low-fat diets in weight reduction programmes. However the dietary principles promoted in recent popular diet books advocating high-protein, low-carbohydrate diets are not supported by the existing evidence.

Fat quality and high-MUFA diets

Similar amounts of different fats contain nearly the same amount of energy, and although monounsaturated fats (MUFA) have less of an obvious influence on cardiovascular disease risk, insulin resistance and cancer than saturated or polyunsaturated fats, MUFA increase body weight more than polyunsaturated fatty acids (PUFA).

Alcohol

Alcohol provides energy that displaces more nutritious foods, suppresses fat oxidation (thereby allowing more dietary fat to be stored), promotes passive overconsumption of fat, and increases the risk of losing control over otherwise restrained behaviour. Alcohol has also been associated with obesity in epidemiological studies. Consequently energy intake from alcohol should be limited.

Exercise

Increased daily physical activity and exercise are important components of weight-control programmes. To induce a weight loss physical activity is not very effective by itself when compared with a hypocaloric diet. However, patients should gradually increase their physical activity to help maintain weight loss. Adequate levels of activity are at least 45–60 minutes of moderate-intensity physical activity on most days of the week. Sustainable and enjoyable changes in physical activity patterns must be made along with a lifelong commitment to health.

Drugs for treatment of obesity

Drugs currently available for the treatment of obesity, or drugs with weight reducing properties used for the treatment of type 2 diabetes or for smoking cessation, can be grouped within three categories: those that alter nutrient metabolism, those that reduce food intake, and those that increase energy expenditure. Those approved in the UK are Orlistat, which is a lipase inhibitor, and Sibutramine, which is an appetite suppressant.

Lipase inhibitors (Orlistat)

Orlistat is a specific inhibitor of intestinal lipase, an enzyme secreted from the exocrine pancreas and responsible for enzymatic fat digestion. It is recommended for use with a diet providing less than 30% of energy from fat. The most frequent adverse effects of Orlistat are flatulence, flatulence with discharge, oily spotting, faecal urgency and incontinence, oily stools, and steatorrhoea. Additionally, the unabsorbed fat binds some fat-soluble vitamins and other nutrients and prevents their absorption. A simple vitamin supplement and increased intake of fruit and vegetables counteracts this effect.

Sibutramine

Sibutramine decreases food intake in humans by increasing meal-induced satiety and exerts a weak thermogenic effect both acutely and during long-term use. It is generally well tolerated and has few side effects, which include dry mouth, headache, insomnia, and constipation and a mild increase in blood pressure and heart rate.

Surgical treatment of obesity

Weight management programmes fail in a substantial proportion of severely obese patients, and surgery is the treatment of choice for well-informed and well-motivated obese patients with acceptable operative risks. The malabsorptive intestinal bypass (jejuno-ileal) has a high rate of complications and cannot be recommended. Gastric bypass has been shown to prevent the progression to frank type 2 diabetes. In a Swedish study of 2000 matched obese patient pairs, one pair member was surgically treated, the other a control. After 8 years the weight loss was 20 kg in the surgical group, while the controls had gained 0.7 kg. The weight loss achieved by surgery has pronounced effects on cardiac structure and function, quality of life, rates of employment, and healthcare costs.

KEY POINTS

- Even a quite normal BMI with abdominal fat accumulation can be responsible for hypertension, hyperlipidaemia, type 2 diabetes, and cardiovascular disease
- The increase in obesity has an important impact on the global incidence of cardiovascular disease, type 2 diabetes mellitus, cancer, osteoarthritis, infertility, birth complications, work disability, and sleep apnoea
- Obesity has a more pronounced impact on morbidity than on mortality, but a BMI of $40 \, kg/m^2$ is associated with a decreased life expectancy of around 10 years
- In only a minority of cases is obesity caused by genetic factors
- Most cases of obesity are due to an inadequately functioning appetite regulation and energy metabolism
- Weight gain and obesity may be triggered in susceptible individuals when the energy density and fat content of the diet is too high, meal times are irregular, daily physical activity is limited
- An unlimited supply of cheap, tasty foodstuffs and larger food portions also help to promote overweight and risk of obesity
- Prevention and treatment of obesity requires a reduced energy intake and increased expenditure by physical activity
- It is recommended that energy intake be lowered by a reduction in energy density and portion sizes of meals, and the avoidance of energy-dense drinks
- The optimal diet is reduced in fat, with increased content of fibre-rich carbohydrates, and protein from meat and dairy products
- Currently approved weight-loss drugs improve the mean weight loss and increase the proportion of subjects who achieve more than 5–10% weight loss
- Surgical treatment may be indicated for morbidly obese subjects at high risk

8.6 PROTEIN ENERGY MALNUTRITION OR UNDERNUTRITION

Introduction

The epidemiology of protein energy malnutrition (PEM) and other forms of malnutrition is covered in more detail in chapter 13. Malnutrition has been defined as a change in nutritional status that carries a high risk of illness, dysfunction, or death, and includes dietary excess but in this section the term malnutrition is taken to mean undernutrition. Commonly used descriptive terms for undernutrition such as chronic energy deficiency (CED) or protein energy malnutrition (PEM), may imply causality in a way that is now recognized as simplistic or false, as children are the first to suffer deprivation due to their high requirements for growth and their dependency. Many classifications have been devised for childhood malnutrition, such as weight for age, and more recently weight for length or height. Growth failure is marked by 'thinness and shortness', sometimes called 'wasting and stunting', but growth faltering is not always due to simple under-feeding, but also to infections. Borderline malnutrition may be common enough to escape notice and a stunted underweight child, living among similarly sized age peers, might well appear to be thriving.

Stunting has been described as an adaptation to longstanding underfeeding but there are limits to such adaptation beyond which health suffers. Variation in height, especially during the early years of life, owes more to nutritional and socioeconomic factors than to ethnic variability. Biological variation in height and body build is generally accepted, but extremes are likely to be detrimental. In practice we assume that anthropometric variables are normally distributed, the normal range extending from −2.0 to +2.0 Standard Deviations from the mean. Undernutrition is therefore defined as >2.0 SD below the reference mean. However the risk of an adverse outcome rises significantly the greater the deviations from the mean.

Anthropometric indicators and reference standards

There is a link between nutrient or energy deficiency and malfunction. Lack of fuel compromises basal metabolism, physical activity, and energy storage. Tissue repair, growth and structural support fail in the absence of substrate, as do many enzymatic processes when micronutrients are deficient. The major fuel stores are in adipose tissue (fat) and lean body mass (protein) and anthropometry offers a simple way of estimating the size of these stores. Total body weight is often used as an indicator of the size of fuel stores, but correcting for height allows a better estimate of the lean and fat mass extra to that in essential structures. An estimate of the partition of fuels between superficial adipose tissue and fat-free mass can be made by measuring skinfold thickness. Weight for height in children is a better prognostic indicator than weight for age alone. Table 8.6 shows the WHO classification of malnutrition.

Deficiency of fuel stores in children is known as protein energy malnutrition (PEM), and in adults as 'chronic energy deficiency' (CED). The term 'protein' is excluded from the descriptive term in adults on the basis that protein requirements are relatively less important after growth has ceased. Wasting indicates that malnutrition is recent, whether weight loss is due to illness or simple under-feeding, and stunting indicates long-term undernutrition. 'Kwashiorkor' indicates nutritional oedema which carries a poor

Table 8.6 Classification of malnutrition (WHO 1999)

	Moderate malnutrition		Severe malnutrition	
Symmetrical oedema	No		Yes	
	SD score	% reference mean	SD score	% reference mean
Weight for height	>−3.0 to <−2.0	≥70% & <80%	<−3.0	<70%
Height for age	>−3.0 to <−2.0	≥85% to <90%	<−3.0	<85%

Table 8.7 Commonly used anthropometric indicators

Indicator	Cut off point for moderate malnutrition	Evidence base for use as indicators
Weight for age	80% of reference mean/~ −2.0 SD	Risk of death rises when weight for age <70% and further at <60%
Weight for height	80% of reference mean/~ −2.0 SD	Risk of death rises at weight for height <70%
(Length) height for age	90% of reference mean/~ −2.0 SD	Risk of death rises at length for age < 90%, rarely used as single index
Body mass index (kg/m²)	18.5 and 17 for men & women in developing countries	Used in adults; borderline values usually supported by evidence of physical incapacity.
Mid upper arm circumference (MUAC) age 1 to <5 yrs	<12.5 cm	Correlates with weight for age < 80% i.e. MUAC used as a swift screening test
MUAC in adults	<23 cm and <19 cm in men & women in developing countries	Evidence base less convincing, used as a proxy for low BMI
Symmetrical oedema		Associated with increased risk and therefore defines severe malnutrition

prognosis, and all oedematous children are defined as severely malnourished. The child with typical kwashiorkor also has variable underweight, 'psychosis', dyspigmented skin and hair, with a classical history of recent weaning or exposure to infection or other stress. Other common features are dry or moist skin peeling, and enlargement of the liver.

Table 8.7 shows indicators used for nutritional assessment of children and adults, with cut-off points that define moderate malnutrition.

The pathogenesis

The main features of uncomplicated PEM and CED are weight loss and wasting caused by negative energy balance, due to factors such as malabsorption, increased energy losses in urine and increased energy expenditure because of infection or malignancy, and from fever. The major causes of negative balance are low intakes of low energy dense foods, exacerbated by infection-related anorexia.

Nutritional oedema is commonly triggered by infection. Reactive oxygen species (ROS), which can cause damage to cell structure and function, are generated during the cellular response to infection. The adverse effects of ROS are normally held in check by antioxidant mechanisms, many of which are dependent on micronutrients such as vitamins A, C, and E, zinc, selenium, and copper. Iron, especially free iron, which increases during inflammation, may act as a pro-oxidant. In PEM, oxidant damage to structural lipids causes cell membranes to become permeable to sodium and potassium, which then leak into the extracellular spaces causing oedema, a hallmark of kwashiorkor. Micronutrient deficiencies therefore play a critical role in predisposing the child with PEM to kwashiorkor. An insufficient supply of amino acids from the diet also leads to reduced protein synthesis by the liver and hence a lower concentration of circulating plasma proteins including albumin and retinol-binding protein.

Stunting is a common form of undernutrition, affecting around 45% of children in developing countries. Certain amino acids, specifically leucine, and various micronutrients such as zinc, copper, molybdenum and possibly vitamin A exert an influence on linear growth. Beneficial effects of zinc supplementation on stunted children have been reported but dietary 'quality' (implying dairy produce, fruits and green vegetables) is more important for growth than any specific nutrient. Catch-up in linear growth during nutritional rehabilitation rarely starts until weight recovery is well under way.

Causes of undernutrition

The risk of underfeeding can begin in fetal life, and is most common during the last trimester of pregnancy. In the first few years of life factors increasing risk of undernutrition include lactation failure, a low energy dense weaning diet, infection and contaminated water. Kwashiorkor was first thought to be due to the low protein content of maize weaning porridge, but infections and low energy intakes from low energy dense foods are now considered important. CED is often linked to HIV. Malnutrition is highly prevalent in hospitals in developing countries, with other severe infections such as typhoid or tuberculosis, or lack of access to suitable feeds. In affluent countries toddlers with PEM usually present with faltering weight gain, and oedema is extremely rare. Children refusing food or eating alternative diets may also present with marginal PEM. Anorexia nervosa and bulimia can present in adolescence, sometimes with severe weight loss (see section 8.7). CED may also occur in deprived groups such as the homeless and the isolated elderly.

Effects

The magnitude of effect of malnutrition on health depends on the timing and duration of nutritional stress. The immediate effect, when low birth weight is due to intrauterine growth retardation, is a high neonatal death rate due to hypoglycaemia, hypothermia and infection. Malnutrition increases vulnerability to other illnesses especially infection. Malnutrition is rarely recorded as a cause of death, although it contributes to the case fatality of many illnesses. Severe malnutrition, especially if accompanied by oedema, has a high case fatality rate.

Prolonged stunting has an adverse effect on cognitive development. The survivor of early malnutrition may recover completely, remain stunted, or have a delayed adolescent growth spurt. Delayed growth and final short stature in women contribute to obstruction in labour, and thereby to high maternal mortality. Adult stunting is also associated with low birth weight. If there is then nutritional excess in adult life, the survivor is at increased risk of chronic diseases such as diabetes or heart disease.

Prevention of malnutrition

Fetal nutrition depends not only on maternal nutrient and energy intake but also on expenditure, and women should be encouraged to avoid heavy work during pregnancy. Exclusive breastfeeding is recommended for six months, except when milk supply fails to meet the growth requirements of the infant. The tradition of prolonged breastfeeding persists in developing countries with 40–50% of mothers still breastfeeding 20–23 months after birth. A current dilemma is the early infant feeding of babies whose mothers are HIV positive or who have died (see chapter 6). Dietary diversification depends not only on access to a variety of foods, but also on willingness to adapt dietary and culinary traditions.

Local manufacture of commercial weaning foods in several countries has reduced their cost, despite the cost of micronutrient fortification. Since convenience foods, ie those prepared without needing to boil water, are fuel efficient and less prone to contamination, their social marketing is likely to prove cost beneficial. Education about safe feeding practices is also important, and should be integrated into school curricula. The immediate benefit of school meals or snacks for older children is increased alertness rather than weight change. Prevention of malnutrition in older people depends more on socioeconomic and educational development and on fairer distribution of global resources, than on household or individual circumstances.

Specific situations and population groups at risk of malnutrition

Famines

Famine is defined as a sharp increase in mortality due to diseases related to acute starvation (see chapter 13). Famine can be a consequence of severe crop failure, often exacerbated by isolation and transport problems, but widespread starvation can occur even when food is available because of sharp increase in food prices, hoarding, and lack of resources to purchase food. Early coping strategies include foraging for wild foods, selling possessions, and reducing physical activity. Typically, young men move away to find work and eventually destitute people will leave home. There is a gradual deterioration of general nutritional status in these people and falling immunization rates. By the time starving people begin to congregate in camps they are vulnerable to infectious diseases, and mortality begins to rise. Early intervention aims to interrupt this progress before irrevocable damage has been done. There is a global and national responsibility to avert famine, by facilitating development, encouraging good governance and preventing war.

Refugees

Conflict has now overtaken climatic disaster as the trigger for large-scale migrations within a country or to another, with people fleeing from danger or seeking food and security. Global estimates indicate that over 10 million people are currently refugees. Food distribution to refugees or in emergency situations may take several forms. A general ration would aim at satisfying total nutritional requirements, using acceptable foods as far as possible, collected in bulk and prepared by the family. This is the preferred method of feeding since it respects autonomy, prevents cross-infection and reduces stress. On-site feeding may be required for at-risk groups, especially young children. There is also therapeutic feeding of malnourished children. When feeding is based on dry foods there is a risk of micronutrient deficiency, especially when refugees are unable to forage or grow vegetables. Vitamin A supplementation is critical and fortification of dry rations with niacin, thiamin and vitamin C is recommended, followed by early facilitation of access to fresh foods.

Hospital malnutrition

Nutritional status on point of admission to hospital has implications both for management and outcome. Undernutrition is associated with prolonged admission. Some conditions, such as renal failure, are associated with increased risk of micronutrient deficiency due to dietary restriction. Surgical patients are also at increased risk of deficiency when for example nutrient absorption has been compromised by gastric by-pass or gut resection. Malnutrition may slow down the metabolism of drugs, and also affect the response to treatment of infections. The prevention of malnutrition (before entry to hospital) is part of primary care for the elderly and other vulnerable groups. Those at risk should be comprehensively assessed at admission, and all attempts to improve the quality of hospital meals encouraged.

Alcoholism

Alcoholism is a global problem, the nutritional consequences of which are worse when superimposed on an already impoverished diet (see chapter 4). A daily intake of 5 to 7 units of alcohol supplies up to 10% of energy requirements as 'empty calories'. Signs of CED will be evident when protein energy intake is compromised. Deficiency of some micronutrients is also common in alcoholics, particularly for folic acid, thiamin, pyridoxine, and vitamin A.

Groups with a high risk of malnutrition in affluent countries

Poverty is linked with malnutrition in affluent countries, and micronutrient deficiency is commonly associated with obesity both in children and the elderly, in the latter linked to cognitive impairment. Refugees into a country are vulnerable soon after their arrival before support structures have been established. Their nutritional status depends on their country of origin, and the time spent in poorly appointed transit camps. Food insecurity in refugees has been reported from the UK. Stunting observed in children from third world countries is likely to be reversible depending on their age.

The single homeless are at special risk, especially when alcohol provides a high proportion of the energy intake, or when appetite is reduced by addiction. The elderly, especially those in residential care or with a recent history of hospital admission, are more likely to be malnourished than the general population. Sarcopenia is a type of muscle loss commonly seen in the elderly, which contributes to weight loss and weakness.

KEY POINTS

- The term protein energy malnutrition (PEM) includes other commonly used terms such as undernutrition, stunting, wasting, marasmus, kwashiorkor, chronic energy deficiency (CED)
- An important factor in the high prevalence of malnutrition in young children is the high nutritional requirement for growth
- Wasting and stunting (thinness and shortness) may be due to different deficiencies
- The major immediate causes of PEM are low intakes of low energy dense foods, exacerbated by infection related anorexia
- PEM in children and CED in adults are similar conditions
- PEM and CED are typified by wasting (underweight for height); both may be complicated by oedema; in children this is known as kwashiorkor
- Moderate malnutrition is common, oedematous malnutrition is rare but has a high fatality
- Undernutrition increases vulnerability to infections, and can have long-term consequences on cognitive development, final stature, problems in childbirth, and increased risk of chronic diseases
- Other specific situations of risk for undernutrition include: famine which occurs when people lose their access to food; refugees from war or famine congregate; hospital malnutrition which occurs in both rich and poor countries; alcoholism; and with poverty, eg among immigrants, the unemployed, the homeless, and following domestic disruption

8.7 EATING DISORDERS

An eating disorder may be defined as a persistent disturbance of eating (or eating-related behaviour) which impairs physical health or psychosocial functioning, or both, and which is not secondary to any general medical disorder or any other psychiatric disorder. The most well recognized eating disorders are anorexia nervosa and bulimia nervosa. These disorders share many features and together they are a major source of ill health among young women, and, increasingly, young men, in Western societies. In addition, there are eating disorders in which the person does not meet the diagnostic criteria for anorexia nervosa or bulimia nervosa. These are the 'atypical eating disorders'. In this chapter, the characteristics of these three groups of eating disorder will be described. Though important, the prevention of eating disorders is beyond the scope of this section.

Anorexia nervosa
Definition

Features required to make a diagnosis of anorexia nervosa are: active maintenance of an unduly low weight (15% below a person's expected weight for their age, height and sex, or a body mass index below 17.5); attitudes and values concerning body shape and weight, including 'relentless pursuit of thinness' and a 'morbid fear of fatness'; and the tendency to judge self-worth largely in terms of shape and weight rather than on the basis of performance in domains such as relationships, work performance or sporting activities. Amenorrhoea is typically present in female anorexic patients. Low weight of anorexia nervosa is achieved in several ways, including strict dieting, excessive exercising, and in some, self-induced vomiting or laxative misuse. The US DSM-IV (Diagnostic and Statistical Manual IV) psychiatric classification distinguishes between two sub-types. The restricting sub-type excludes regular binge-eating or purging behaviour. A person with anorexia nervosa can alternate between sub-types at different times in their illness.

Epidemiology

The average prevalence of anorexia nervosa (actual number of cases at a certain point in time) in Western societies is 280 per 100,000 young females, with higher rates in female dancers and athletes, such as distance runners and gymnasts. A typical estimate of the incidence of anorexia nervosa in females is 8 per 100,000 of the population per year; in males the value currently lies at about 0.5 per 100,000 per year.

Development

The onset of anorexia nervosa is generally in adolescence, although childhood-onset or pre-pubertal cases are observed. In children, boys represent 20–25% of referrals. Occasionally, anorexia nervosa does not begin until adulthood. Often it starts as normal dieting which then gets out of control.

Clinical features

Weight loss is primarily achieved through a severe reduction in food intake. People with anorexia nervosa have greater knowledge about the caloric and macronutrient content of foods but lack awareness of micronutrient contents.

In most cases hunger persists but the perception and reporting of hunger are often distorted. Denial of hunger may be experienced as rewarding and a mark of personal self-control. The consequences of starvation, such as a slow rate of gastric emptying, can make food intake unpleasant as eating only a little results in bloating but normalizing the amount and pattern of eating helps to rehabilitate hunger and satiety.

Frequent intense exercising is common and also contributes to the low body weight. Laxative and diuretic misuse and self-induced vomiting may also be practised.

There is disturbance of body image, all or parts of the body being seen as larger than their actual size. Patients often have limited recognition of their disorder. Other psychological symptoms resulting from semi-starvation include depressed mood, irritability, social withdrawal, loss of sexual libido, preoccupation with food, and eventually, reduced alertness and concentration, heightened sensitivity to cold and a variety of gastrointestinal symptoms such as constipation, fullness after eating, bloatedness and vague abdominal pain, restlessness, lack of energy and early morning wakening.

Amenorrhoea, if sustained, is associated with osteopenia, possibly progressing to osteoporosis and risk of bone fractures, and is often irreversible. Acute complications for males or females include dehydration, electrolyte disturbances (due to purging), cardiac compromise with arrhythmia, gastrointestinal mobility disturbances, renal problems, infertility, hypothermia, and other evidence of hypometabolism.

Causation

Dieting is a general vulnerability factor for both anorexia nervosa and bulimia nervosa and is more likely in those who are heavier and dissatisfied with their body, although relatively few young women who diet develop an eating disorder. Other risk factors, many of which are shared with other psychiatric disorders, include personality traits of perfectionism, negative self-evaluation, and adverse childhood experiences such as victimization or abuse.

Genetic factors are implicated by family studies. Eating disorders are largely confined to countries that have an abundance of food, that hold a thin body shape as ideal, and in which dieting is commonplace. Peers and family may also be influential in victimizing those not conforming to shape or weight ideals or aspirations. Sociocultural factors appear to channel women's dissatisfaction and distress to focus on body shape and size, providing an outlet for individual pathology, with thinness being relentlessly pursued by those who see no better way to solve their problems. Social withdrawal isolates the person from his or her peers, encouraging further self-preoccupation. Many patients report that exerting strict control over eating is in itself intensely rewarding. However, the most potent maintaining factor is likely to be the extreme concerns about shape and weight.

Management

Patients with anorexia nervosa are usually persuaded to seek help by concerned relatives or friends, and as a consequence they attend reluctantly. There are two aspects to treatment: establishing healthy eating habits and a normal weight through a combination of education, support, encouragement and nutritional counselling, on an inpatient, day patient or outpatient basis; and addressing those factors liable to result in relapse using treatments such as parental counselling, family therapy, interpersonal psychotherapy or cognitive behavioural therapy. Drugs have a limited role. Short-acting minor tranquillizers may occasionally be used to reduce the anxiety experienced prior to eating, and if depressive symptoms persist following weight restoration, antidepressant drugs may be prescribed.

Course and outcome

The proportion of individuals with anorexia nervosa who fully recover is modest. Less than 50% of cases can be rated as having a good outcome. For about a quarter, outcome is poor with weight never reaching 85% of recommended weight for height. Around two-thirds of patients continue to have morbid food and weight preoccupations. Up to a quarter of the patients develop bulimia nervosa. Anorexia is associated with a major increase in mortality. In general, adolescents have better outcomes than adults, and younger adolescents better outcomes than older adolescents.

KEY POINTS

- The judgement of self-worth primarily in terms of shape and weight is a core feature of anorexia nervosa
- The disorder is much more common in females than males, with onset generally in adolescence
- Weight loss is primarily achieved through a severe reduction in food intake
- The goals of treatment are establishing healthy eating habits and a normal weight, and addressing those factors liable to result in relapse
- A variety of treatment approaches are used but the proportion of individuals who fully recover is modest

Bulimia nervosa

Definition

Bulimia nervosa was first clinically described in 1979, viewed as an unusual variant of anorexia nervosa. Three features are required to make a diagnosis of nervosa: the presence of frequent bulimic episodes, on average at least twice a week for three months, involving the consumption of unusually large amounts of food, the size of binges typically between 1000–2000 kcal; the use of compensatory behaviour to control body shape and weight, self-induced vomiting and laxative or diuretic misuse; and the presence of attitudes and values concerning shape and weight similar to those found in anorexia nervosa, although body weight is often in the normal range as the effects of the overeating and weight control behaviour tend to cancel each other out.

Epidemiology

People with bulimia nervosa are typically older than those with anorexia nervosa, most presenting in their late teens and early twenties. Bulimia nervosa is found in all social classes, and in greater numbers than anorexia nervosa.

Development

Many patients with bulimia nervosa present with a history of disturbed eating stretching back into adolescence, and around a third have previously fulfilled diagnostic criteria for anorexia nervosa. The slightly later age of onset suggests the importance of other personal issues or life stressors, such as leaving home, for the development of the disorder. This also has implications for the maintenance of the disorder and how it is treated.

Clinical features

There are many similarities with anorexia nervosa but two important differences are in body weight and frequency of binges which are a source of great shame and they are kept hidden from others, leading to under-reporting.

Sustained depressive and anxiety symptoms are a prominent feature of bulimia nervosa. Rigid control over eating is associated with multiple self-imposed dietary rules: when food should be eaten or not eaten; exactly what should be eaten or not eaten; and the overall amount of food that should be eaten. Binges are often precipitated by breaking these rules.

The majority of patients have few physical complaints. The most commonly presented are irregular or absent menstruation, weakness and lethargy, vague abdominal pain, salivary gland enlargement, and significant erosion of the dental enamel on the palatal surface of the upper front teeth from self-induced vomiting. The most serious physical complications are apparent in those who frequently vomit or take laxatives or diuretics.

Causation

Many of the putative risk factors for anorexia nervosa are also risk factors for bulimia nervosa. Some differences can be classed in two groupings of factors: exposure to dieting and related risk factors, including parental and childhood obesity, and critical family comments about weight, shape or eating; and a number of general risk factors for psychiatric disorders including parental psychiatric disorders such as depression, alcohol and substance abuse during childhood, low parental contact but high parental expectations, neglect and abuse.

Total immersion in the binge distracts the person from emotional distress but this relief is temporary, and negative affect plays an important role in binge eating. Eating induces negative feelings, such as guilt, as binge eating becomes out of control. Purging relieves guilt and discharges anger and may eventually replace bingeing as a means of reducing tension. But purging evokes feelings of shame and self-disgust, devaluing the self-view and fostering the negative affect that triggers binge eating. This cycle is a target of treatment.

Management

Most people with bulimia nervosa are ashamed of their eating habits, and keep them secret for many years. If they present for help they may complain of features associated with the disorder rather than the disorder itself. Consultation seeking is more common than in anorexia nervosa as bingeing and purging have less perceived benefit than does food avoidance and low body weight for anorexia nervosa.

Several psychotherapies are effective in improving the symptoms of bulimia nervosa but most evidence is available on cognitive behavioural therapy, and it is generally impressive and replicable. Pharmacological treatment is used more in bulimia nervosa than in anorexia nervosa but only antidepressants have any beneficial effect.

Course and outcome

Around three-quarters of patients who complete treatment make a full and lasting recovery. Follow-up of at least 5 years indicates that between a third and a half of those with bulimia nervosa at outset still had an eating disorder, and between 10–25% still had bulimia nervosa.

KEY POINTS

- Bulimic episodes (bouts of out of control over-consumption) are accompanied by compensatory behaviour (such as self-induced vomiting)
- The prevalence is increasing and is characteristic of females in their late teens and early twenties
- While sharing some clinical features with anorexia nervosa, patients with bulimia nervosa differ in respect of body weight and frequency of bulimic episodes
- Increased exposure to dieting and general risk for psychiatric disorder contribute to the development of bulimia nervosa
- Reducing and eliminating binge eating and purging are primary treatment goals
- Cognitive behavioural therapy is a very effective therapeutic approach

Atypical eating disorders

Around half of the cases of eating disorders in the community are neither anorexia nervosa nor bulimia nervosa. These patients are said to have an atypical eating disorder.

Eating disorder not otherwise specified (EDNOS)

Many patients with EDNOS have symptoms similar in form to anorexia nervosa and bulimia nervosa but fail to meet their diagnostic criteria either because a particular feature is missing (partial syndrome) or because they do not quite meet the specified level of severity (sub-threshold case). These variants of anorexia nervosa and bulimia nervosa are likely to have similar risk and maintaining factors to those described above, and they appear to respond similarly to treatment.

Binge eating disorder (BED)

The research diagnostic criteria for binge eating disorder differ from those of bulimia nervosa in the frequency and length of binge episodes, and do not include the core psychopathology of shape and weight concern, only the significant distress over the binge eating. Studies suggest rates of 2–3% in the adult population, higher in obese samples, with BED present in 5–10% of those seeking treatment for obesity in the USA. However, the association between BED and obesity is not invariable. Binge eating disorder is seen in an older age group (most presenting between age 30–50), and is more common in men than either anorexia nervosa or bulimia nervosa (20–25% of cases are male).

Both cognitive behaviour therapy and interpersonal psychotherapy appear extremely effective in reducing binge eating and maintaining this relief. Pharmacotherapy, primarily anti-depressants, also reduces the frequency of binge eating.

KEY POINTS

- Atypical eating disorders represent around half of the cases of eating disorders in the community
- Patients with eating disorders tend to migrate between the diagnostic categories of anorexia nervosa, bulimia nervosa, and the atypical eating disorders
- Patients with binge eating disorder (BED) have neither intense shape and weight over-concern nor use purging behaviours after bingeing
- Many different approaches show success in treating BED

8.8 ANAEMIA

Introduction

Anaemia is the term given to a condition in which the haemoglobin concentration of blood is sufficiently low to impair the oxygen carrying capacity of the blood. This in turn will compromise the oxygen delivery to tissues, with a number of clinical and physiological effects. Anaemia is defined by a haemoglobin concentration below the age appropriate range for healthy individuals (Table 8.8).

Anaemia is the result of abnormalities in red blood cell production, or accelerated destruction of red blood cells, or excessive blood loss. In a nutrition context the most important route to anaemia is through a failure to produce an adequate number of normal red blood cells, which can occur if there is inadequate availability of a nutrient essential for their production. Anaemia can be classified according to the average size of red blood cells in the circulation, and this also gives a clue to the underlying cause. Thus, microcytic, normocytic and macrocytic anaemia are terms used to describe anaemia with small, normal or large sized red blood cells. Typically microcytic anaemia is due to iron deficiency but the anaemia of vitamin B_1 or copper deficiency is also microcytic. Macrocytic anaemia is most commonly due to a deficiency of folate or vitamin B_{12}, whilst normocytic anaemia is characteristic of the anaemia sometimes seen in chronic disease states such as cancer or chronic infection.

Table 8.8 Minimum acceptable levels of haemoglobin (Hb) according to age

Age (years)	Hb (g/L)
0.5–6.0	110
>6–14	120
Boys >14	130
Girls >14	120
Male adult	130
Female adult	120
Pregnancy	110

Prevalence

The most common cause of anaemia worldwide is nutritional iron deficiency and the World Health Organization estimate that 2 billion of the world's population (largely in developing countries) currently have marked iron deficiency anaemia. Whilst iron deficiency is certainly the most common cause of anaemia worldwide, and anaemia prevalence is used as a proxy for iron deficiency, the contribution that other nutrient deficiencies, malaria, and other parasitic infections make to the global burden of anaemia is important.

Anaemia is a serious public health problem worldwide throughout the lifecycle, and this is clearly shown in Table 8.9. Pregnant women and young children are most at risk; recent estimates suggest that in South East Asia for example, about 67% of children 0–5 years old and 76% of pregnant women are anaemic.

Effects of anaemia

Presenting features of anaemia (of any aetiology) typically include tiredness, breathlessness during physical exertion, and paleness. Whilst mild anaemia in many individuals is of little health consequence (due to a number of compensatory mechanisms such as increased cardiac output, diversion of blood flow to vital organs and increased release of oxygen from haemoglobin), severe anaemia exceeds the body's ability to adapt resulting in impaired oxygen delivery to the tissues. This in turn has deleterious effects on a number of important body functions.

Work performance

At all ages anaemia results in reduced oxygen carriage to the tissues with an adverse effect on oxidative metabolism. A reduction in work capacity due to anaemia has been reported in agricultural labourers in several different countries, engaged in a variety of tasks. In female tea pickers in Sri Lanka and in male Indonesian rubber plantation workers who had hookworm infection, reduced productivity was directly related to the severity of anaemia. Since the cause of the anaemia was overwhelmingly due to iron deficiency, following iron supplementation iron deficient subjects showed improved performance, with the greatest progress seen in subjects who had the most severe anaemia.

Table 8.9 Prevalence of anaemia by age group

	Developing countries (per cent)	Industrialized countries (per cent)
0–4 years	43	17
5–14 years	53	10
Non-pregnant women	44	12
Pregnant women	57	18
Men	34	5
Elderly	50	11

Source: ACC/SCN 2000

In developing countries women are also engaged in hard physical work, even when pregnant. In these harsh environments anaemia in pregnancy is commonly associated with higher rates of low fetal birth weight and perinatal death. Furthermore an anaemic mother is more likely to die from haemorrhage at the time of delivery. The precise aetiology of such severe anaemia is uncertain because these women are at risk from multiple nutrient deficiencies as well as malarial anaemia.

Iron deficiency anaemia

Iron deficiency is the commonest nutritional deficiency worldwide, particularly affecting young children and women of reproductive age (WHO 1992). The areas worst affected include sub-Saharan Africa, South and Southeast Asia and the West Pacific. Rates of iron deficiency anaemia in women range from around 40% in Africa to 65% in South Asia. Iron deficiency is also associated with poverty in the USA and the UK but even when the adult diet is high in flesh foods, the weaning diet may be deficient in iron. Iron deficiency in young children may be due to avoidance, for religious reasons, of commercial weaning foods containing meat. Macrobiotic vegetarian diets have also been causally linked with iron deficiency, although reports are conflicting. 'Junk food' diets have been incriminated in iron deficiency in adolescents.

Since iron is essential to the synthesis of the oxygen carrier haemoglobin, the size and haemoglobin density of the red blood cell is reduced by deficiency. Iron deficiency anaemia is therefore characterized by red blood cells with a low mean cell volume (MCV) and lower mean cell concentration of haemoglobin (MCHC). The rate of production of red cells (erythropoiesis) is not affected by iron deficiency.

The earliest sign of iron deficiency in an otherwise healthy individual is reduced stores, with low bone marrow iron, and low serum ferritin. As iron status deteriorates, the rate of iron transport falls, but red cell function remains satisfactory for a while. Anaemia is evidence that inadequate iron is reaching the developing red blood cells in the bone marrow.

Some indicators of iron status give confounding results. The ferritin apoprotein behaves like an acute phase protein so that, in acute infection or inflammation, its serum concentration may rise to normal or even elevated levels, even when the body is iron deficient. High values for serum ferritin may also co-exist with anaemia in children with kwashiorkor.

Causes of iron deficiency

As with other nutrients, iron status depends on the balance between intake and losses. Dietary iron deficiency is especially common where the main dietary source is non-haem iron in plant foods, which is absorbed less well than haem-iron. Avoidance of meat by adults is more commonly due to poverty than culture, flesh foods being eaten on special occasions. In meat-free diets, cereals are a major iron source, especially when consumed as fortified breakfast cereals, and dark green vegetables and pulses also make a useful contribution.

The dietary reference values for the USA and those published by WHO/FAO include an increment in iron intake during pregnancy and lactation. The cumulative effect of perinatal blood loss and short birth interval increases the risk of iron deficiency. In the humid tropics, persistent low grade blood loss due to intestinal parasites, such as hookworm and whipworm, may also be a factor as well as less dramatic blood loss from (urinary or intestinal) schistosomiasis.

The major iron store in the newborn is in haemoglobin itself, and babies are born with a high haemoglobin concentration. Catch-up growth, during the early months of suckling, on a diet which is naturally low in iron, leads to an increased risk of iron deficiency in infancy and this is exacerbated by weaning onto foods with low iron availability.

Effects specific to iron deficiency anaemia

Cognitive development

Iron is active in neurotransmitter systems in the brain and the effects of deficiency depend on the maturity of the affected individual. The relationship between iron deficiency and impaired performance in mental and motor tests in children is well established. Brain iron content increases throughout childhood and reaches its maximal levels in young adulthood between the ages of 20–30 years. Compelling evidence demonstrates that infants with iron deficiency anaemia fare less well in an array of psychomotor tests than non-anaemic age-matched counterparts. Even though measurable indices of body iron status can be normalized in these children by giving iron supplements, cognitive function is still impaired some 10 years later in those subjects who were severely iron deficient in childhood.

Immune function

The role of iron in infection is complex, since it is a nutrient for both host and pathogen, especially for intracellular organisms such as malaria, and also a potential toxicant. Studies in iron deficient but otherwise healthy humans have shown reduced production of myeloperoxidase (a precursor to bacterial killing) by neutrophils, reduced bactericidal activity of macrophages, and also a reduction in T lymphocyte number and proliferation. These abnormalities are corrected by iron repletion. The adverse effect of iron deficiency on the cellular response is more marked than its effect on humoral immunity. More importantly, anaemic children with malaria were reported to deteriorate if given oral iron. Iron is not given currently by injection, and iron supplementation of formula milks is more modest. The question whether iron treatment during acute malaria increases the severity of illness has not been resolved. Prudence, however, dictates that iron treatment to anaemic children be postponed until malaria has been treated, and that community supplementation should be postponed until after the malaria season.

Treatment of iron deficiency anaemia

People with confirmed iron deficiency are generally treated with oral iron as a ferrous salt. Treatment should continue until stores are replete, estimated to be three months after normalization of haemoglobin concentration. Supplementation is generally recommended in pregnancy with a daily dose of 60 mg of elemental iron for 6 months, and higher dosage for mothers presenting late for antenatal care. Disappointing results of supplementation programmes may be due to multifactorial anaemia as well as poor compliance. In high risk areas combined treatment with folic acid is more effective, especially in Asia and Africa, and multiple micronutrient supplementation is also promoted, despite some reports of a reduced haematological response, eg when iron supplementation is combined with zinc. An enhanced response to iron supplementation has been attributed to synchronous vitamin A supplementation in vitamin A deficient subjects. Iron deficiency may coexist with malnutrition and infection in young children.

Prevention of iron deficiency anaemia

In areas at risk of iron deficiency, fortification of staple foods is a cost-effective strategy. Even when fortification appears to be effective and cost beneficial, the long-term success of the strategy depends on legislation and active participation of an informed community. In western countries, the majority consumes a diet in which iron is highly bioavailable. Fortification of bread flour and commercial breakfast cereals with iron and other nutrients is long established and accepted although it has been suspended in some European countries.

Anaemia caused by other micronutrient deficiencies

By contrast with the microcytic anaemia of iron deficiency, in deficiency of folate and vitamin B_{12}, which are both necessary for cell proliferation, the process of erythropoeisis is faulty and circulating red cells are fewer in number and unusually large (macrocytic). A disturbance in globin synthesis can occur in riboflavin deficiency, which is manifested by fewer circulating red cells of normal or reduced size and haemoglobin concentration. The rare anaemia of copper deficiency is microcytic and hypochromic. In multiple deficiency a mixed picture is common.

Folate and vitamin B_{12} are involved in DNA and protein synthesis and in some amino acid interactions. Anaemia of folate deficiency is characterized by macrocytosis and the presence of large nucleated red cell precursors (megaloblasts) in the marrow, because of impaired synthesis of purines and pyrimidines for DNA synthesis. Folate deficiency can affect regeneration of gut epithelia, provoking secondary malabsorption. Periconceptional folate deficiency may result in neural tube defects. Malaria increases requirements for folate in order to replace red cells destroyed by parasitization, and in developing countries anaemia is more common in the malaria season. Iron and folate deficiency together with malaria contribute to the high prevalence of anaemia in pregnancy, and thereby to fetal growth retardation in poor tropical areas.

Dietary folate deficiency is due to low intakes of folate-rich foods such as green leafy vegetables, pulses, and cereals, especially when requirements are increased, eg during pregnancy or in malaria and other haemolytic conditions. Low folate intake is relatively common in some high income countries, although frank anaemia is largely restricted to pregnant women and the elderly.

Vitamin B_{12} is unique among vitamins in that deficiency may arise from an isolated defect in absorption. The vitamin is only available in foods of animal origin. Vitamin B_{12} deficiency in high income countries is most common in the elderly, primarily as a result of impaired absorption, but is seen in all ages in populations in developing countries, where the consumption of animal foods is often extremely limited. Severe and prolonged deficiency is associated with a mixed motor and sensory neuropathy, which may be irreversible. Neurological signs may be aggravated by administration of folate. The anaemia resembles that of folate deficiency, and it is important to make the distinction.

Riboflavin deficiency interferes with iron absorption in animals, and riboflavin deficiency often tracks with poor iron status in humans, although a causal link has not been well established. Recent work on vitamin A has demonstrated interference with iron absorption, and haemoglobin concentration has been seen to rise after correction of vitamin A deficiency.

Copper is widely distributed in foods, being found in the germ of grains, in legumes and shellfish. Deficiency is most commonly due to artificial parenteral diets, or increased losses as in dialysis. Deficiency may also arise due to inborn errors of copper metabolism. The anaemia of copper deficiency is microcytic because caeruloplasmin, which oxidizes ferrous to ferric iron for storage or transport to the red cell, is copper dependent (see the *Sight and Life* website for available downloads concerned with nutritional anaemia).

KEY POINTS

- Anaemia is the result of abnormalities in red blood cell production, or accelerated destruction of red blood cells, or excessive blood loss
- Microcytic, normocytic and macrocytic anaemia are terms used to describe anaemia with small, normal or large sized red blood cells
- The most common cause of anaemia worldwide is nutritional iron deficiency and the World Health Organization estimate that 2 billion of the world's population (largely in developing countries) currently have marked iron deficiency anaemia
- Deficiencies of other micronutrients, including folate, vitamins B_2, B_{12} and A, and copper, can also lead to anaemia under some circumstances
- Iron deficiency is strongly linked with diets low in haem-iron and high in phytate, which have low bioavailability of iron
- Dietary iron deficiency is exacerbated by blood loss due to intestinal parasites
- Work capacity can be impaired in anaemia of any aetiology
- In young infants and children iron deficiency anaemia is also associated with motor and cognitive delay

FURTHER READING

ACC/SCN 2000 United Nations Administrative Committee on Coordination/Standing Committee on Nutrition in collaboration with the International Food Policy Research Institute. Fourth report on the world nutrition situation. SCN, Geneva (refer to UN ACC/SCN publications for annual reports on the world nutrition situation)

Department of Health 1998 Report on Health and Social Subjects 48. Nutritional Aspects of the Development of Cancer. Report of the Working Group on Diet and Cancer Committee on the Medical Aspects of Food and Nutrition Policy. The Stationery Office, London

Doll R, Peto R 2003 Epidemiology of cancer. In: Warrell D A, Cox T M, Firth J D, Benz E J Jr (eds) Oxford textbook of medicine, 4th edn. Oxford University Press, Oxford, p 193–218

Fairburn C G, Brownell K D (eds) 2002 Eating disorders and obesity. A comprehensive handbook, 2nd edn. Guilford Press, New York

Joint WHO/FAO Expert Consultation 2003 Diet, nutrition and the prevention of chronic diseases. WHO Technical Report Series 916. WHO, Geneva

Riccardi G, Rivellese A, Williams C 2003 The cardiovascular system in nutrition and metabolism. In: Gibney M J, Macdonald I A, Roche H M (eds) Nutrition and metabolism. The Nutrition Society Textbook Series. Blackwell Publishing, Oxford

World Health Organization 1999 Definition, diagnosis and classification of diabetes mellitus and its complications: report of a WHO consultation. WHO Geneva

World Health Organization 2000 WHO Consultation on Obesity. Obesity: preventing and managing the global epidemic. WHO Technical Report 894. WHO, Geneva

World Cancer Research Fund 2007 Food, nutrition, physical activity and the prevention of cancer: a global perspective. American Institute for Cancer Research, Washington

WEBSITES

International Association for the Study of Obesity
www.iaso.org
International Obesity Taskforce
www.iotf.org
World Health Organization
www.who.int.org
British Psychological Society
http://www.bps.org.uk/eatingdisorders/files/ED.pdf
UK Eating Disorders Association
http://www.edauk.com/
Royal College of Psychiatrists
http://www.rcpsych.ac.uk/info/eatdis.htm
Sight and Life
www.sightandlife.org

CHAPTER 9

Nutrition and the Hard Tissues

OBJECTIVES

By the end of this chapter you should be able to:

- understand the dynamic nature of skeletal metabolism
- define osteomalacia, rickets and osteoporosis
- discuss the role of vitamin D and calcium nutrition in skeletal health
- appreciate the role of other nutrients in skeletal health
- give definitions for dental caries, erosion, abrasion and periodontal disease
- describe the indices used for the measurement of dental caries
- describe the epidemiology and trends of dental caries in Western and other countries
- outline the structure of the tooth
- explain the mechanisms of the decay process
- summarize evidence for the role of dietary sugars and fluoride in the causation and prevention of decay
- compare the relative cariogenicity of various sugars and other carbohydrates
- summarize the interaction of protective effects of fluoride and destructive effects of sugars

9.1 INTRODUCTION

This chapter concerns the physiology and nutritional factors affecting the hard tissues of the body. The first section deals with bones and their two main nutrition related disorders, osteoporosis, and osteomalacia or rickets, and the second section with teeth and their main diet related disorder, dental caries.

9.2 BONE STRUCTURE AND CHANGES

Bone composition

Bone has several functions. It provides: mechanical support and protection for internal organs; a function in acid–base balance; defence against some toxins such as lead, which can be adsorbed to bone; and production of blood cells (haematopoiesis).

The human adult skeleton weighs approximately 3–4 kg, and is about 10% water, 60% inorganic material (minerals), and 30% organic matrix which consists largely (95%) of a single protein, type I collagen. The minerals consist chiefly of calcium, phosphate and carbonate in a crystalline form called hydroxyapatite. Deficiency or excess of these components in bone may contribute to loss of bone strength and to fractures.

There are two main types of bone cells, osteoclasts and osteoblasts, which have opposite functions. Osteoclasts are responsible for bone resorption and osteoblasts for bone formation.

Types of bone

The skeleton is composed of two types of bone, cortical or compact bone, which forms the outer shell of bones and accounts for about 80% of skeletal mass, and trabecular or spongy or cancellous bone, which forms the interior scaffolding of bone and accounts for as much as 70% of bone surface area and metabolic activity. The spaces between the trabeculae contain red marrow which is responsible for the formation of blood cells (haematopoiesis).

Bone changes

Bone is a metabolically active tissue. Although the total amount of bone tissue in an adult is relatively static, about 5–10% of existing bone is replaced through 'remodelling' each year. Bone growth, and change in bone shape in children occurs by a mechanism called 'modelling' through differences between bone formation and resorption.

The 'calciotropic hormones' regulate the process of bone formation and resorption. These include parathyroid hormone (PTH) which stimulates bone resorption, but can also stimulate bone formation; vitamin D and its metabolites which influence mineral supply; sex steroids (oestradiol and testosterone) which decrease bone remodelling; glucocorticoids, of which the predominant effect is to inhibit bone formation; and growth hormone, insulin-like growth factors and thyroid hormones which increase bone remodelling.

The fetal skeleton is initially composed mainly of unmineralized cartilage, and mineralization occurs mainly during the last 10 weeks of pregnancy at a rate of more than 100 mg calcium/day. This continues after birth as the size and shape of bones changes during growth. Skeletal mass increases from about 100 g in the neonate to about 3000 g in an adult (peak bone mass) at about age 35. Over 90% of peak bone mass is achieved by age 18, and so children and adolescents are a particularly important target for interventions to increase bone mass for later life. Bone mineral content declines in the elderly, and is particularly rapid in women after the menopause, caused in large part by a reduced ovarian production of oestradiol. Peak bone mass is the most important predictor of bone mineral content in later life.

Genetic and lifestyle factors influence bone mineral accrual during growth, including exercise, calcium intake, general nutritional status, smoking and use of medications such as corticosteroids and some contraceptives.

Pregnancy and lactation increase calcium requirements, which are met by increased efficiency of calcium absorption from the diet and by maternal bone mineral loss. Calcium requirements of the fetus are relatively small (approximately 30 g) in comparison with lactation (up to 1 g of calcium per day for milk production) which is largely obtained through skeletal mineral loss. This does not appear to have any long lasting effect on bone mineral content or on later fracture risk.

A wide variety of genetic and acquired diseases such as collagen disorders, cancer and infections can influence the skeleton. The two most common diseases affecting the skeleton are (a) osteoporosis, and (b) osteomalacia or rickets due to vitamin D deficiency, in both of which nutrient supply plays a role. Disorders which influence intake or gastrointestinal absorption of nutrients (such as anorexia nervosa, coeliac disease and inflammatory bowel disease) may also cause skeletal disease due to deficient nutrient supply, drug therapy, immobility, endocrine disturbances and the response to inflammation.

9.3 SKELETAL FRACTURE

Skeletal fractures occur as a result of excessive stress or poor bone health, mainly reduced mineral content. Fractures are most common in children and in the very elderly. In children these involve mainly long bones, are more common in males, and are only weakly associated with bone mineral content, while in the elderly they classically occur in bones which have a high proportion of trabecular bone (the wrist, hip and spine), are more common in women, and are strongly associated with low bone mineral content (osteoporosis). The healthcare costs and morbidity associated with these fractures are substantial.

Obese individuals have a lower fracture risk than lean individuals as fat provides 'padding' during falls and they have higher bone mineral density due to increased production of oestrogens in fatty tissue, and to mechanical strains induced by excess body weight. Anorexia nervosa results in marked loss of bone mineral content and an increased risk of fracture during later life.

9.4 OSTEOPOROSIS, OSTEOMALACIA AND RICKETS

Osteoporosis

Osteoporosis is characterized by low bone mass and 'microarchitectural' deterioration of bone, resulting in an increased risk of fracture. The World Health Organization (WHO) defines osteoporosis as a bone mineral density value less than 2.5 standard deviations below that expected for young adults, and osteopenia when bone mineral density is between 1 and 2.5 standard deviations below the young adult mean. However many osteoporotic fractures occur in individuals who do not fulfil these criteria for a diagnosis of osteoporosis.

At least 30% of postmenopausal women in Western countries are defined as having osteoporosis according to WHO criteria. However, differences in the length and width of bones as well as non-skeletal factors, such as frequent falling, poor muscle strength, low body mass and poor vision, also influence fracture risk. Many of these risk factors may be influenced by nutritional status.

Treatment aims to increase bone mineral density, reduce bone remodelling, and decrease the risk of falls. Measures include avoidance of smoking, increasing dietary intake of calcium, ensuring adequate vitamin D status, and exercise and a variety of drugs such as bisphosphonates, oestrogens, selective oestrogen receptor modulators and intermittent parathyroid hormone.

Osteomalacia

Osteomalacia results from defective mineralization of bone matrix (osteoid). The commonest cause is vitamin D deficiency. Other causes include disorders of phosphate metabolism, genetic defects, and excessive intake of nutrients such as fluoride.

Rickets

Rickets is osteomalacia that occurs when bones are still growing. Rickets has been an important cause of childhood illness and deformity for many centuries. Following the industrial revolution, the combination of urbanization, pollution and poor diet resulted in increased prevalence of the disease in England. Rickets continues to be an important disease in the developing world, and is still seen in developed countries, particularly in non-Caucasians.

Children with rickets classically present with knock-knees or bowed legs, muscle weakness, and short stature. In breast-fed infants, rickets can develop within the first few months of birth, particularly when the mothers of these infants have vitamin D deficiency. These infants may have craniotabes (soft areas of the skull causing a 'ping-pong' ball sensation on pressure), thickening of the wrists and ankles, and enlargement of the costochondral junctions (rachitic rosary). Fractures and other deformities can occur. Children with rickets also have poor muscle development and tone. The skeleton is poorly mineralized, and the growth plates are widened (cupped) and irregular on x-ray. As in adult osteomalacia, there is an excess of unmineralized osteoid. Infants with rickets may develop respiratory infections, and are more likely to have tuberculosis. Many of the clinical features of rickets resolve within a short period after administration of adequate amounts of vitamin D but pelvic deformities can lead to later difficulties during labour.

In the early part of the 20th century it was discovered that rickets could be cured by a fat-soluble nutrient or sunshine exposure. An unfortified infant diet contains a very small amount of vitamin D, although there are small amounts in milk and egg yolk. Causes of osteomalacia and rickets include

---

Box 9.1 Factors contributing to vitamin D insufficiency

1. Deficiency of sunlight-derived vitamin D
   - Failure to go out-of-doors
   - Limited UV-B exposure in wintertime
   - Countries with limited UV-B exposure
   - Decreased skin exposure due to traditional dress
   - Use of sunscreen creams
   - Ageing
   - Darker skin colour
2. Gastrointestinal disease
   - Pancreatic disease (fat malabsorption)
   - Coeliac disease
   - Other malabsorption syndromes
3. Anticonvulsant drug therapy
4. Defective renal production of $1,25(OH)_2D$
   - Renal insufficiency
   - Genetic vitamin D pseudodeficiency rickets

---

high dietary intakes of phytate; increased skin pigmentation or traditional dress; calcium deficiency; genetic or acquired disorders of phosphate metabolism or vitamin D metabolism; and deficiency of the enzyme alkaline phosphatase (Box 9.1).

9.5 THE ROLE OF CALCIUM AND VITAMIN D IN BONE (SEE CHAPTER 5)

The risk of poor bone mineralization is greater in modern society than for our distant ancestors. The genetic constitution of modern humans has changed little over the past 10,000 years, but the environment has altered markedly. Cultivated plant foods such as cereal grains have far less calcium than do other vegetable food sources and dietary calcium intake was probably twice as great in pre-agricultural humans. Modern humans get less exercise and far less sunshine exposure than did our evolutionary ancestors. There is very little vitamin D in the unsupplemented diet of most modern humans.

Increasing calcium intake through supplements or dairy foods results in a reduction in bone resorption within two hours, and a decrease in serum PTH after several weeks of intervention. Several studies have shown that calcium supplementation alone or with vitamin D reduces the risk of osteoporotic fracture in elderly men and women living in institutions or at home. Calcium supplementation appears to have less influence on bone loss in the years immediately after the menopause, possibly due to the overriding importance of oestrogen deficiency during this time.

Children and adolescents are a particularly important target for interventions to increase bone mass. Randomized controlled trials of calcium or dairy supplementation in children for periods up to 3 years found a greater bone mass accrual in the order of 1–7%, possibly due to a reduction in the rate of bone remodelling.

Calcium supplementation and adequate protein intake has important therapeutic value in osteoporosis and combined supplements of calcium and vitamin D are often recommended to patients with osteoporosis. Most calcium supplementation studies which have shown a skeletal effect have used intakes of at least 1000 mg per day. Maintenance of body weight is critical, since moderate weight loss and low body weight are associated with loss of bone mass and risk of fracture. However, excessive calcium intake can result in hypercalcaemia, renal insufficiency or renal stones, and impaired absorption of other nutrients such as iron, phosphorus and zinc.

9.6 PROTEIN, ACID–BASE BALANCE AND BONE

A diet high in protein results in increased urinary calcium excretion. This was thought to indicate increased bone resorption to buffer the acid load resulting from protein catabolism, but more recent studies suggest that increased excretion may be due in large part to increased efficiency of dietary calcium absorption. Plant proteins result in less acid production than animal proteins but evidence that intake of animal protein is harmful to the skeleton is not strong. Increasing protein intake may increase bone mineral density and decrease the risk of falling in some populations, particularly in the elderly.

It is overly simplistic to consider animal protein as a single nutritional entity. Whereas purified protein products (such as casein) that are used in many studies result in increased urinary calcium loss, more recent studies using meat as a protein supplement have shown little effect on urinary calcium excretion. The relevance of protein intake may also vary by age and nutritional status. Elderly persons with osteoporotic hip fracture are often undernourished and low body weight is an important risk factor for fracture. Protein and calcium supplementation in randomized control trials improves clinical outcome after hip fracture, increases muscle strength and improves bone mineral density.

There is evidence that a diet high in fruit and vegetables is associated with a slightly reduced fracture risk. The relationship between the alkalinizing effect of fruit and vegetable intake on the one hand and the acidifying effect of meat intake on the other hand has received considerable attention. However, most studies have not shown significant differences in skeletal health or fracture risk between vegetarians and meat eaters. The intake of fruit and vegetables is associated with lifestyle factors such as smoking, alcohol consumption and exercise and statistical correction for these confounders is often different. It is premature to draw conclusions about the role of fruit and vegetables in the prevention of fracture risk until the results of randomized intervention trials are available.

9.7 THE ROLE OF OTHER VITAMINS ON BONE

Excessive intake of vitamin A causes increased concentration of calcium in the blood (hypercalcaemia), increased bone resorption and skeletal disease, but vitamin A intake within the general population is not clearly related to skeletal health. Deficiency of B vitamins, particularly folate, riboflavin and vitamin B_6, leads to increased plasma homocysteine, which may be associated with low bone mineral density and increased fracture risk. Vitamin C is necessary for collagen synthesis and cross-linking; scurvy (severe vitamin C deficiency) is associated with bone pain, subperiosteal haemorrhages and fractures around the growth plates but is now rare except in food faddists or in extreme malnutrition. However, there is some evidence that milder vitamin C deficiency may affect skeletal health, particularly in smokers. Supplementation with vitamin K_2 has been reported to increase bone mineral density and reduce the rate of osteoporotic fracture. The importance of dietary vitamin K as a determinant of fracture risk is uncertain.

9.8 THE ROLE OF OTHER MINERALS ON BONE

A diet high in sodium increases urinary calcium excretion and so excessive sodium intake should be avoided by individuals with increased fracture risk. Bone mineral consists largely of calcium phosphate, and phosphorus supply is therefore essential for skeletal development but excess phosphorus intake lowers urinary calcium excretion and impairs absorption of calcium from the diet. Phosphorus is present in a wide variety of foods, and is also added to foods and cola drinks as polyphosphates or phosphoric acid. The possible harmful effect of a high phosphorus diet on the skeleton may be more relevant when calcium requirements are high during puberty. The form of ingested phosphorus is also important: polyphosphates may have a greater deleterious effect on calcium balance than orthophosphates.

Fluoride increases the activity of osteoblasts and substantially increased fluoride intake is associated with severe skeletal disease (fluorosis). Fluoride therapy in patients with osteoporosis increases trabecular bone mineral density, but this is associated with an increased rate of fracture rather than a decrease. Many elderly people consume zinc deficient diets and zinc undernutrition may increase the risk of osteoporosis. Several studies have reported that women with postmenopausal osteoporosis had elevated urinary zinc levels compared to healthy controls, and that in this population group urinary zinc excretion was associated with bone resorption.

9.9 THE ROLE OF OTHER DIETARY COMPONENTS ON BONE

Phyto-oestrogens are widely promoted as a 'natural' alternative to oestrogen replacement therapy to minimize the risk of osteoporosis in post-menopausal women. Isoflavones are phyto-oestrogens which have weak oestrogen-like properties and are found in high concentrations in foods such as soya. Several studies have reported a positive association between bone mineral density and intake of soya foods in Chinese and Japanese postmenopausal women but the association is less clear in populations with lower habitual soya intake.

Alcohol abuse and dependence may compromise bone quality and increase risk of fracture, due to a direct toxic effect of alcohol on bone osteoblasts, insufficient intake of other nutrients, vitamin D deficiency, decreased sex hormone secretion and increased risk of falls. There is less evidence that moderate alcohol consumption is associated with fracture risk.

Most studies have found no association or a weak increase in fracture risk with excessive consumption of caffeine-containing beverages. Although caffeine decreases slightly the efficiency of calcium absorption, this would be offset entirely by addition of two tablespoons of milk to a cup of coffee.

Studies in teenagers have reported that a high intake of carbonated cola-type drinks is associated with a low bone mineral density and a higher prevalence of fracture, which may be due to other associated lifestyle or dietary factors but the phosphorus content and caffeine content of some carbonated drinks may contribute to risk.

9.10 TEETH

Teeth are important for enhancing facial appearance as well as for eating and speaking. Dental diseases inflict considerable pain and anxiety and are more costly to health care services than the cost of treating cardiovascular diseases and osteoporosis. Nowadays, people are retaining their teeth well into older age and it is a realistic expectancy that teeth are for life. Man has two dentitions. The deciduous dentition begins to appear in the mouth at about 6 months of age, consists of 20 teeth and is shed by early adolescence and is replaced by the permanent dentition (between the ages of about 6 and 21 years) which consists of 32 teeth.

Dental diseases include enamel developmental defects (eg hypoplasia and fluorosis), dental tissue loss (eg erosion, abrasion and attrition), periodontal disease (gum disease) and dental caries. Enamel defects may occur while the teeth are forming; the two main types are fluorosis, caused by excess ingestion of fluoride during tooth development, and hypoplasia, which has many causes including infections, drug side effects, congenital defects, dental trauma and dietary deficiencies.

Dental erosion is the loss of dental mineralized tissues by acids from diet and/or the environment and by regurgitation (eg in bulimia). Other forms of tooth wear include attrition due to grinding of the tooth surfaces and abrasion, often due to over harsh brushing of the teeth. The age-related loss of dental tissue is accelerated by elements of the modern lifestyle, including an increase in consumption of acidic drinks, such that approximately 50% of young people aged 4–18 have signs of erosion to their teeth.

The most common periodontal diseases are gingivitis, which is inflammation of the gums, and periodontitis which involves the periodontal ligament and eventually the alveolar bone, leading to increased mobility of the teeth and their eventual loss. About 10–15% of the population in industrialized countries have severe chronic periodontitis. Plaque on teeth adjacent to the gingivae initiates an inflammatory response in the connective tissue which can lead to collagen destruction and anaerobic bacteria build up. Response to plaque may be modified by dietary and hormonal factors (eg pregnancy) and diseases such as diabetes. The disease progresses more rapidly in undernourished populations. A deficiency of vitamin C has been historically associated with periodontal disease as it is essential for collagen formation, hence the integrity of the periodontal ligament, blood vessel walls and alveolar bone matrix. Topical application of folate is effective in preventing gingivitis in pregnant women. However nutrition and diet are generally not important in the prevention or treatment of periodontal disease, the main focus of which is plaque removal. The main causes of tooth loss are dental caries in children and periodontal disease in adults. As the latter has only a minor relationship with nutrition, the main focus of this chapter section is on dental caries.

9.11 DENTAL CARIES

Dental caries was rare until the 19th century when the prevalence and severity rose rapidly, 'poor teeth' being the most important cause of rejection of volunteers for service in the Boer War. The first surveys of the dental health of children in the UK between 1906 and 1908 showed that 90% of children were affected by decay with an average of four decayed teeth per child and, as consumption of sugars increased, reached its peak in the late 1950s and 60s. Interruptions to this trend occurred during the First and Second World Wars when the prevalence of dental caries fell by 40% and 30% respectively in the UK, due to a fall in sugars consumption. Since the 1970s dental decay has declined dramatically, largely due to the introduction of fluoride in toothpaste. In 1973 the average number of teeth affected with dental caries per 14-year-old child was 7.4, falling to 4.7 in 1983 and to 2.0 in 1993 but these improvements have now levelled off and in inner city populations levels are increasing slightly.

The severity of dental decay is measured using the dmft/DMFT (primary dentition/permanent dentition) index, which is a count of the number of teeth that are Decayed, Missing or Filled. These indices are widely used throughout the world for monitoring levels of dental decay.

Dental decay is very strongly related to social class with highest levels in the most socially disadvantaged. Pre-school children from manual social classes are more likely to be frequent consumers of confectionery and sugared soft drinks and more likely to be users of dummies and reservoir feeders. 59% of older people from manual working backgrounds are edentulous compared with 38% from non-manual backgrounds. Regional differences exist in levels of decay with the highest levels being reported in Northern Ireland and Scotland and the lowest levels being reported in London and the South East.

9.12 THE DECAY PROCESS

Dental caries is the localized loss of dental hard tissues as a result of acids produced by bacterial fermentation of sugars in the mouth and its development is influenced by the structure of the tooth, the salivary flow rate and composition and the presence or absence of fluoride.

Theories of causation

Several older theories of causation include worms, vitamin D deficiency and an autoimmune disease. Only the chemo-parasitic theory (also known as the 'acid theory') has persisted and is now widely accepted by dental scientists worldwide. Experiments showed lactic acid was the main acid produced during fermentation and that the centre of carious lesions was acidic; thus lactobacillus was viewed as the main class of cariogenic bacteria. It is now thought that mutans streptococci initiate caries and that lactobacilli become involved at a later stage when the low pH conditions produced by mutans streptococci favour their growth.

The structure of the tooth and the decalcification process

To understand the action of bacterial acids on the teeth an appreciation of the tooth structure is required. The teeth are composed of three mineralized tissues – enamel, dentine and cementum (Fig 9.1). Dentine forms the bulk of the tooth and is covered on the roots by a thin layer of cementum and on the crown by hard enamel. The teeth are supported by the alveolar bone of the maxilla or mandible, covered in epithelium which around the necks of the teeth is called the gingivae (gums). The teeth are held in the alveolar bone by the periodontal ligament, allowing the teeth to move slightly. Enamel contains no cells, nerves or blood vessels and is insensitive, but the dentine is very sensitive to many stimuli. The nerves and blood vessels supplying the dentine come from the pulp that forms the soft centre of a tooth, supplied by nerves and blood vessels from the alveolar bone via the apical foramen of the tooth roots. Dental enamel consists of crystals of hydroxyapatite, a crystalline compound composed of calcium and phosphate in a thinly dispersed organic matrix.

The role of dental plaque

An essential factor in the aetiology of dental caries is dental plaque, a white, slightly glutinous layer, which builds up on the surfaces of teeth when they are not cleaned. Micro-organisms then multiply to make up about 70% of plaque while the remaining 30% consists of the plaque matrix made up of polymers derived from dietary sugar by enzymes secreted by the plaque micro-organisms. These polymers are glutinous and form an energy store

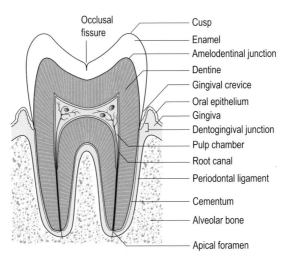

Figure 9.1 Vertical section through a permanent molar tooth (diagram drawn by D. S. Brown and reproduced with permission).

from which bacteria feed during long breaks between the host's meals. Dental plaque is usually found in areas around the teeth which are least easily cleaned, mainly in the pits and fissure of the occlusal (or chewing) surfaces between adjacent teeth (proximal surfaces) or along the gingival margin of the tooth on the buccal (outer) or lingual (inner) surfaces of the teeth. Diet has an important influence on plaque composition; a diet high in sucrose encourages the growth of acid-tolerant bacteria such as mutans streptococci.

Dietary sugars diffuse into the dental plaque where they are metabolized by plaque microorganisms to acids which reduce the pH of dental plaque and dissolve the mineral phase of enamel, thus beginning the caries process. Enamel hydroxyapatite usually begins to dissolve around pH 5.5. When the pH rises above this value remineralization of enamel may occur. Saliva promotes remineralization as it contains bicarbonate which increases pH and encourages deposition of mineral in porous areas where demineralization of enamel or dentine has occurred. If the pH in the mouth remains high enough for sufficient time then complete remineralization may occur. However, if demineralization dominates the enamel becomes more porous until finally a carious lesion forms. High levels of calcium and phosphate in plaque will help resist dissolution of the enamel. The development of caries is also influenced by the composition of the tooth (the structure of the enamel can be altered by the diet while the teeth are forming), the quantity and composition of saliva (eg calcium and phosphate content and buffering power) and the time for which dietary sugars are available for fermentation.

The Stephan curve

Stephan, in the 1940s, used microelectrodes to show that the resting pH of plaque was around 6.5–7 but, on exposure to sugars (glucose or sucrose), fell rapidly within a few minutes, to around pH 5, followed by a slow recovery to baseline pH over the next 30–60 minutes. pH plotted against time is generally referred to as a 'Stephan curve' (Fig 9.2) and has been commonly used

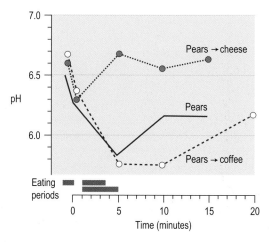

Figure 9.2 Stephan curves produced by eating either cheese or sugared coffee after tinned pears in syrup. From Rugg-Gunn et al 1975 (reproduced with permission).

to measure the acidogenic potential of a range of foods as an indirect measure of their cariogenic potential. However, this takes no account of protective factors in foods, the resistance of enamel and salivary factors that influence the caries process, and needs to be interpreted alongside data from other types of study including animal studies and epidemiological surveys.

Different food combinations result in different patterns in plaque pH. For example cheese following a sugary snack almost abolishes the fall in plaque pH that usually results from sugars consumption, probably due to the stimulation of saliva by its strong flavour and low carbohydrate content. Other foods that are good stimuli to salivary flow include peanuts and sugar-free chewing gum. If consumption of sugary foods is restricted to mealtimes, the risk of caries can be reduced.

9.13 PROMOTING AND PROTECTIVE FACTORS FOR DENTAL CARIES

Many factors can promote dental decay including: poor oral hygiene; high *Streptococcus mutans* counts; and an excess intake of dietary sugars. Several factors are known to be protective, most notably fluoride exposure (both dietary and non-dietary) and restricted intake of sugars, and also a number of other dietary factors including milk, cheese and xylitol.

Diet can affect the teeth while they are forming, before they erupt into the mouth (a pre-eruptive effect) and, once erupted, by a local direct effect. In developing countries, in the absence of dietary sugars, undernutrition is not associated with dental caries but coupled with a high intake of sugars undernutrition results in levels of caries greater than expected for the level of sugars intake. Despite considerable past interest in the pre-eruptive effect of diet on tooth decay, today the post-eruptive local effect of diet in the mouth is considered to be much more important.

Factors promoting dental caries
Dietary sugars

In the past, a positive correlation between sugar intake and levels of dental caries between countries was found. Today, the relationship is less strong in countries with high sugar intake since these countries are on the upper flattened part of the sigmoid relationship curve. However, sugar availability still accounts for over a quarter of the variation in dental caries levels.

A marked increase in dental caries occurred in populations that have undergone the 'nutrition transition', that is where traditional diets that were low in free sugar have been replaced by a westernized diet high in free sugar. High sugar consumers with higher than average levels of dental caries include confectionery workers, sugar cane cutters and children taking long-term sugared liquid medicines. Groups of people with a low sugar intake show low level of caries including children in institutions where strict dietary regimens low in sugar are followed and also in children with Hereditary Fructose Intolerance, a condition in which fructose, and therefore sucrose must be avoided. During the Second World War the reduction in sugar availability in many countries was related to a reduction in caries.

There have been two human intervention studies of special importance. First, the Vipeholm Study was conducted in a mental institution in Sweden shortly after the Second World War in which 964 mostly male patients were divided by wards into one control group and six test groups, given high sucrose intakes at meals only, or at and between meals, in non-sticky (sucrose solution, chocolate) or sticky forms (caramels, toffees, sweet bread). It was concluded that: sugars consumption even at high levels is associated with only a small increase in caries increment if taken up to four times a day as part of meals; consumption of sugars between meals as well as at meals is associated with a marked increase in caries; and caries activity disappears on withdrawal of sugars from the diet. The highest caries increment was observed in the group that consumed 24 sticky toffees throughout the day.

The second human intervention study took place in Turku, Finland, in the 1970s with the aim of investigating the effect over two years on dental caries of nearly total substitution of sucrose in a normal diet with either fructose or xylitol. The xylitol group had 56% fewer cavities than the sucrose group, but a similar number of cavities formed in the sucrose and fructose groups. Xylitol was therefore less cariogenic than the sucrose or fructose, due to the inability of plaque micro-organisms to metabolize xylitol to acids.

Both amount of sugars intake and the frequency with which it is eaten are important for caries development and the two variables are strongly associated – reducing one of these variables will result in a reduction in the other.

Starches

There is little evidence from epidemiological studies that the intake of staple starchy foods is associated with dental caries, in contrast to a much closer relationship between caries and sugar availability on a worldwide basis. The intake of starch increased in Norway and Japan during the years of the Second World War yet the occurrence of caries was reduced. Starchy foods generally produce less of a decrease in plaque pH compared with sugar, and wholegrain starchy staples may also have properties that protect the teeth from decay and require more mastication, thereby stimulating secretion of saliva, increasing its buffering capacity.

Other carbohydrates

Modern diets contain an increasing array of carbohydrates other than starches and sugars including maltodextrins, glucose syrups (collectively known as glucose polymers) and non-digestible oligosaccharides such as oligofructose and gluco-oligosaccharides. The latter are increasingly being used in foods as they are pre-biotics, encouraging the growth of favourable colonic bacteria. Less is understood on the cariogenic potential of these carbohydrates.

Fruit

There is little evidence from epidemiological studies to show fresh whole fruit to be an important factor in the development of dental caries, and in fact apples have long been used as a symbol of oral health. Some plaque pH studies have found fruit to be acidogenic, but less so than sucrose; however, these take no account of the protective factors found in fresh fruits or of the fact that they provide a good stimulus to salivary flow.

Many fruits are acidic – eg citric acid in citrus fruits, oxalic acid in rhubarb, tartaric acid in grapes and malic acid in apples – which has led to concern that fruit consumption may contribute to erosive tooth wear. Fruit juices are more erosive than whole fruits since the latter provide a good stimulus to salivary flow.

Minerals

Some trace elements increase dental caries although their influence is relatively small. Higher selenium intakes are related to higher caries prevalence.

Factors protective against dental caries
Fluoride

Fluoride increases the resistance of the teeth to decay in several ways. First, if ingested during the development of the enamel, it becomes incorporated into the enamel crystal structure and replaces the hydroxyl groups in hydroxyapatite to form fluoroapatite which is more stable and resistant to demineralization. Second, remineralization of enamel in the presence of fluoride results in the porous lesion being remineralized with fluoroapatite rather than hydroxyapatite and thirdly, fluoride inhibits bacterial sugars metabolism which results in less acid production. Fluoridation of drinking water can reduce dental caries by 50% but does not eliminate dental caries. The benefits of water fluoridation have been observed even in populations where use of other sources of fluoride such as fluoride toothpaste is widespread. Despite a marked protective effect of fluoride on caries prevalence, a relationship between sugars intake and caries still exists in the presence of fluoride.

The link between water fluoride content and dental caries prevention was first established in the USA in the early 20th century and its effectiveness has now been demonstrated in over a hundred surveys in more than 20 countries including the UK. Where water fluoridation has been discontinued levels of dental caries have subsequently increased: a 25% increase in dental caries was observed in some areas of Scotland over 5 years after removal of water fluoridation.

Fluoridation of drinking water can substantially decrease dental caries but an excess of fluoride during the development of the teeth may cause 'dental fluorosis', an enamel developmental defect ranging from small white diffuse opacities to severe pitting and staining of enamel in more severe cases. For front teeth the period when there is greatest risk of fluorosis is between two and five years. Severe fluorosis is rare in the UK and cases have usually been linked with excessive fluoride ingestion from eating toothpaste or misuse of fluoride supplements. Severe fluorosis including skeletal fluorosis is observed particularly in countries that have very high levels of fluoride in water supplies, such as in areas of India, Thailand, in the Rift Valley of East Africa and in many Arab states.

The optimal level of fluoride in water is the level at which a substantial caries reduction is observed with a negligible prevalence of enamel fluorosis. In temperate climates including the UK the optimum concentration of fluoride is 1.0 mg/L while in warmer climates it might be nearer 0.6 mg/L. Water fluoridation is endorsed by science and health organizations including the International Dental Federation, the International Association for Dental Research and WHO. Despite this expert endorsement there are small groups of people who strongly oppose water fluoridation on the grounds of perceived health risks and imposed treatment of the water supply. In addition to water, suitable vehicles for artificial fluoridation are salt and milk although neither of these is used extensively. Dietary fluoride provides a local effect on the teeth whilst in the mouth and a systemic effect on the teeth after digestion and absorption. Fluoride in toothpaste and mouth rinse provides a mainly topical effect as these are not supposed to be swallowed.

Other dietary factors

Other trace elements are protective against dental caries although their influence is of relatively small importance. These include dietary molybdenum, strontium, boron and lithium. Other dietary components and foods such as phosphates, calcium, casein and polyphenols, milk and cheese may also have cariostatic properties. Other foods such as honey, chocolate and liquorice all contain factors that protect against dental caries but the benefits of these factors is overridden by the negative effect of the high sugars content of these foods or in the case of liquorice the dark staining effects. Sugar-free foods that stimulate salivary flow are caries protective and include sugar-free chewing gum.

KEY POINTS

- The skeleton is composed of cortical bone, which is a dense form of bone comprising about 80% of skeletal mass, and trabecular bone which forms the interior scaffolding of bone
- In the adult skeleton most metabolic activity in bone occurs by the process of 'remodelling' or bone turnover which maintains the structure and homeostatic functions of the skeleton
- Osteoporosis is a disease characterized by low bone mass and microarchitectural deterioration of bone, which results in an increased risk of fracture
- Nutritional intervention during childhood and puberty may increase peak bone mass and reduce the risk of fracture in later life
- Most studies report that a low intake of animal protein is associated with lower bone mineral density and increased fracture risk
- Combined supplement of vitamin D and calcium reduces fracture incidence in elderly people
- The prevalence and severity of dental caries in industrialized countries has decreased since the late 1970s but improvements have now halted in younger age groups

- In many developing countries, the prevalence of decay is increasing with a rise in sugar intake
- Dental caries is strongly related to social class with a higher prevalence in lower social classes
- Dental caries occurs due to demineralization of the dental mineralized tissues by acids derived from the bacterial metabolism of dietary sugars to acids
- Plaque on the tooth surface is largely composed of bacterial cells and extracellular glucans
- Changes in plaque pH on consumption of a food provide a measure of acidogenic potential which is an indirect measure of cariogenic potential
- Diet influences the teeth while forming but this effect is of less importance than the local intra-oral effect of diet on the teeth
- Evidence from many different types of study has shown that both the frequency and the amount of intake of sugars are related to dental caries
- Some foods protect against decay – these include milk, cheese, some plant foods and foods that stimulate salivary flow
- Fluoride is a highly effective caries-preventive measure but it does not eliminate dental caries

FURTHER READING

Dietary Reference Intakes for Calcium, Phosphorus, Magnesium, Vitamin D, and Fluoride (1997); report accessible via *www.nap.edu*

Rugg-Gunn A J, Edgar W M, Geddes J A M, Jenkins G N 1975 The effect of different meal patterns upon plaque pH in human subjects. British Dental Journal 139:351–356

Rugg-Gunn A J, Nunn J H 1999 Nutrition, diet and oral health. Oxford University Press. Oxford

World Health Organization 1996 Fluorides and oral health. WHO Technical Report Series No 846. WHO, Geneva

CHAPTER 10

Diet and the Gastrointestinal Tract

OBJECTIVES

By the end of this chapter you should be able to:

- summarize the main features of digestion and absorption
- describe the most common chronic diseases which affect the intestinal tract, their epidemiology and clinical presentation, aetiology and pathophysiology
- discuss the role of diet in their management
- discuss current understanding of food allergies and intolerance

10.1 INTRODUCTION

The primary function of the gastrointestinal tract is to facilitate digestion and the absorption of nutrients, although it also makes an important contribution to the body's immune function. Intestinal function is modulated by gastrointestinal peptide hormones and an enteric nervous system (ENS). The GI tract comprises the mouth, pharynx, oesophagus, stomach, small intestine (duodenum, jejunum and ileum), the large bowel or colon, and the rectum and anus (Fig 10.1). Digestion is initiated in the mouth, continues in the stomach, and is completed in the small intestine. This process is aided by the presence of enzymes in saliva and gastric juices, and those secreted into the small intestine, as well as bile salts released by the gall bladder. Undigested material travels to the large bowel, where bacterial fermentation can occur, with the production of stool which is excreted via the rectum.

The immune system of the gastrointestinal tract has a number of different roles. Following ingestion of food or beverage the general trend is towards suppression of immunity to allow the digestion of substances foreign to the body, in other words, *oral tolerance*. However, active immunization may also follow the feeding of antigen and this is typically in the form of harmless secretory IgA antibody. In some circumstances there is, however, induction of potentially pathogenic immune reactions.

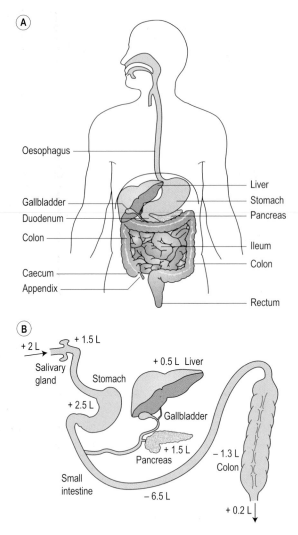

Figure 10.1 The gastrointestinal tract (A) and movement of fluid through different regions (B). L = litres. (The daily amounts and sites of fluid secretion and absorption are from data in Ma & Verkman 1999.)

Gastrointestinal disorders can arise in a variety of circumstances, including exposure to pathogens, or particular food items, or nutrient deficiencies. Diet is often the only practicable therapy that patients are offered.

10.2 DIGESTION AND ABSORPTION

The gastrointestinal tract comprises different regions of activity in terms of digestion and absorption. Figure 10.2 depicts a diagrammatic representation of a cross-section across the intestinal wall, illustrating the relationship between the absorptive surface area and the blood and lacteal system that carry the products of digestion away from the gastrointestinal tract. The major components of the diet are starches, sugars, fats and proteins. These

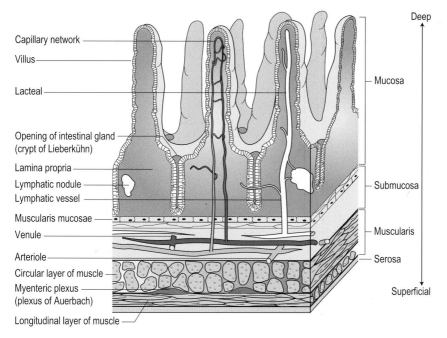

Capillary network

Villus

Lacteal

Opening of intestinal gland
(crypt of Lieberkühn)

Lamina propria

Lymphatic nodule

Lymphatic vessel

Muscularis mucosae

Venule

Arteriole

Circular layer of muscle

Myenteric plexus
(plexus of Auerbach)

Longitudinal layer of muscle

Deep

Mucosa

Submucosa

Muscularis

Serosa

Superficial

Figure 10.2 Cross-section of intestinal wall. (Redrawn with permission from Figure 24-18 in Tortora & Anagnostakos 1990. Reproduced with permission of John Wiley & Sons, Inc.)

have to be hydrolysed to their constituent smaller molecules for absorption and metabolism. Starches and sugars are absorbed as monosaccharides; fats are absorbed as free fatty acids and glycerol (plus a small amount of intact triacylglycerol); proteins are absorbed as their constituent amino acids and small peptides. Table 10.1 summarizes the sites of nutrient absorption along the gastrointestinal tract.

Digestive processes in the mouth

Chewing both grinds the food and also mixes it with saliva, which contains α-amylase and proteolytic enzymes that initiate digestion of dietary starch and protein. Lipid digestion also begins in the mouth, initiated by lipase secreted by the tongue (lingual lipase).

Digestive and absorptive processes in the stomach

Swallowing transfers a food bolus from the mouth to the oesophagus and thence to the stomach. Following a meal, gastric secretory activity follows three well-defined phases:

- the cephalic phase, during which the sight, aroma and anticipation of food stimulates the parasympathetic intestinal nervous system, leading to gastric acid and gastrin secretion
- the gastric phase, associated with increased acid and pepsinogen secretion
- the intestinal phase, which occurs towards the end of liquidization of food in the stomach.

DIET AND THE GASTROINTESTINAL TRACT

Table 10.1 Regional anatomy of the intestine and sites of nutrient absorption

Region	Functions performed	Mucosal surface	Nutrients digested	Nutrients absorbed	Major site of absorption	Electrolytes absorbed
Mouth	Grinding food to smaller particle size Moistening food (saliva) Initial digestion by lipase and α-amylase Initiation of safety mechanisms	Small folds	Small amount of protein, starch	Small amounts of glucose, peptides and amino acids	No	No
Stomach	Intestinal defence (eg acid secretion) Homogenizing food to smaller particle size Moistening food (gastric secretions) Further enzyme secretion Gastric emptying meters delivery of nutrients to the small intestine Feedback of satiety messages	Rugae and pits	Protein, lipid	Insignificant amounts	No	No
Small intestine	Completion of digestion by pancreatic enzymes Absorption of digestion products of carbohydrate, protein and fat Absorption of water and electrolytes Absorption of minerals and micronutrients Feedback of satiety messages	Rugae, villi and microvilli	Protein, lipid, carbohydrate	Amino acids, peptides, fatty acids, glucose, fructose, galactose	Carbohydrate, fat, protein, water, electrolytes	Sodium, potassium, calcium, magnesium, chloride, phosphate
Colon	Final salvage of water and electrolytes Mucin breakdown Conversion of bilirubin to urobilinogen Cholesterol catabolism Organic acid production ('acetate buffer')	Rugae and pits	Dietary fibre – digested by bacteria and fermented to short-chain fatty acids	Acetate, propionate, and butyrate and carboxylic acids	Short-chain fatty acids, water, electrolytes	Magnesium and calcium in form of soaps with fatty acids

Both dietary triacylglycerol and protein are hydrolysed by enzymes secreted in the gastric juice. Gastric lipase hydrolyses triacylglycerol to release free fatty acids. Gastric acid denatures dietary protein and facilitates hydrolyses by pepsins, which are generated from precursor pepsinogens.

Gastric emptying

The rate of gastric emptying is influenced by the amount of food eaten during a meal, and nutrients present in the food, but the control is exerted by neural or hormonal signals arising in response to nutrients in other parts of the gut. The effect is really one of feedback inhibition so that the rate at which the products of digestion in the stomach are allowed to move into the small intestine is regulated by the rate at which they are further digested and absorbed in the small intestine. Thus the presence of nutrients in the duodenum exerts an inhibitory effect on gastric emptying through the *duodenal brake*. Furthermore, the presence of nutrients in the ileum exerts a similar inhibitory effect on gastric emptying, known as the *ileal brake*. For example, fat in the meal that reaches the ileum inhibits gastric emptying, through effects on sensory receptors. Such an effect is mediated by neural and hormonal factors. Luminal lipid stimulates release of the regulatory peptide hormones cholecystokinin (CCK), neurotensin, peptide YY (PYY) and glucagon-like peptides (GLP), which collectively inhibit gastric motility.

In addition to the complex neural and hormonal signals, gastric distension is a very powerful inhibitory signal that increases feelings of fullness and satiety and slows down eating.

Digestive and absorptive processes in the small intestine

As the semi-liquid products of digestion in the stomach (called chyme) pass through the pyloric sphincter into the small intestine they are exposed to the digestive activity of intestinal secretions as well as the emulsifying activity of bile, produced in the gall bladder. Two hormones, secretin and cholecystokinin, are released into the duodenum, and these elicit the secretion of pancreatic enzymes and bile. Enzymes secreted by the pancreas act upon proteins, lipids and starch. The digestion of protein is achieved by proteases including trypsin, chymotrypsin, elastase and carboxypeptidases, and their combined actions lead to the production of free amino acids and short peptides.

The digestion of lipids, which was initiated in the stomach, continues in the small intestine with the formation of mixed micelles that have a hydrophobic core and hydrophilic outer surface. Pancreatic lipases hydrolyse lipids with the release of free fatty acids. The pancreatic secretions are relatively alkaline and thereby neutralize the acidity of the chyme. Intestinal motility facilitates the passage of food and the products of digestion down the gastrointestinal tract by the action of waves of contraction, called peristalsis. These waves of contraction begin in the oesophagus and run through the gastrointestinal tract.

Digestion and absorption of carbohydrate

In the small intestine carbohydrate digestion continues with the further hydrolyses of starch by pancreatic amylases to yield a mixture of glucose oligomers.

These are further hydrolysed by the brush-border glucosidases to glucose, maltose and isomaltose. Disaccharides are hydrolysed to their constituent monosaccharides by disaccharidases on the brush border of the enterocytes. Uptake of glucose and galactose into the enterocytes takes place via the same active (sodium-linked) transporter (SGLT1), while fructose, some other monosaccharides and sugar alcohols are carried by passive transporters. Glucose can also be transported by a second glucose transporter, GLUT2, which responds to an increased dietary load of carbohydrate. Most carbohydrate absorption takes place in the duodenum, upper jejunum and proximal ileum.

Digestion and absorption of protein

The endopeptidases of gastric and pancreatic juice hydrolyse proteins to yield oligopeptides and hydrolyses continues by aminopeptidases secreted by the intestinal mucosa and pancreatic carboxypeptidases, to yield free amino acids and di- and tripeptides. Transport into the enterocytes occurs via transporters specific to particular amino acids. Intracellular peptidases complete the hydrolyses of small peptides, and the resultant amino acids pass into the bloodstream. Some relatively large peptides enter the bloodstream intact, either by passing between cells or by uptake into mucosal cells and this is the basis of food allergy.

Digestion and absorption of fat

The process of fat digestion is one of progressive emulsification of dietary fat and hydrolyses of triacylglycerol to free fatty acids and monoacylglycerols. The final product of fat digestion is the micelle which is taken up by the enterocyte. Short chain fatty acids enter the villus microcirculation, but most of the fatty acids are re-esterified to triacylglycerol in the enterocyte, packaged into chylomicrons and secreted into the lymphatic system. Cholesterol and fat-soluble vitamins are absorbed dissolved in the hydrophobic core of the micelles. Free fatty acids can diffuse freely across the cell membrane.

Events in the colon

The colonic microflora produce short chain fatty acids (SCFA), acetate, propionate and butyrate, by fermentation of resistant starch and non-starch polysaccharides. Butyrate is a preferential fuel for the colonic mucosa, and promotes colonocyte differentiation. It may thus have a significant role in preventing colon cancer. Water uptake is stimulated by SCFA absorption and this is likely to be one of the major mechanisms for water and electrolyte salvage in the large intestine.

Water and electrolytes

The human small intestine absorbs 6.5 to 7.5 litres of water each day. Water absorption is proportional to the amount of substrate and electrolyte that moves across the membrane and the direction of water movement is governed by solute movement. In cholera, excessive secretion of chloride into the colon is accompanied by water secretion and diarrhoea, leading to dehydration and eventually death, unless treated.

Sugar alcohols, used as sweeteners, such as xylitol, lactitol and sorbitol, are poorly absorbed and will enter the colon with water, for fermentation. If the colonic fermentation capacity is exceeded then diarrhoea ensues because the excess water carried into the colon with the sugars cannot be absorbed. Other causes of osmotic diarrhoea include dietary fibre such as guar gum, probiotics such as fructose oligosaccharide and beans that contain large quantities of stachyose, all of which are substrates for bacterial fermentation.

The role of the gastrointestinal tract in the regulation of feeding (see chapter 2, section 2.11)

Energy balance is maintained by both short- and long-term mechanisms to regulate energy intake and expenditure. Some reference has already been made to the ways in which the presence of food in different parts of the gastrointestinal tract can generate signals that feed back to regulate gastric emptying. Short-term control of appetite is regulated by the gastrointestinal tract as well as by the metabolic response to ingested nutrients. The gastrointestinal tract provides regulatory feedback signals that arise from direct effects of absorbed nutrients in the circulation, from neural signals from the gut and liver, and from hormonal signals. The taste of food, as well as the smell before eating, stimulates secretion of gastric juice and intestinal motility. The importance of taste in controlling sensations of hunger and satiety is seen in patients receiving long-term tube-feeding who experience constant feelings of hunger although nutritionally replete.

During eating, food stretches the stomach and induces a complex series of signals that lead to cessation of eating. The mechanism is due to stretch, not gastric pressure, and works through direct inhibition of the stimulating effect of pleasurable tastes on eating. Once in the small intestine nutrients in foods are detected by receptors in the intestinal mucosa which leads to the sending of signals to the brain that control eating. For example, the presence of fat in the intestinal lumen is sensed by receptors that lead to the secretion of the hormone cholecystokinin, which elicits inhibition of eating.

Absorbed nutrients may also elicit signals that modulate eating behaviour. For example, in adequately nourished subjects, the intravenous infusion of lipid stimulates dopamine activity and this is associated with increased satiety ratings and feelings of fullness. However, despite the existence of mechanisms to induce feelings of satiety and control eating these can be overridden centrally such that, for example, it is often possible to consume an appetizing dessert even following a heavy meal.

10.3 DISEASES OF THE GASTROINTESTINAL TRACT

Food has a complex relationship with the integrity and function of the gastrointestinal tract. Dietary inadequacies can impair normal development, structure and function, leading to malabsorption and secondary nutrient deficiencies. The gastrointestinal tract can also be profoundly adversely affected by exposure to certain foods or nutrients, sometimes in association with a genetic susceptibility. Additionally, the use of appropriate dietary measures may be central to treatment of gastrointestinal disease. This part of the chapter will consider chronic gastrointestinal diseases and the role of diet in their aetiology and treatment.

Coeliac disease

Coeliac disease is a form of food intolerance which affects around 1 in 200 individuals and is defined as lifelong gluten intolerance which usually responds to gluten withdrawal. The protein gluten is found in wheat, barley and rye. Ingestion of the gluten causes villous atrophy of the jejunum and subsequent malabsorption. Coeliac disease produces atrophy of the small bowel mucosa, which leads to impairment of the digestion and absorption of nutrients. The atrophy and subsequent malabsorption of nutrients can be corrected by following a gluten-free diet.

There are two ages of peak incidence, one when the infant is weaned on to gluten-containing foods and a second in the third or fourth decade of life. Factors such as early gluten exposure and breast feeding pattern are thought to be important determinants of the different prevalences of this condition throughout the world.

Pathology

Coeliac disease usually affects the jejunum, but in some cases lesions may extend as far as the distal ileum. Intestinal crypts in affected regions are elongated and open out on to a flattened mucosal surface where there is villous atrophy. These structural changes decrease the amount of epithelial surface available for digestion and absorption.

Clinical features

Coeliac disease in childhood is characterized by weight loss or failure to thrive, anaemia, lassitude and diarrhoea. It may be accompanied by abdominal pain, steatorrhoea, blood loss and dehydration. Adult disease may also present with more subtle and variable symptoms such as anaemia, bone disease, neurological abnormalities and abnormal liver function. A suspicion of coeliac disease may be confirmed by the presence of serum antibodies to the main antigens in coeliac disease, such as the wheat glycoprotein gliadin. However definitive diagnosis demands a jejunal biopsy confirming total or partial villous atrophy.

Aetiology

Intolerance to gluten is the defining feature of coeliac disease. The major protein fractions of gluten are gliadin and glutenin. Genetic factors are now known to be important in the pathogenesis of coeliac disease; subjects who have human leukocyte antigen (HLA) DQ2 or DQ8 are at increased risk of developing the disease. Coeliac disease is associated with other autoimmune disorders including type 1 diabetes, thyroid disease and rheumatoid arthritis.

This is important because certain cases of coeliac disease may only be diagnosed by the appearance of the other autoimmune condition; in addition many believe that a gluten-free diet improves the control of the associated disease.

Nutritional deficiencies

As a result of damage to the gastrointestinal mucosa the production of digestive enzymes is impaired with an associated reduction in digestive capacity. Additionally, secondary to intestinal villous atrophy there may be a significant reduction of mucosal surface area causing malabsorption of macro- and micronutrients and associated nutritional deficiencies. Iron deficiency anaemia is common and in cases where there is prolonged severe diarrhoea, deficiencies of sodium and potassium may develop. When malabsorption is severe enough to cause steatorrhoea there may be impaired absorption of calcium and fat-soluble vitamins. Calcium absorption may also be compromised by defective calcium transport, and low bone mineral density and osteoporosis are common chronic features of the disease. Low serum folate concentrations are common and may be accompanied by elevated plasma homocysteine. B_{12} deficiency may develop secondary to folate deficiency or if the distal ileal mucosa is affected. Improvements in nutritional status are generally seen in response to a gluten-free diet but in some cases nutritional intervention may be necessary.

Treatment

Patients typically respond well to exclusion of gluten from the diet, which requires the strict exclusion of wheat, barley, rye and oats. However, gluten is often a component of processed foods and this may not always be evident from the list of ingredients. The British Society of Gastroenterology and Coeliac UK suggest that patients with coeliac disease should, in addition to following a gluten-free diet, be advised to consume 1500 mg of calcium per day to reduce the risk of osteoporosis.

Complications of undiagnosed coeliac disease or failure to comply with dietary exclusion of gluten increases risk of intestinal lymphoma, carcinoma of the oesophagus or colon, osteoporosis and general malnutrition.

Inflammatory bowel disease

Inflammatory bowel disease comprises Crohn's disease (CD), and ulcerative colitis (UC). Both are chronic inflammatory disorders with similar clinical features, but whereas CD may occur anywhere in the gastrointestinal tract UC is confined to the colon. Both diseases occur predominantly in the northern hemisphere, throughout North America and Northern Europe. CD tends to present in adolescence or during the third decade whilst UC occurs around the fourth to fifth decade. There is a second peak for both conditions around the eighth decade.

Crohn's disease

Crohn's disease is a chronic inflammatory disorder of the alimentary tract, characterized by episodes of relapse and remission. It most commonly affects the terminal ileum and colon. Ulceration of the mucosal wall with oedema and inflammation of the bowel in between give the mucosal surface the cobblestone appearance that is typical of this disease. If the condition becomes well established the bowel wall may thicken and the lumen narrow, predisposing the individual to strictures and intestinal obstruction.

Clinical features

The main presenting symptoms of Crohn's disease in adults are abdominal pain, diarrhoea and weight loss and in children, fever and lethargy and failure to thrive. Biochemical characteristics include raised inflammatory markers such as C reactive protein or other acute phase proteins and a raised platelet count. Patients become anaemic and plasma albumin concentrations may be reduced.

Aetiology

The aetiology of Crohn's disease is not well understood but genetic and environmental factors are likely to be important. Individuals who have a first-degree relative with Crohn's disease have a 2–3× increased risk of developing the disease compared with the rest of the population. Certain dietary patterns, smoking and the use of the contraceptive pill have all been linked with the development of Crohn's disease. A number of dietary factors have been investigated as potential determinants of risk for Crohn's disease but the quality of the studies has been generally poor and the results inconclusive. For example, some studies have reported that patients with Crohn's disease consume greater quantities of refined sugar foods than controls, but low sugar diets have not been shown to modulate disease activity. Epidemiological data from Japan show that increased incidence of Crohn's disease tracks with an increased fat consumption, as well as an increase in the ratio of n-6 to n-3 fatty acids in the national diet, suggesting a role for fat in the aetiology of this condition.

Nutritional deficiencies

Nutritional deficiency is a common complication of Crohn's disease. Because of its relapsing and remitting nature, deficiency states may develop insidiously over a number of years, remaining undetected until they are multiple and severe. Much of the evidence suggests that poor dietary intake is not the major cause of deficiencies, but rather that the pathophysiology of the disease and the use of certain medications compromise nutritional status. For example, the absorptive area of the small intestine may be considerably reduced as a result of inflammation or following surgery. Iron deficiency anaemia is a frequent complication in Crohn's disease and may develop secondary to gastrointestinal blood loss and small bowel malabsorption or resection. Extensive intestinal ulceration leads to loss of albumin and iron as a result of leakage of blood and plasma from inflamed mucosa. A fistula in the gastrointestinal tract may cause a short circuit, reducing the length of tract available for digestion and absorption.

Damage to the ileum can specifically reduce the absorption of vitamin B_{12} and damage or loss of the terminal ileum will impair reabsorption of bile salts, which can lead to malabsorption of fat-soluble vitamins. Other factors may contribute to a deterioration in fat-soluble vitamin status, including the use of antibiotics, which interfere with the profile of intestinal flora and reduce the availability of vitamin K from bacterial production. The inflammatory condition can elicit a fall in the production of retinol binding protein, which is a negative acute phase protein, and this compromises transport of retinol from the liver into the plasma.

Corticosteroids are commonly used in the treatment of active Crohn's disease, the use of which can reduce calcium absorption and increase its urinary excretion. This is thought to be the main cause of poor bone mineral density in these patients. The use of sulphasalazine causes competitive inhibition of folate absorption and the use of cholestyramine impairs absorption of nutrients through binding in the gastrointestinal tract.

Inflammation leads to increased production of cytokines, eicosanoids, catecholamines and glucocorticoids which give rise to a catabolic response, protein breakdown and negative nitrogen balance. This is a reason for the apparent increase in protein requirements in patients with Crohn's disease.

Even though the disease process itself has such an important effect on nutritional status in patients with Crohn's disease, many patients eat inadequately because they develop anorexia or sitophobia (fear that eating may produce symptoms). Changes in taste may be caused by deficiency of trace elements such as zinc, copper and nickel or as a result of drug therapy. Strictures may cause abdominal pain and vomiting.

Dietary treatment

Dietary therapy has proved valuable in the treatment of patients with Crohn's disease, either as a primary treatment for the condition or for the correction of associated nutritional deficiencies.

The first stage of dietary therapy involves the use of enteral feeding to achieve remission, whilst the second stage involves the maintenance of remission. Enteral feeds include elemental diets, which are liquid mixtures of essential and non-essential amino acids, glucose, lipid, vitamins, minerals and trace elements; semi-elemental diets, which are peptide-based; and polymeric diets, which include whole proteins. All types of enteral feeds can be effective in producing remission in patients with Crohn's disease, with evidence of a reduction in pro-inflammatory cytokines. Once remission is achieved there are a number of methods used in clinical practice to ensure against further relapse. Different centres have developed specific maintenance diets for Crohn's disease patients, including the low-fibre, fat-limited exclusion diet (LOFFLEX) developed by the gastroenterology research unit at Addenbrooke's Hospital, Cambridge, but there is little evidence that any of these diets offers particular advantages.

Ulcerative colitis

Ulcerative colitis is an inflammatory disease that affects the mucosa of the colon starting from the anus and extending proximally but which, unlike Crohn's disease, does not affect the small intestine.

Clinical features

The characteristic symptoms of UC are diarrhoea and rectal bleeding with the passage of mucus. The colonic mucosa in UC is inflamed and swollen with an increased blood flow. In more severe cases ulceration arises. Ulcers are initially small and discrete but may coalesce and enlarge, extending more deeply in to the lamina propria. Long-term UC carries a markedly increased risk of developing colon cancer probably as a consequence of chronic inflammation.

Blood loss may lead to anaemia and hypoalbuminaemia, which may be severe enough to cause peripheral oedema. Abdominal pain is common and is usually worse after meals. Anorexia leads to weight loss. Severe diarrhoea may cause loss of water and electrolytes leading to dehydration, hypomagnesaemia and hypocalcaemia.

Aetiology

The cause of UC is not known. Although its onset often appears to follow gastroenteritis no specific pathogen has yet been discovered. In contrast to normal individuals, the bacterial flora of the colon in patients with UC is highly unstable and can vary considerably over short periods of time. It has been suggested that mucosal inflammation arises from an immune reaction to the resident colonic microflora.

It has also been suggested that butyrate, which is a product of bacterial fermentation in the colon and which is the primary fuel for colonocytes, is taken up into colonocytes less efficiently in patients with UC. This could be due to increased concentrations of hydrogen sulphide and mercaptides, products of bacterial fermentation, and which are present in higher concentrations in the large bowel of patients with UC. However, there is no evidence that the administration of butyrate by enemas leads to an improvement of symptoms in UC.

As in Crohn's disease there is a strong familial tendency but so far no specific gene has been identified that increases susceptibility to UC.

Treatment

The pharmacological treatment of UC is similar to that of CD with corticosteroids being the cornerstone of management. Drugs releasing 5-aminosalicylic acid are very helpful and patients who become steroid dependent or resistant may require immunosuppressive agents such as azathioprine.

Unlike Crohn's disease patients, dietary intervention is not used as primary therapy. Enteral feeds may be used to improve nutritional status but unlike Crohn's disease they do not reduce colonic inflammation. Supplementation with omega 3 or omega 6 fatty acids in the hope of reducing inflammation has not proved successful.

Irritable bowel syndrome

The most frequently encountered disorder of the gastrointestinal tract is irritable bowel syndrome (IBS) which, in the western world, accounts for up to 50% of referrals to gastroenterologists. Prevalence is estimated at being between 10 and 15%. It is more likely to occur in women than men (2:1) and is not age dependent.

Pathology and clinical features

Patients typically present with a history of abdominal pain accompanied by a change in bowel habit, which may be diarrhoea or constipation. Other symptoms include flatulence, bloating, a feeling of incomplete evacuation, urgency, straining and mucus. No abnormality however can be found to account for these symptoms after radiology and endoscopy of the gastrointestinal tract and standard haematological and biochemical screening. Stool culture reveals no pathogens. The diagnosis therefore is by negative exclusion of other pathology.

Aetiology

Despite its high prevalence in Western countries IBS is the least well understood of all gastrointestinal conditions. Treatment is often ineffective and symptoms may continue for years. Many patients seek treatment from homeopaths and alternative practitioners. Confusion about IBS is compounded because it is not a single discrete entity but a syndrome made up of several quite separate conditions that may produce abdominal pain with or without a change in bowel habit. The lack of pathological findings has led many authorities to believe IBS is primarily a psychological condition. Early studies suggested that IBS might be the result of insufficient intake of dietary fibre, and associated long GI transit times. However there appears to be little discernible difference in the fibre intake of healthy individuals and IBS sufferers and there is little evidence that an increased intake of fibre alleviates the symptoms of IBS. Fibre supplements are now generally reserved for cases when IBS is associated with constipation.

The gastrointestinal tract is continuously exposed to a wide range of foreign bacteria, chemicals and foods, many of which have the capability of acting as antigens and provoking immune responses. The gastrointestinal immune system is major factor in the defence of the organism against these agents. Some foods evoke an allergic reaction in susceptible individuals, and this is the basis of food allergy but no evidence of classical food allergy has been demonstrated in IBS. In contrast to classical IgE-mediated allergy, where small quantities of allergens provoke symptoms of pain, diarrhoea and vomiting within an hour, food reactions in patients with IBS are provoked by much larger quantities of food and may take several hours or days to begin. This has prompted a search for non-immune mechanisms of food intolerance. Some beverages, such as coffee, tea and wines, may provoke symptoms because of constituent chemicals such as caffeine and ethanol. However, this is not true for the majority of food intolerances in patients with IBS and it has been suggested that abnormal colonic fermentation may underlie their reactions.

Prospective studies have shown that the development of IBS is much more likely after bacterial gastroenteritis or a course of antibiotics. These events may damage the colonic flora and lead to abnormal fermentation of food residues entering the caecum.

Dietary treatment of IBS

Nutrient deficiencies may develop as a result of the exclusion of foods or food groups from the diets of patients with IBS. For example, low intakes of calcium and vitamin D are reported in patients who exclude dairy products from their diets. A high fibre diet is used in the treatment of IBS patients presenting with constipation. A diet with low fibre content can reduce gas production and symptoms in patients that present with diarrhoea, bloating urgency and pain. In some patients a low fibre diet is supplemented with a synthetic, non-fermentable fibre, and this provides a diet that can increase stool bulk, and thereby reduce the risk of developing constipation, without the side effects of excess fermentation often experienced with a high-fibre diet.

Exclusion diets may be used for the treatment of patients with IBS who present with symptoms of food intolerance. A core exclusion diet is followed for a period of two weeks, and individual foods may be reintroduced every two days. Foods that do not trigger symptoms can be incorporated back into the diet. Approximately 25% of Europeans with symptoms of IBS test positive for lactose intolerance but not all patients with lactose intolerance respond to a low lactose diet, probably because these patients are intolerant to other constituents of cow's milk. As diets are always restrictive and difficult to follow, there is interest in the possibility of improving symptoms in IBS by manipulating the gastrointestinal flora with the use of probiotics. Probiotics are normally live bacteria, which have been found to be beneficial to the host by affecting the microbial balance. Although some patients have reported benefit, at present the evidence for a beneficial role for probiotic bacteria in the treatment of IBS is limited.

10.4 FOOD ALLERGIES AND FOOD INTOLERANCE

Introduction

Adverse reactions to ingested food cause a wide variety of symptoms, syndromes and diseases for which the general descriptive terms 'sensitivity', 'allergy' and 'intolerance' are often used.

The terms *food intolerance* and *food sensitivity* are used in a general way for all reproducible, unpleasant reactions to a specific food or food ingredient, which are not psychologically based. The reaction may have a clearly defined metabolic, pharmacological or immunopathological basis, or may have no known mechanism. The provoking agent may be a single food or ingredient, but sometimes – particularly in IgE-mediated food allergy – many different foods are involved.

In *food allergy* there is reproducible food intolerance, evidence of an abnormal immunological reaction to the food and a plausible mechanism implicating an immunological process. A careful history and often a double-blind placebo-controlled food challenge are necessary to confirm or refute the diagnosis of a food allergic reaction.

Psychologically-based food aversions comprise both psychological avoidance, when the subject avoids food for psychological reasons, and psychological intolerance, which is an unpleasant bodily reaction caused not directly by the food but by emotions associated with the food. Psychological intolerance normally does not occur when the food is given in an unrecognizable form.

Diagnostic approaches
Elimination diets and challenge studies

The relationships between exposure to certain foods and patient symptoms can be examined through the use of elimination diets and provocation tests. The most robust approach involves double-blind placebo-controlled food challenges, using objective measures of response. These might include measures of respiratory function, intestinal permeability tests, and the extent and severity of skin rashes. The effects of eliminating specific foods from a diet can be tested systematically with such objective tests. The most common foods eliciting a reaction are cow's milk, egg, wheat, peanuts and tree nuts, soy, and less often, fish and shellfish.

Laboratory tests for the diagnosis of food intolerance

A number of tests are available to aid in the diagnosis of food intolerance. These involve exposing the individual to selected antigens and examining the short term response, qualitatively and quantitatively. For example:

- *Skin prick tests:* A skin prick test involves the placing of a small amount of a suspected allergen on the skin and introducing it into the epidermis by gently pricking the skin surface. A positive reaction is manifested as the development of a wheal, the diameter of which can be measured to grade the reaction. A positive test can confirm that the patient is atopic.
- *Atopy patch test (APT)*: Atopic eczema in infancy and childhood is often caused or aggravated by common food allergens such as milk, egg and wheat. The APT test involves the application of suspected allergens to the patient's back under a dressing that is allowed to remain in contact with the skin for 48 hours. The area is then visually examined for reddening.
- *Endoscopic studies and intestinal biopsy*: This procedure is often used in patients with a variety of slow-onset gastrointestinal symptoms, such as frequent loose stools or features of unexplained iron deficiency, osteoporosis, weight loss, slow gain in height, and other features of malnutrition. It requires the collection and examination of a small piece of the intestinal lining.

Presenting features of food intolerance and food allergies

A wide range of conditions in childhood have been associated with food allergies and intolerance including eczema, wheeze, mood changes, epilepsy, failure to thrive, diarrhoea, vomiting and gastrointestinal blood loss. Prevalence estimates for adverse reactions to foods range from 3–7.5% in childhood. The prevalence of food intolerance in adults seems to be lower, but many adults with food allergic reactions have a history of adverse reactions to foods in childhood. Many of the symptoms reported in children are reported in adults, but additionally, there is evidence to suggest that migraine in adults might be linked with food intolerance. Some food-provoked symptoms in adults are gastrointestinal in origin. They include nausea, bloating, abdominal pain, constipation and diarrhoea. These features are similar to those of the irritable bowel syndrome. The symptoms may arise either because of abnormal motility or because an individual has a lower pain threshold to sensations accompanying normal contraction or distension of the gut. Many people who avoid specific foods and have an unsubstantiated self-diagnosis of food allergy suffer from the irritable bowel syndrome.

Approaches to dietary treatment

Symptoms and clinical features may conform to well-recognized phenomena or to a disease associated with a specific food. This will be suspected from the patient's history and confirmed by a small number of tests. Examples include asthma and rhinitis associated with salicylate intolerance; flatus and diarrhoea induced by sugar alcohols such as sorbitol; an increase in milk consumption unmasking a disease presenting in an anaemic child with failure to thrive and a positive family history. In other patients, food intolerance will form part of a wider differential diagnosis. Dietary treatment typically takes the form of elimination of the relevant foods, if they can be identified.

Example of food allergy: milk

Cows' milk is taken as an example of a food that can evoke different reactions, with different underlying mechanisms. Antibodies to cow's milk proteins are found in the sera of most children and about 10–20% of healthy adults. There is, however, a wide spectrum of adverse responses to the consumption of cow's milk in childhood, both in terms of the symptoms and the timing of their appearance, which might be immediate or take over 24 hours to appear.

- *Atopic eczema:* Eczema can occur in exclusively breastfed infants, and this can be due to the transfer of absorbed food antigens from the mother's diet to her milk. Food intolerance and enhanced immune responsiveness to foods are also features of atopic eczema in adults but the antigens concerned are usually fish, shellfish, eggs, peanuts and tree nuts and milk sensitivity does not seem to be important.
- *Cow's milk intolerance with malabsorption syndrome:* The classical milk-induced malabsorption syndrome with a flattened intestinal mucosa and failure to thrive seems to be on the decline. Infants and children are more likely to suffer from vomiting, diarrhoea, eczema, urticaria and angioedema, recurrent otitis and constipation.
- *Cow's-milk-sensitive colitis:* Typically, an infant with food-sensitive colitis presents before the age of 1 year, with loose stools containing mucus and blood. An elimination diet and clinical monitoring with rectal biopsy shows a pattern of improvement similar to that seen clinically. These infants respond well to elimination of the cow's milk from their diet or from the mother's diet if they are still breastfed. Most children can tolerate cows' milk by the age of 2–3 years.

Treatment of milk allergy

The treatment of cow's-milk-induced allergic systems is the complete elimination of milk and of milk-derived products. Extensively hydrolysed infant formulae are tolerated by a high proportion of infants who suffer from the less severe form but amino acid based formulae are used in more severe cases.

Lactose intolerance

Lactose is a disaccharide which is exclusively present in milk and milk products, where it is the main sugar. It is a major source of energy in the young infant. Lactose is hydrolysed in the small intestine by a lactase to give glucose and galactose. Galactose is then rapidly converted into glucose in the liver. Lactase activity naturally falls from levels in infancy to adult levels between the ages of 3 and 5 years in 75% of the world's population, while 25% of the population, mainly in the Far East, appears to maintain infant levels of lactase in adulthood.

Adverse reactions to the ingestion of lactose in a lactase-deficient person include nausea, bloating, abdominal pain and diarrhoea. The post-weaning drop in intestinal lactase activity may occur as early as 2 years in some races, or at 5 years in Caucasians, so that schoolchildren occasionally may be intolerant of lactose. Since lactose malabsorption may be the norm in some ethnic groups, lactose malabsorption and even lactose intolerance will often coexist with other diseases. As with other states of food intolerance, the strict diagnosis of lactose intolerance relies on objective measurements of the clinical effects of the withdrawal and reintroduction of lactose. The only effective treatment of lactose intolerance is a diet with low lactose content. Foodstuffs high in lactose, such as fresh milk, powdered milk and milk puddings, should be avoided but most lactose-intolerant patients can tolerate about 10 g of fermented milk products such as yoghurt, in which the lactose content has been reduced. Lactose-reduced milk and milk products are commercially available.

KEY POINTS

- The gastrointestinal tract is the site of digestion and absorption of dietary carbohydrates, fat and protein, and of the absorption of vitamins, minerals and trace elements
- Digestion of nutrients begins in the mouth and continues in the stomach and the small intestine; the products of digestion are absorbed mainly in the duodenum and jejunum
- The gastrointestinal tract plays a role in the regulation of feeding, through direct effects, and neural and hormonal signals
- Chronic diseases of the intestine are associated with complex interactions between diet, the intestinal microflora and intestinal mucosal immunity
- Diet may be of significant value in modifying intestinal damage and the clinical course of these diseases
- Manipulation of the gastrointestinal flora may provide a way of treating these disorders
- Some foods elicit adverse reactions described in terms of allergy or intolerance
- Food intolerance and allergy can be difficult to diagnose and treat

FURTHER READING

Bender D A 2008 Introduction to nutrition and metabolism, 4th edn. CRC Press, Boca Raton, FL

Brostoff J, Challacombe S 2002 Food allergy and intolerance, 2nd edn. WB Saunders, London

Camilleri M, Spiller R 2002 Irritable bowel syndrome diagnosis and treatment. WB Saunders, Edinburgh

Ma T, Verkman A S 1999 Aquaporin water channels in gastrointestinal physiology. Journal of Physiology 517:317–326

Thomas B 2001 Manual of dietetic practice, 3rd edn. Blackwell Science, London

Tortora G, Anagnostakos N P 1990 Principles of anatomy and physiology. Harper and Row, New York, p 760

CHAPTER 11

Diet and Genotype Interactions: Nutritional Genomics

OBJECTIVES

By the end of this chapter you should be able to:

- describe the process of gene expression
- explain how diet can modulate gene expression and how genotype may influence nutrient requirements
- discuss the importance of diet–gene interactions in determining disease risk

11.1 INTRODUCTION

Early studies of nutrient requirements typically sought to characterize the biochemical and clinical effects of nutrient depletion and repletion. More recently the focus has shifted towards an understanding of nutrient intake profiles associated with optimum health. What is clear is that individuals respond differently to the same intake of specific nutrients and that what constitutes adequacy in one person may be inadequate in another. Additionally, dietary intake profiles considered to increase risk of chronic disease are associated with different levels of risk in different individuals. Genetic factors are central to these inter-individual differences. Developments in molecular biology techniques have led to great progress in our understanding of the role of genetic constitution (genotype) in determining individual responses to food. They have also helped us to understand how nutrients affect the way in which the information in genes is used to produce specific proteins, in other words how the genes are expressed (phenotype). The term nutritional genomics is used to describe the study of nutrient–gene interactions.

11.2 A MOLECULAR APPROACH TO UNDERSTANDING NUTRIENT–GENE INTERACTIONS

The principles of gene expression

The information necessary for the synthesis of every individual protein in an organism is encoded by genes along the length of DNA. Large numbers of different genes are linked together and assembled to form chromosomes, the number of which varies from species to species. There are 46 chromosomes in humans and it has been estimated that there are about 25,000 human genes.

In order to understand the way in which proteins can be encoded by DNA it may be useful to refer again to the structure of DNA and RNA, described in section 4.4, under Protein synthesis. Briefly, DNA is a double helical structure of two polymers of nucleotides, each comprising a sugar, a phosphate and one of four bases (adenine, guanine, cytosine and thymine). The order of bases in a length of DNA codes for the order of amino acids to be incorporated into a protein. This code (the genetic code) is read in groups of three bases (codons). In RNA the sugar is ribose, rather than deoxyribose, and RNA contains the base uracil instead of the thymine in DNA. In the cell nucleus the synthesis of a particular protein is directed by the sequence of bases on a specific region of DNA which acts as a template to transcribe the sequence of bases into a complementary strand of messenger RNA (mRNA). This is possible because pairs of bases can form specific bonds with one another, namely adenine with thymine and cytosine with guanine (Fig 11.1). Transcription produces a molecule of mRNA, which is transferred from the nucleus to the cytoplasm. The information in the mRNA is then translated (used to specify the sequence of amino acids) into a polypeptide, a process that takes place on ribosomes. Once the polypeptide chain of a protein has been synthesized it will fold into its three-dimensional structure and may undergo further post-translational modifications to the fully functional protein (Fig 11.2).

Regulation of gene expression

Regulation of gene expression by nutrients and other factors can, in principle, occur at any level from the initial transcription of genomic DNA through to the final modifications of the finished protein product.

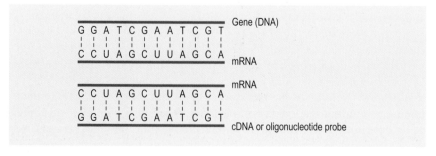

Figure 11.1 Coding of mRNA from DNA and complementarity of cDNA, or oligonucleotide, probes in the detection of mRNAs.

Transcriptional and post-transcriptional regulation

The primary control of gene regulation occurs at transcription by acting on the regulatory promoter region of the gene. The promoter consists of short lengths of bases (motifs) in the gene, which are recognized by specific proteins called transcription factors, defined as proteins that are required to initiate or regulate transcription. These transcription factors bind to the DNA and exert their influence on transcriptional activity. Nutrients can either have a direct influence on the transcription factors by acting as ligands, or indirectly by influencing the expression of other transcription factors, which in turn bind to the target gene promoter.

Retinol (vitamin A) provides a good example of how a nutrient can influence transcription. Once in its target cell, retinol is converted to isoforms of retinoic acid which are transferred to the nucleus and act as ligands for the transcription factors, retinoic acid receptor (RAR) and retinoic X receptor (RXR). These transcription factors bind to a part of DNA called the retinoic acid response element (RARE), found in a number of genes, and thereby increase transcription of these genes (see chapter 5, section 5.3).

Post-transcriptional regulation is evident where changes in the cytoplasmic levels of mRNA are observed without any corresponding changes in the

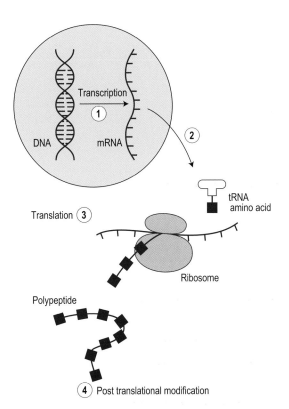

Figure 11.2 (1) Synthesis of single-stranded messenger RNA (mRNA). (2) Movement of mRNA into cytoplasm, binding to ribosome. (3) Transfer RNA (tRNA) molecules carry specific amino acids to the ribosome, in an order determined by the codon sequence on mRNA. (4) Polypeptide chain is released from the ribosome, and may undergo chemical modification.

transcription rates. This can occur at any one of a number of levels, including RNA synthesis, mRNA transport into the cytoplasm and mRNA stability. One example of post-transcriptional regulation of a gene by a nutrient is the effect of iron on transferrin receptor expression. When intracellular iron levels are low, iron regulatory proteins are increased (up-regulated) and bind to the mRNA of the transferrin receptor, thereby increasing stability, and more protein is synthesized.

Translational and post-translational regulation

The process of translation from mRNA to protein can also be influenced by various factors. For example, translation of the iron storage protein, ferritin, is inhibited when iron status is low; the converse is true when iron status is high. Once released from the ribosome, a developing protein can undergo further chemical modifications such as phosphorylation, which will result in changes in the biological function or activity of the protein. This is termed post-translational regulation.

11.3 METHODS AND TOOLS USED TO STUDY NUTRIENT–GENE INTERACTIONS

Measurement of gene expression

All genes are present in the nucleus of each cell of the body but cellular function is determined by which of these genes are active and there are distinct tissue and cell specific gene expression patterns. For example, the insulin gene is expressed in the β-cells of the pancreas and not in adipocytes or hepatocytes. Similarly, the pattern of genes expressed changes during development, and in response to environmental stress as well as to diet and to other stimuli.

Expression of a gene is measured by the detection and measurement of the corresponding mRNA. Tissues or cells may therefore be screened to assess whether a particular gene is expressed, or is being expressed at a particular point in time and which factors influence the expression of that gene.

Three main techniques are available for detecting mRNAs: northern blotting, the ribonuclease protection assay and the reverse transcription polymerase chain reaction (RT-PCR). In northern blotting, RNA extracted from a tissue is separated on the basis of molecular size by electrophoresis on gels and the mRNA of interest identified using a specific probe (piece of DNA or RNA corresponding to the gene of interest labelled radioactively or with other detectable molecule that will bind to the DNA or RNA and allow detection). In the ribonuclease (RNase) protection assay, extracted RNA is incubated with a probe targeted to the specific mRNA and the enzyme ribonuclease A. When the probe is bound to the target mRNA the duplex cannot be digested by the enzyme, and can be detected following gel electrophoresis. RT-PCR is the most sensitive of these methods. It uses a complementary DNA (cDNA) sequence specific to the mRNA of interest and the polymerase chain reaction (system for in vitro amplification of DNA) is then used to produce multiple DNA copies of the original mRNA. The PCR product is separated and identified by electrophoresis.

The expression of a very large number of genes simultaneously can be assessed using DNA microarrays, in which thousands of mRNAs can be detected at the same time using labelled probes to specific mRNAs.

Proteomics

Although the study of genomics (study of the entire genome or genetic composition) is hugely informative in that it tells us what the potential is for protein synthesis in a cell, it does not tell us what proteins are actually present. Proteomics (study of the proteins produced) allows specific patterns of gene expression to be measured at the protein level. The proteome *(PROTein complement expressed by a genOME)* is normally defined as all the proteins that are present in a particular cell/tissue/organism at a particular time. In proteomics, proteins extracted from tissue samples or from cells are separated by gel electrophoresis carried out in two dimensions and localized by staining and image analysis. Individual protein species can then be identified by mass spectrometry.

Transgenics

The term transgenics describes the integration of a gene from one species into the genomic DNA of another organism. This technology can provide important information about the effects of a specific gene on the metabolism and the phenotype of an organism. Techniques are also available to allow us to determine the effects of deletion or 'knock-out' of a specific gene on the function of a tissue or an organism.

RNA interference

Naturally occurring, short stretches of double-stranded RNA molecules are capable of regulating the expression of many genes within a cell and are involved in fundamental processes such as growth and development. Synthetic RNA molecules can be designed for specific genes to study the effects of preventing the expression of the target gene in a particular cell.

11.4 EFFECTS OF NUTRIENTS ON GENE EXPRESSION

Nutrient effects on gene expression can be transmitted indirectly, via hormones for example, or directly, as in the effects of retinoic acid on transcription described earlier. The most obvious changes in response to nutritional state are those associated with fasting and subsequent refeeding. Thus the expression of many genes encoding nutrient transporters and hormones, as well as enzymes involved in metabolic pathways, may be altered on fasting and refeeding. For example, the expression of leptin and of fatty acid synthase is suppressed on fasting and reactivated on refeeding. In addition, particular nutrients such as carbohydrates and lipids may have specific effects.

Thus switching from a high carbohydrate to a high fat diet leads to the suppression of genes encoding proteins associated with fatty acid synthesis while the expression of genes involved in gluconeogenesis is activated (see chapter 4).

The mammalian intestine undergoes major adjustments during its development, particularly at weaning, when the high protein milk diet of relatively constant composition is replaced by a diet of variable composition. Individual nutrients influence the expression of the genes encoding digestive enzymes and specific transporters. For example, monosaccharides such as glucose and fructose increase the number of transporter molecules present in the brush border membrane of gastrointestinal mucosal cells in order to optimize absorption when these nutrients are introduced into the diet.

In recent years, evidence has accumulated to support a link between fetal nutritional status and adult morbidity and mortality. This is known as the 'fetal origins' hypothesis which states that inappropriate nutritional status in the mother at critical times during fetal development can result in disproportionate fetal growth, with the programming of the adult onset of several diseases including coronary heart disease, type 2 diabetes and hypertension. Such a phenomenon implies a long-term programming of gene expression in response to fetal nutritional status.

11.5 POLYMORPHISMS AND THEIR EFFECTS ON NUTRIENT METABOLISM

The most abundant and simplest form of variation in genotype between individuals is a result of mutations at individual points along the DNA sequence, termed single nucleotide polymorphisms (SNPs, pronounced 'snips'). Some polymorphisms do not lead to changes in the amino acid encoded, while others do, which means that some SNPs are more likely to influence protein function than others. Those that do alter protein function are often associated with an inborn error of metabolism, such as phenylketonuria, or glycogen storage disease. The consumption of special diets can usually alleviate the patient's condition.

Most common diseases such as diabetes, obesity and cardiovascular disease are a consequence of complex interactions between multiple genes and environmental/lifestyle factors, particularly diet and physical activity. An individual's susceptibility to such diseases is determined in part by their exact genetic make-up, specifically their SNP profile. For this reason it can be useful to examine associations between SNPs in particular genes, diet, and common diseases.

MTHFR C677T

One example of a common polymorphism that is thought to interact with diet in determining disease risk occurs in the gene expressing the enzyme 5,10-methylenetetrahydrofolate reductase (MTHFR). This enzyme is involved in generating 5-methyltetrahydrofolate, which is central to the metabolism of the amino acid homocysteine. A common SNP referred to as C677T leads to a reduced activity of this enzyme and an increase in plasma homocysteine, which may be a risk factor for cardiovascular disease. Furthermore, people who are homozygous for this polymorphism seem to have a lower risk of colorectal cancer. Importantly, the effects of the polymorphism are observed most readily in people who have a low dietary intake of folate.

Vitamin D receptor (VDR)

In the form of cholecalciferol, vitamin D exerts its biological activity, principally the maintenance of calcium homeostasis to assist in the growth and integrity of bone. To elicit its biological activity it binds to the vitamin D receptor, VDR. A number of mutations of the VDR gene have been identified which are associated with loss of function of the receptor and which result in hereditary vitamin D-resistant rickets.

11.6 DIET, GENOTYPE AND SUSCEPTIBILITY TO DISEASE: THE EXAMPLE OF OBESITY

It is well accepted that interactions between genotype, diet, and other environmental factors are central to disease susceptibility in individuals. Obesity is a good example of such a disease and one in which nutritional genomics has had some early successes. The immediate environmental determinants of obesity include diet and physical activity. Easy access to cheap, palatable, high fat 'fast foods' and increasingly sedentary lifestyles are overwhelming our genetically determined regulatory mechanisms for energy balance.

There are several single gene mutations in laboratory animals which lead to frank obesity – *ob*, *db*, *fat*, *tub* and agouti genes in mice, and the *fa* gene in the rat, and these have proved invaluable in obesity research. Studies in such animal models have made an important contribution to our understanding of the role of leptin in energy balance regulation. This hormone, synthesized predominantly in white adipose tissue, has a central function in the control of appetite (which is inhibited) and energy expenditure (which is stimulated). Mutations in the leptin gene or in its receptor result in either no protein product at all or an abnormally functioning protein, and such effects are associated with obesity in animal models or humans. However, polymorphisms in specific genes or clusters of genes are likely to be of greater importance to the generality of obesity in the human population. It is also likely that dietary factors modulate the effects of specific polymorphisms.

11.7 PERSONALIZED NUTRITION

Given the fact that interactions between diet and genotype influence nutrient handling, flux through metabolic pathways, and risk of important diseases, there is current interest in the possible value of customized dietary advice to individuals. The concept is that specific dietary advice would take into account genotype and lifestyle and thereby optimize health and minimize disease risk. It remains to be seen whether this 'personalized nutrition' approach can substantially impact on the nation's health.

KEY POINTS

- Nutritional genomics, or *nutrigenomics*, describes the study of interactions between individuals and diet at the level of the genome and its protein products
- Nutrients can influence gene transcription by interacting with transcription factors, and by interactions at the post-transcriptional, translational and post-translational levels
- The most common form of genetic variation between individuals is the result of single base changes along the DNA sequence, termed single nucleotide polymorphisms (SNPs)
- Interactions between genotype and environment are central to disease risk in an individual
- Personalized nutrition describes the use of specific dietary advice to individuals, taking into account genotype and lifestyle

FURTHER READING

Bender D A 2008 Introduction to nutrition and metabolism, 4th edn. CRC Press, Boca Raton, FL

Lucock M 2007 Molecular nutrition and the ascent of humankind. Wiley Blackwell, Oxford

Tyers M, Mann M 2003 From genomics to proteomics. Nature 422:193–197

CHAPTER 12

Nutritional Epidemiology and Nutritional Assessment

12.1 EPIDEMIOLOGY

OBJECTIVES

By the end of this section you should be able to:

- define nutritional epidemiology
- summarize its aims and limitations
- outline the concepts of population, exposure, outcome and epidemiological effect
- define validity and repeatability
- interpret results of a study taking into account possible effects of bias, chance and confounding, and the question of generalizability
- summarize criteria for assessing evidence of causality
- explain the main features of different epidemiological study designs, including their strengths and weaknesses

Introduction to the science of epidemiology

Epidemiology is the study of the distribution and causes of disease in populations. It addresses the following type of questions: Why is breast cancer more common in the US than in Japan? Can diets rich in fruit and vegetables reduce blood pressure? Do dietary differences explain social gradients in cardiovascular disease mortality?

In public health and health promotion, epidemiology is important both to provide knowledge for action and to evaluate the effect of interventions. This chapter describes the basic concepts of epidemiology, important aspects to consider when interpreting results, and the most common study types – with examples from nutritional epidemiology.

Important concepts in epidemiology
The population at risk

The population of interest for a particular study is called the population at risk. It can be defined as world regions, countries or districts, but often by specific demographic characteristics such as age and gender, or by very specific characteristics such as the children of mothers that used vitamin A supplements during pregnancy.

The outcome

In epidemiological studies, the term outcome or endpoint refers to the disease or health-related variable being studied. Outcome measures are typically either binary or continuous variables. For example if the endpoint of interest is death, the outcome variable will be binary with two groups (dead and alive), or a population can be divided into diseased versus non-diseased, giving cases (dead or diseased) as opposed to controls (alive or non-diseased). Many of the important outcomes in nutritional epidemiology are on the other hand continuous measures with a continuum of severity rather than an 'all or none' phenomenon, such as blood pressure or body weight.

- *Incidence* is defined as the number of new cases appearing in the study population during a specified period of time. If a population of 100,000 people saw 190 cancer cases over a period of one year, the cancer incidence would be 0.0019 per person year, or 1.9 cancer cases per 1000 person years.
- *Prevalence* is the proportion of a population that is cases at a given point in time. It is a paradox that efforts to improve the survival of those with a disease without curing it will increase the prevalence.

Mortality rates are a special form of incidence rates – the incidence of death – and can have different forms: crude mortality rates relate to the population as a whole. Mortality rates for specific groups, most commonly by gender and age, contribute to a better understanding of death rates. Box 12.1 provides definitions of these terms.

The exposure

An exposure is any factor suspected to modify the risk of the outcome of interest. Exposures include a broad range of factors, from microbiological or chemical agents to all kinds of physical, social or psychological variables. Common exposures in nutritional epidemiology include nutrients, foods or food patterns, and socioeconomic variables.

Many diseases, such as coronary heart diseases and cancer, have a long lag between the onset of the relevant exposure to manifest stages of the disease. This is called the latency period. The relevant dietary exposure affecting the risk of developing cancer may therefore be 10–20 years before the cancer is diagnosed. Without historical data on past exposures, it is sometimes assumed that measurements at a later period may serve as reasonable alternatives, and if dietary habits are stable over time present food intakes certainly can give some indication of intakes in the past. Recall of past exposures

> **Box 12.1** Definitions of incidence, prevalence and mortality rates
>
> **Incidence** =
>
> $$\frac{\text{Number of new cases}}{\text{Total person time at risk}}$$
>
> **Prevalence** =
>
> $$\frac{\text{Number of existing cases at one point in time}}{\text{Population at same place and time}}$$
>
> **Crude death rate** =
>
> $$\frac{\text{Number of deaths (defined place and time)}}{\text{Mid period population (same place and time)}}$$
>
> **Age specific death rate** =
>
> $$\frac{\text{Number of deaths to people in a particular age group (defined place and time)}}{\text{Mid period population (age group, same place and time)}}$$
>
> **Cause-specific death rate** =
>
> $$\frac{\text{Number of deaths due to a particular cause (defined place and time)}}{\text{Mid period population (same place and time)}}$$

is often problematical and so measurements of current exposures are preferred as they are much more amenable to quality control.

In an experiment where an exposure is assigned to the participants, the exposure is often called an intervention. Usually this is hypothesized to be a protective factor such as a treatment or a drug as it would be unethical to expose participants to suspected harmful factors other than over very short periods.

Measures of association and effect

Various statistical methods are used to measure the association between exposure and outcome. For example, relative risk (abbreviated RR) is the measure of effect most commonly used when both the exposure and the outcome are binary variables. This is given by the ratio of risk, or incidence, in the exposed group to the risk in the unexposed group. A relative risk of one indicates that there is no difference in incidence between the exposed and the unexposed. When the relative risk is higher than one, the exposure poses a hazard; while a relative risk lower than one means that the exposure is protective. Another commonly used measure is the attributable risk (AR) which is the incidence among the exposed minus the incidence among the non-exposed.

The odds ratio (abbreviated OR) is an alternative to relative risk. The term *odds* refers to probability based on a ratio rather than a proportion. An example is obesity (the exposure) and gestational diabetes (the outcome). If 50 of 100

Table 12.1 Calculating relative risk (RR), attributable risk (AR) and odds ratio (OR)

	Cases	**Non-cases**	**Total**
Exposed	a	b	a + b
Non-exposed	c	d	c + d
Total	a + c	b + d	

$RR = Risk_{exposed}/Risk_{unexposed} = [a/(a + b)]/[c/(c + d)]$

$AR = Risk_{exposed} - Risk_{unexposed} = [a/(a + b)] - [c/(c + d)]$

$OR = (a/c)/(b/d) = ad/bc$

women with gestational diabetes were obese the odds of obesity among the diabetics are 50:50 (odds = 1), while if 20 of 100 non-diabetics were obese the odds of obesity among the non-diabetics are 20:80 (odds = 0.25). The odds ratio is calculated by dividing the odds of exposure among the cases by the odds of exposure in the non-cases, here:

$$(50:50)/(20:80) = 1/0.25 = 4$$

The odds of being obese among the women with gestational diabetes are therefore four times greater than among the healthy women (see Table 12.1).

Quality of the measurements

The foundation of any scientific study is valid and reproducible measurements. Poorly measured variables, either exposure or outcome, can lead to misleading results and incorrect conclusions. Validity is an expression of the degree to which a measurement assesses the aspect it is intended to measure. The goal for most studies is to generate results that have a wider application beyond the study participants, in other words to get results that are *generalizable* to the whole population at risk. The generalizability of a study is the same as the *external validity*.

Interpretation of results

If an association between exposure and an outcome is observed, this may be due to four different reasons: bias, chance, confounding or a true causal relationship.

Bias

Bias refers to measurement errors or misclassification that lead to results that consistently deviate from the truth. There are many sources of bias that fit into two broad categories: selection bias and information bias.

For example a group of people is invited to participate, but only a subset is willing to take part. Participants who volunteer to take part in studies are likely to be more educated and health conscious than the general population and therefore not fully representative of the study population – the results may misrepresent the true disease burden. An example of information bias is that obese subjects tend to underestimate their energy intake more than non-obese subjects do, and so self-reports of diet in a study of obesity are likely to be biased.

The role of chance

When is a difference most likely to be caused by chance? Chance cannot be eliminated, but statistics provide measures to quantify the element of chance and account for the uncertainty in the results of a study, such as hypothesis testing, significance testing and confidence interval.

Confounding

A confounder is any factor that can cause or prevent the outcome of interest and at the same time is associated with the exposure in a way that distorts the observed exposure–outcome association. For example, the relationship between bladder cancer and coffee drinking can be due to another risk factor for this type of cancer that is also associated with coffee intake. Smokers are more likely to be heavy coffee drinkers and if smoking was the real risk factor for bladder cancer, it is called a confounder, producing spurious effects or hiding real ones.

Confounding can often be adjusted for. In the example above, the data could be analysed separately for smokers and non-smokers.

Causality

Smoking as a risk factor for lung cancer produces one of the strongest relative risks demonstrated for any lifestyle disease, although causation can rarely be proven without doubt. Epidemiology has to be considered together with other types of evidence, such as laboratory-based studies. A set of criteria proposed by Sir Austin Bradford Hill is often used to judge whether one or a series of studies strongly suggests a causal association between a risk factor or intervention and an outcome. These are:

- *Strength* of the association
- *Consistency* of studies
- *Specificity* (ie one particular exposure always should lead to a specific disease but this criterion is probably less relevant as many diseases have multiple causes and some factors contribute to more than one condition)
- *Temporal sequence of cause and effect*
- *Biological gradient* (where the risk increases or decreases progressively with higher exposure)
- *Biological plausibility and coherence*
- *Experiment (reversibility)* (when reducing a factor that increases the disease risk gives a corresponding drop in disease risk)

Epidemiological studies have contributed considerably to present scientific understanding of the relationships between dietary habits, social factors (including cultural and psychological determinants), and health. The failure to demonstrate associations between diet and disease may in many instances be due to the imprecision of the measures of diet rather than to the absence of an association.

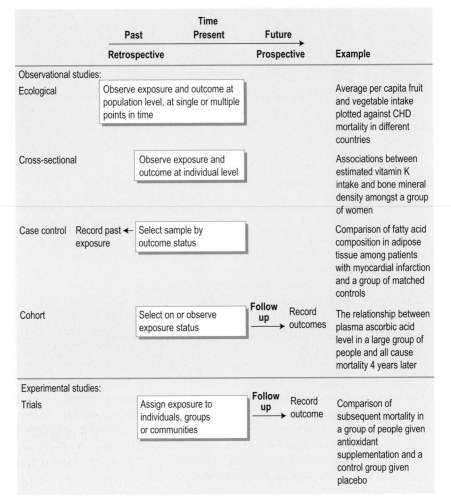

Figure 12.1 A schematic overview of epidemiological study designs and their main characteristics.

Epidemiological study designs

Figure 12.1 gives a schematic overview of the main study designs. Study designs differ according to whether the researchers observe natural processes (observational studies) or are attempting to influence the exposure (experimental studies), and according to the time order of collecting information in exposure and outcome, either at the same time or with a time difference.

Observational study designs

These include:

- *Ecological studies* in which the exposure and outcome measures are matched at a group or population level instead of at the individual level, either between populations or in the same population compared over time.
- *Cross-sectional studies* in which both the outcome and exposure status are determined simultaneously, and so it is impossible to distinguish if one

appeared before the other. For example if it is found that people with high blood cholesterol eat more low fat foods than the general population, this may be due to a dietary change following diagnosis.

- *Case-control studies* in which patients that have developed a specific disease or condition (the cases) are compared with healthy controls who are representative of the population these cases come from (the controls).
- *Cohort studies* in which a group of people is followed over time to record which individuals develop the outcome of interest, usually a disease or a cause-specific death.

Experimental study designs

- *Randomized controlled trials* assess the effects of an intervention or treatment by comparing it with an established treatment or placebo (inactive treatment).
- *Community intervention studies* with interventions designed to promote health at the community level, using mass media, supermarkets, workplaces or other settings believed to offer cost-effective means of influencing population behaviour. Such intervention studies may involve a control group, or consist of an uncontrolled before-and-after design.

Systematic reviews

With the ever-increasing flow of newly published articles, gathering and evaluating the evidence is a massive task for any researcher, not to mention health practitioners. Systematic reviews summarize the results of similar studies. Meta-analysis is a sub-category of systematic reviews. Results from several independent studies are combined and analysed. When meta-analyses are well conducted, they provide an unbiased and more precise estimate of the effect of interest. The Cochrane Collaboration (http://www.cochrane.org/) was founded in 1993 with an aim 'to help people make well-informed decisions about health care by preparing, maintaining and ensuring accessibility to systematic reviews'. The main emphasis of the Cochrane Collaboration is on the effects of health care interventions.

Nutritional epidemiology

Epidemiology has expanded from its early focus on infectious diseases into the aetiology of chronic diseases, which are characterized by low incidence, long latency periods and multiple causes. Although dietary aspects are very relevant exposures to consider for chronic diseases, there are two groups of challenges that are particularly important in nutritional epidemiology:

- the complex nature of diet as exposure
- the difficulties in measuring this exposure.

Diet is not a simple behavioural variable such as smoking, but a series of variables, including nutrients, non-nutrients, single food items and food groups. Recently, increased attention has also been given to physical characteristics of a food, meal composition and food patterns, just adding to this list of exposure variables to consider. Dietary variables are also very challenging to analyse because these are strongly correlated; for instance, persons with a high intake of vitamin C often also have high intakes of fibre, β-carotene and other antioxidants. This is because foods rich in one nutrient may be rich in other nutrients.

Dietary determinants of disease are often risk factors; they increase the probability that a particular disease or malign condition will develop. To widen the range of exposure to study, investigators often seek to select populations with diverse diets, for instance by including special groups within a population such as vegetarians or by studying diet–disease relationships across different countries. Nutrient intake–outcome relationship may be complicated by intermediate factors such as biological availability. Some of the variability in results can be explained by particular genotypes having different responses to exposures from the rest of the population. The other main challenge is the difficulty in measuring any dietary variable. Diets vary from day to day and change over time and the composition of foods also varies over time so that to get a true average of dietary habits over time, it is necessary to repeat measurements.

Considerable effort has been put into developing biomarkers of dietary intake. Biochemical measures are objective compared to self-reporting of diets and could potentially replace dietary assessment methods. Such markers are measurements of nutrients in different body fluids and tissues that can be related to dietary intakes but many biomarkers are expensive to use in large populations and are still not an alternative to dietary assessment methods in many observational epidemiological studies.

KEY POINTS

- Population is the population of interest for a particular study question
- Outcome is the disease or health-related variable being studied
- Exposure is any factor that may influence the risk of the outcome
- Measure of association and effect is the quantified relationship between exposure and outcome
- Validity is the degree to which a measurement assesses the aspect it is intended to measure
- Reproducibility is the degree to which a measurement produces the same result when used repeatedly under given conditions
- An observed exposure–outcome association can be due to four factors: bias, chance, confounding or a true causal relationship
- Bias – systematic deviation of results from the truth – takes two main forms: selection bias (related to the sample) and information bias (related to the data)
- Chance – random variation may produce a plausible or implausible finding

- Confounding – confusion between two processes – may distort study findings
- Causality can rarely be proven, but if bias, chance and confounding have been considered and the Hill criteria are broadly met, then causal inference is appropriate
- The essential question a study seeks to answer guides the decisions regarding the study sample, how exposure and outcome are measured and the preferred study design
- The external validity (generalizability) of a study depends on its design and execution
- Observational study designs (ecological studies, cross-sectional studies, case-control studies and cohort studies) permit examination of the world as it is, including its hazards
- Experimental studies (trials) are powerful tools for testing health-related hypotheses (usually treatment or prevention)
- The effects of diet can be studied at a number of levels: nutrients, non-nutrients, foods and food patterns
- Dietary variables are strongly interrelated. It may be difficult to single out the relevant variable
- Between-population comparisons offer a useful means for investigating dietary effects on health by widening the range of exposures

12.2 NUTRITIONAL ASSESSMENT

OBJECTIVES

On completion of this section, you should be able to:

- summarize the purposes for which each of the currently-used measures of nutritional status has been developed, and the scope of their individual usefulness and their limitations
- outline the broad choices of different types of available measures, comprising (a) dietary estimation; (b) anthropometric measurements; (c) biochemical status indices; and, to a lesser extent, (d) functional and clinical evidence of adequacy
- summarize the common criteria for usefulness and reliability of these indices and measures, and list some of the common pitfalls that must be avoided during planning, practical work and interpretation
- understand why dietary assessment needs to be carried out
- describe the various methods of dietary assessment used at national, household and individual level
- appreciate the strengths and weaknesses of the different approaches to dietary assessment at national, household and individual level
- recognize the contexts in which it is appropriate to use specific methods

- understand how to take into account the measurement errors associated with dietary assessment when interpreting results from dietary surveys
- understand the different uses of various anthropometric measures used to assess nutrition status
- understand the equipment used and techniques of measurement
- appreciate how inaccuracies in recording can be minimized
- understand the use of measurements to calculate indices of nutritional status
- compare the measurements and indices to the most appropriate reference
- summarize the available choices of tissue and body fluid samples that may be selected and collected for biochemical status assessment
- describe common problems of interpretation of biochemical markers
- describe the inter-relationships between the biochemical and other indices of nutritional status, to be used in conjunction with each other for a composite and integrated picture of status and nutritional adequacy.

Introduction to nutritional assessment methods

Measures of nutritional status are usually valuable as they may be predictive of health outcomes. The major categories of nutritional assessment include: (a) dietary, (b) anthropometric, (c) biochemical status and (d) functional and clinical status.

In this section, the main focus will be on the first three categories, although the importance of category (d) is always implicit in the discussion. The functional tests are most useful as research tools to investigate causal links, whereas the biochemical indices are most useful in population surveys and individual nutritional investigations. Clinical signs may be less specific for particular nutrients than are biochemical tests.

One of the most important growth areas in current nutritional research effort is the development of useful 'intermediate markers' between diet and health outcomes, since many of the latter may develop over long periods, and indeed over a lifetime.

Dietary assessment
The objectives of dietary assessment

The exact purpose of the assessment, what is to be measured, in whom, over what time period, and how the measurements are to be collected will determine which technique is most appropriate for a given purpose.

Methods of dietary assessment

There are five stages at which food availability and consumption can conveniently be measured (Fig 12.2) – these range from national statistics to

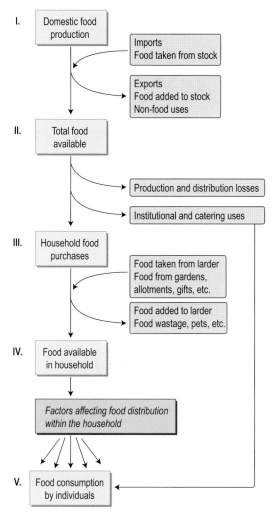

Figure 12.2   Points in the food supply chain at which it is convenient to measure food availability or consumption.

individual consumption. Information from the finer levels of measurement (individual, household or institution) can be built up to provide a picture of consumption at regional or national level.

Assessment at regional or national level

Domestic food production (I)

Most governments require farmers and food producers to report how much food they produce. This is part of ongoing food surveillance which provides an overview of the adequacy of the national food supply.

Total food available (II)

Of far greater usefulness in estimating a country's food supply are food balance data (or 'food disappearance data' or 'consumption level estimates') published by the United Nations Food and Agriculture Organization (FAO) and then summarized in longer time series. These values reflect domestic food production plus imported food (including food aid), food taken from storage, minus food exported or added to stocks or used for non-food purposes (eg sugar used in the brewing industry, grain fed to livestock). When the totals are divided by the number of people in the population, the result is expressed as food 'available' per person. It is also possible to estimate the nutrient content of the food available and to estimate the availability of energy and nutrient per person. These data are widely used for making comparisons between countries to learn about the extent of hunger at the national level (see chapter 13) as well as the relationships between diet and disease. The data are limited in that: they provide an estimate for the country as a whole, not for different population groups; no account is taken of waste or losses of food; the consumption estimates give higher values than those derived from other types of surveys.

Assessment at household level (III and IV)

There are four main techniques used to assess food consumption at the household level: food accounts, inventories, household recall, and list recall.

Food accounts

The main food provider is asked to keep a record of either the quantity or cost (or both) of all household food acquisitions (purchases, gifts, food from gardens or allotments, payments in kind, takeaway foods eaten at home, etc). In Britain, the National Food Survey (NFS) was conducted annually for over half a century from 1950 to March 2001. Since April 2001, the data have been collected in the Expenditure and Food Survey. This combines the former NFS and Family Expenditure Survey. The latter provided much more detailed socioeconomic and demographic data about each household than the NFS, and the new survey allows for better analysis in relation to variations in household characteristics.

Inventory method

This is similar in nature to the food account method, in that respondents are asked to keep records of all foods coming into the house. In addition, a larder inventory is carried out at the beginning and end of the survey period. The method has the advantages of providing a direct measure of the amount of food and nutrients available for consumption within a single household.

Household record

The foods available for consumption (whether raw or processed) are weighed, or estimated in household measures, allowing for preparation waste (eg discarded outer leaves, peel, trimmed fat, etc). Any food consumed by visitors is estimated and subtracted from the total, and an allowance is made for food waste (food prepared but not consumed), either by collecting the waste directly (which is likely to underestimate the true waste) or by estimating the proportion of the total prepared food believed to be wasted. The technique is useful in countries where much of the diet is home produced.

List recall

This is a structured survey in which the respondent is asked to recall the amount and cost of food obtained for household use over a given period, usually one week. In addition to food purchases and acquisitions, it takes into account the use of food. It can therefore be used to provide an estimate of food costs as well as net household consumption of both foods and nutrients. The technique is well suited to populations in which most food is purchased rather than home-produced. It is relatively quick and cheap, as it requires only a single interview. Problems persist concerning foods eaten away from home, consumption of food by visitors, and distribution of nutrients within families.

Assessment at the level of the individual (V)

There are two main approaches to individual dietary assessments, prospective and retrospective. Prospective methods involve collecting or recording current diet, while retrospective methods require subjects to recall either recent or past diet. Generally speaking, any measurement of diet will be biased in some way by the measurement process itself. There are therefore no entirely objective measures of an individual's food consumption or nutrient intake except in the controlled conditions of a laboratory.

The main advantage of prospective methods is that they provide a direct measure of current diet. Retrospective methods require subjects to recall aspects of their diet. This may involve remembering the type and amount of all individual items consumed over a specified period of time (eg 24-hour recall), or creating a mental construct of 'usual' consumption involving recollection of both the frequency of consumption of specific foods or food groups and the amounts consumed. The main advantages of the retrospective methods are that they are quick to administer compared with prospective methods but many sources of bias affect retrospective dietary assessments, such as memory errors, presence of an observer, daily variation in diet and irregular eating habits (Table 12.2).

Prospective methods

- *Duplicate diet method*: This technique requires subjects to weigh and record their food consumption at the time of eating. At the same time, they weigh and put aside an exact duplicate portion of each food consumed. These samples are then analysed chemically for their energy and nutrient content.
- *Weighed inventory method*: The weighed inventory is one of the most widely used techniques. Subjects keep a record of all food and drink consumed. Each food item is weighed immediately prior to consumption using portable food weighing scales.
- *Household measures technique*: The method is similar to the weighed inventory, except that subjects record portion sizes in household measures (cups, bowls, spoonfuls, etc.) rather than weighing their food

Retrospective methods

- *24-hour recall*: A trained interviewer asks subjects to recall and describe every item of food and drink consumed over exactly 24 hours.

Table 12.2 Strengths and limitations of measurements of individual food consumption

Method	Strengths	Limitations
Prospective methods General features:	Current diet	Labour intensive
	Direct observation of what is eaten	Requires literacy and numeracy skills
	Duration of survey can be varied to meet requirements for precision of estimates of food consumption or nutrient intake	Subjects need to be well motivated
		Usual consumption pattern may change due to:
		– inconvenience of recording
		– choice of foods which are easy to record
		– beliefs about which foods are 'healthy' or 'unhealthy'
		Overweight subjects tend to under-report true consumption levels
		Coding and data entry errors are common
Duplicate diet	Direct analysis of nutrient content of food (not dependent upon food composition tables)	Very expensive
	Required in metabolic balance studies	Intense supervision needed
		Usual diet may not be consumed
Weighed inventory	Widely used, facilitates comparisons between studies	Food composition tables used to estimate nutrient intake
	Precision of portion sizes	
Household measures	No scales needed	Loss of precision compared with weighed inventory
Retrospective methods General features:	Inexpensive	Biases caused by:
		– errors in memory, perception and conceptualization of food portion sizes
		– presence of observer
	Quick	Daily variation in diet not usually assessed
	Lower respondent burden than required for prospective methods	Dependent on regular eating habits
	Can assess current or past diet	Food composition tables used to estimate nutrient intake
Diet history	Assesses 'usual' diet	Over-reporting of foods believed to be 'healthy' (eg fruit)
24-hour recall	Very quick	Prone to underestimate intake due to omissions
	Can be repeated to gain measure of daily variation and improve precision	Single observation provides poor measure individual intake
Food frequency and amount questionnaire	Suitable for large-scale surveys	Requires validation in relation to reference measure
	Can be sent by mail or email	Literacy and numeracy skills needed if self-completed
	Short version can focus on specific nutrients with few food sources	

- *Diet history:* The diet history is used to assess 'usual' diet over the recent past. Typically, an interviewer trained in the diet history technique begins by carrying out a 24-hour recall of diet. This is then elaborated, and subjects are asked to describe the range of foods that would be likely to be consumed, the frequency of their consumption, and typical amounts. Differences between weekdays and weekends are clarified, and seasonal variations elaborated.
- *Food frequency questionnaire:* Food frequency questionnaires (FFQ) are pre-printed lists of foods on which subjects are asked to indicate the typical frequency of consumption and to state in household measures the average amount consumed on the days when the food is eaten.

Anthropometric assessment

Anthropometry is a relatively quick, simple, and cheap means of assessment of nutritional status. This involves the physical measurement of some or several aspects of human body size, which, when related to normative values, are taken to be outcomes of nutritional exposure (World Health Organization 1995).

Uses, advantages and limitations

Anthropometry is the most commonly used method of nutritional assessment due to the relative cheapness and portability of equipment needed, the high accuracy and precision relative to dietary methods, and the relatively low level of training required. All of the measurements given in Table 12.3 are appropriate for the assessment of undernutrition, while waist and hip ratios are useful in the assessment of overnutrition.

The most common anthropometric measures of undernutrition in children are weight and height, either individually or combined, relative to reference values. The two preferred indices are height for age and weight for height, since they can be used to discriminate between acute and chronic undernutrition. Although weight for height can be used to assess overnutrition in children, the body mass index (BMI) is now the most widely used measure for this purpose, although it is a less sensitive marker of body fatness than skinfold thickness (see chapter 8).

Types of anthropometric measurements

The most basic measurements, height (or length) and weight, are fundamental to all nutritional anthropometric studies, since they give the simplest measure of attained skeletal size (height or length), and of soft tissue mass (weight). Arm and calf circumferences are used as proxies for soft tissue mass. Decline in height with increasing age among the elderly has been noted in studies throughout the world. Demispan (distance between index–middle finger web and the sternal notch) has been shown to be a reliable and reproducible alternative indicator of stature in the elderly.

Skinfolds are used as proxies for body fatness although they are measures of subcutaneous fatness only. Since body fatness is largely comprised of both subcutaneous and visceral fat, the use of skinfolds assumes that the partitioning

Table 12.3 Recommended measurements for nutritional assessment

Age group (years)	Practical field observations	More detailed observations
0–1	Weight, length	Head and arm circumference, Triceps and subscapular skinfolds
1–5	Weight, length, height, arm circumference	Triceps and subscapular skinfolds
5–20	Weight, height, arm circumference	Triceps, subscapular and medial calf skinfolds Calf circumference
Over 20	Weight and height	Arm and calf circumference Triceps, subscapular and medial calf skinfolds Waist and hip circumferences (overnutrition only) Demispan (elderly subjects)

of subcutaneous to visceral fat does not vary across nutritional states. This assumption is likely to be wrong, given that visceral fat and subcutaneous fat have recently been shown to be biologically distinct.

Waist and hip circumferences gives a composite measure of fatness, both subcutaneous and visceral. Lower limb skinfold and circumference measures are valuable, since it cannot be assumed that measures of the upper body are also representative of the lower body, but these are used mainly for research purposes.

Equipment, standardized methods, indices

The most commonly used item of equipment is the weighing scale, which must have a high degree of accuracy, and should where possible measure to within 10 grams. While beam balances have traditionally fulfilled the criteria of precision and accuracy needed, inexpensive digital bathroom-type scales that have a load cell as sensor are equal in accuracy and precision to the beam balance. The second most common item of equipment is the stadiometer, which is an instrument for measuring height. This can either be attached to a wall, or be a rigid measuring rod, against which subjects can be aligned vertically. With children up to the age of 2 years, the convention is to measure recumbent length using an infant measuring board. Circumference measurements are best carried out using a flexible steel tape, calibrated in centimetres with millimetre gradations. Other types of tape, including cloth and fibreglass tapes, are apt to stretch with repeated use, and therefore become less accurate. Skinfolds can only be measured using skinfold calipers, of which the Harpenden skinfold caliper is the most widely used.

Weight should be measured with the subject wearing the minimum amount of clothing either decently possible or culturally acceptable. The weight of clothing should be subtracted, since this can add at least 0.4 kg to the measurement. Height is measured with the subject's back to the measuring device, feet together, with heels, buttocks and back touching the scale. The head is placed in the Frankfort plane (an imaginary line passing through the external ear canal and across the top of the lower bone of the eye socket, immediately under the eye) the headpiece is brought down onto the head, and the measurement read off the measuring rod. Recumbent length will always give a greater measurement than a standing measurement. Recumbent length is measured in young children either because they are too young to stand, or because they cannot stand still in the appropriate pose long enough for a measurement to be made. Many growth references show discontinuity in values at about 2 years of age, reflecting a difference from recumbent pose to a standing one. Revised references by the World Health Organization correct for this.

Circumferences must be measured with the tape while applying a constant tension, ensuring that there is no indentation of the skin. Either squeezing or slackness will give erroneous measurements. When arm circumference is measured, the arm should be relaxed. The left arm is used by convention, although significant differences between right and left arm have been demonstrated, larger measurements existing in the arm of habitual use. Waist circumference is taken at the narrowest point between the lower costal rib border, and the iliac crest. If there is no narrowing, then the measurement is made at the midpoint between these two landmarks. Hip circumference is made at the level of the greatest posterior protuberance of the buttocks. The gluteal muscles should be relaxed.

Skinfold has the greatest error rate of all anthropometric measurements, and extreme care is needed with this category of measurement. The skinfold site should be carefully located and marked. The right side of the body is always used, irrespective of the handedness of the subject, except where it is not possible to do so because of injury. The skinfold is picked up at the marked site, and is held between the thumb and forefinger, care being taken not to incorporate the underlying muscle tissue in the grasp. This can be difficult to identify, especially in muscular or obese subjects. The calipers are applied about 1 cm above where the skinfold has been grasped; care needs to be taken not to place the calipers either too deeply or too shallow into the skinfold, since this is a major source of potential measurement error.

Among the elderly, demispan is measured by tape, taking the distance between the index–middle finger web and the sternal notch. Among incapacitated adults, recumbent measurements of arm and waist circumferences have good precision and correlation with measurements taken in the standing position. However, hip circumferences are generally lower in the recumbent position, while suprailiac skinfold is less precise.

Accuracy of measurements

Even poorly conducted anthropometry is far more reproducible (precise) and valid (accurate) than the majority of techniques used to measure individual dietary intake. However, there is a need to measure accurately, and be aware of the pitfalls of anthropometry. This set of techniques is more simply carried out than many other measurements of nutritional status, and there is often a tendency to delegate measurement to less-qualified individuals. But all potential anthropometrists should receive adequate training from an expert or supervisor to reach an accessible level of expertise prior to survey, and maintain this level of expertise throughout.

Indices and reference standards for anthropometric nutritional assessment

Adults

The most commonly used measure of undernutrition and overnutrition in adults is the Body Mass Index (BMI) which is calculated from the weight in kilograms divided by the height in metres, squared. Adult undernutrition has been labelled chronic energy deficiency, and BMI cut-offs for this are: 17–18.5, grade I CED; 16–17, grade II CED; below 16, grade III CED. BMI cut-offs of 25, 30 and 40 are used internationally to define mild, moderate, and severe obesity respectively, although various nations may have differently defined criteria. The cut-off of 25 is called overweight by some. In addition, waist circumferences and waist:hip ratio are simple measures of central distribution of body fatness.

Children

Large scale anthropometric surveys associated with public health surveillance in industrialized nations first led to the generation of growth curves for children, and distribution curves for adults, for use in health monitoring. These subsequently came to be used in nutritional assessment globally.

In order to estimate nutritional status of children from anthropometry, values of measurements such as height and weight must be related to normative values. This is done by comparing individual values using percentiles, percentage of the mean or median reference value for age, and/or Z (standard deviation) scores. There is rough correspondence between Z scores, centiles, and percentage of median reference value. As a very general rule of thumb, 90% of median reference value for height for age is roughly similar to the 3rd percentile, and $-2Z$ scores height for age; 80% of median weight for age is roughly equivalent to the 5th percentile, and $-1.5Z$ scores of weight for age; while 80% of median reference value of weight for height is roughly equivalent to the 3rd centile and $-2Z$ scores of weight for height.

The use of growth references developed in industrialized nations for the use of nutritional assessment of individuals in less developed nations has been widely debated. Studies showing that the growth patterns in height of well-fed, healthy preschool children from globally diverse populations are broadly similar have led to the acceptance by the World Health Organization of the United States National Center for Health Statistics 1977 reference curves for height and weight for international use in the late 1970s. A revised international growth reference based on well-off children from six developed and developing countries was published by the World Health Organization in 2007.

Biochemical assessment

Biochemical assessment ideally forms part of a coordinated set of nutritional investigations that may also include diet estimates, anthropometry, functional and clinical investigations. These are used to distinguish between deficiency, adequacy and overload of one or more nutrients.

Biochemical markers of nutritional intake and status

Biochemical markers are specific diagnostic compounds that can be measured in accessible human body fluids and tissues such as blood, urine, saliva, hair and nails. They are selected on the basis that they can be used as predictors for the different levels of nutrient intake and of tissue status adequacy that occur in human individuals and populations. Biochemical markers are potentially useful for the following reasons:

- they can be measured with high specificity, accuracy and objectivity
- they can represent the integral effect of dietary intakes of nutrients from food and supplements over short or long periods of time
- they are usually nutrient-specific and are rapidly responsive to the correction of nutrient deficiencies
- in a few cases such as urinary sodium, potassium, nitrogen, fluoride and iodide, dietary nutrient intakes can be predicted more accurately from biochemical indices than from diet assessment.

Nutrient indices measured, and feasibility of predicting intakes from indices

Many blood and urine nutrients exhibit 24-hour and seasonal cycles, which can be a source of misinterpretation. Therefore, representative surveys need to span a range of collection times. Secular changes over longer time periods, attributable to changing climatic conditions or changing lifestyles, food imports, etc, need to be monitored by periodic or regularly repeated surveys.

The fundamental aim of biochemical monitoring is to define whole body adequacy for specific nutrients. However, the practicalities of assessment limit the researcher to readily-accessible fluids and surface tissues. The relationship between these and the critically-vulnerable internal organs is a complex one. Biochemical status indices for individual nutrients are as follows:

Protein and essential amino acids
There are no good indices for tissue protein status. The most commonly-used index is serum (or plasma) albumin, measured by a dye-based assay, or by a more specific and reliable immunoassay, which is lowered in conditions such as kwashiorkor (see chapter 8) but is also reduced by the acute phase reaction, and severely malnourished children commonly have infections. A more reliable index of inadequate protein supply may be the plasma amino acid profile, since the 'essential' amino acids, notably the branched-chain amino acids, are lowered when dietary protein is inadequate. Protein intakes can be monitored fairly accurately by nitrogen excretion rates.

Essential fatty acid status (and fatty acid profiling)
Although plasma fatty acid concentrations are often used as markers of intake, interpretation is difficult because of diurnal variation; concentration of fatty acids in red blood cell membranes shows a better relationship with intake.

Fat-soluble vitamins
Vitamins A and E are commonly measured in serum or plasma, together with the carotenoid pigments, by high performance liquid chromatography. Plasma

retinol is a good (ie discriminatory) status index only when body stores are low; a high level is indicative of adequate status, but a low level may be a consequence of acute-phase infection/inflammation processes. Plasma vitamin E (tocopherol) levels are usually expressed as a ratio to cholesterol or total lipids, since the vitamin E content of plasma is highly dependent on its lipid content.

Vitamin D status is assessed by the concentration of 25-hydroxyvitamin D in serum or plasma. Levels vary enormously between the seasons and with variable sunlight exposure. Older people in the UK, especially those in institutions such as nursing homes, are especially vulnerable to inadequate status. Their Reference Nutrient Intake (RNI) for adequate status is $10\,\mu g/day$, but few older people in the UK achieve this intake.

Vitamin K status is measured (crudely) by the rate of blood clotting, or more sensitively and specifically by 'PIVKA' (protein induced by vitamin K absence or antagonism) and recently by vitamin K serum or plasma levels, or the degree of under-carboxylation of osteocalcin in plasma.

Water-soluble vitamins

Vitamin C status is usually measured by serum or plasma vitamin C concentrations or (in older studies) by buffy coat (total mixed white cells) vitamin C. The latter is more closely related to body stores and long-term status, but requires a cumbersome assay. Despite confounding influences of acute phase processes in some studies, plasma vitamin C correlates relatively well with recent intakes (~1–2 weeks) of the vitamin from foods and supplements.

Of the B-vitamins, thiamin (B_1), riboflavin (B_2) and pyridoxine (B_6) status levels are commonly assessed by the activation coefficients of specific erythrocyte enzymes that require these vitamins as part of their essential cofactors: transketolase for thiamin; glutathione reductase for riboflavin, and erythrocyte amino acid aminotransferases for the vitamin B_6 coenzymes. For vitamin B_6, plasma pyridoxal phosphate concentration is often preferred. Folate, vitamin B_{12}, biotin and pantothenic acid are commonly assessed by serum or plasma concentrations. Red cell folate is a better index of long-term folate intakes and body-stores than plasma or serum folate are, but it is more difficult to measure. Niacin status is usually assessed by its urinary breakdown products: N-methyl nicotinamide (NMN) or pyridones. Several B vitamins can be assessed by their erythrocyte concentrations, which some investigators now prefer, since they are relatively free from acute phase effects. Several B vitamins have associated functional indices (eg homocysteine or methylmalonic acid) which are discussed below.

Mineral nutrients

Some of the essential minerals can be monitored by 24-hour urine collections (eg Na, K, I, Se); while others are best studied in blood serum or plasma (eg Mg). Some are best studied in relation to their functional effects, such as on bone-related enzymes and turnover markers (eg Ca, P) and the Se-enzyme, glutathione peroxidase, usually in whole blood or red cells (Se). Zn can be assessed by plasma zinc levels, but this index is strongly (negatively) affected by acute phase effects. Plasma analytes (eg thyroid-stimulating hormone, thyroglobulin, T_4 and T_3 thyroid hormones and their ratios) are also indicators of iodine status.

Functional indices

Nutrient-sensitive functional status indices such as plasma homocysteine (for folate, vitamin B_{12} and vitamin B_6 status); plasma methylmalonic acid (for vitamin B_{12} status) and oxidative damage markers (such as malondialdehyde or F2-isoprostanes) which are modulated by the so-called 'antioxidant' nutrients are useful to predict disease risk, or as intermediate end-points for intervention studies.

Acute phase reactions

Blood nutrient levels are influenced by intake and tissue stores, but also the common acute phase reaction (caused by infection and inflammation) which increases or decreases some blood nutrients. It is, therefore, important to avoid making nutrient status measurements when an infection is clearly present as indicated by acute phase proteins such as C-reactive protein.

Markers of dietary intake: inorganic elements, vitamins, macronutrients

Some nutrient related biochemical indices are influenced primarily by the corresponding nutrient intakes, but the majority is not, because variable absorption, homeostatic control or turnover and excretion perturb the intake–status relationships. These can be grouped as follows:

- status measurements that are fairly reliable predictors of intake: eg nitrogen, Na, K, I, F from urinary excretion rates
- the biochemical markers that only predict intake categories (eg high, medium or low) but cannot provide an accurate quantitative estimate of intakes. These include plasma vitamin C and carotenoids; red blood cell levels of B-vitamins
- markers that are generally useless as indicators of intake include plasma levels of many mineral elements, such as calcium, sodium, potassium and copper. By contrast, plasma iron, zinc, magnesium and selenium can provide some useful status information.

In conclusion, biochemical markers of nutrient intakes and tissue status are potentially powerful tools, but are often subject to mis-use and mis-interpretation.

KEY POINTS

- Nutritional status can be assessed using dietary, anthropometric, biochemical and clinical methods
- There is a wide variety of methods for assessing diet. The method chosen should be appropriate for the purpose and circumstances of the work being carried out
- All methods for dietary assessment include errors. It is important not to take the measurements of food consumption and nutrient intake at face value, to understand the likely sources of error and

to appreciate how the errors may influence the interpretation of apparent associations (or apparent lack of associations) between diet and health

- Anthropometry is the most frequently used means of assessing nutrition status of a population and each age group has its own most appropriate anthropometric measures
- The ease of collection of anthropometric measurements should not mask the considerable potential for error in collection
- The measurements are typically compared to those obtained for 'healthy' populations. These normative reference standards are continually being updated and reviewed
- Biochemical indices of nutrient status may, in certain cases, reflect recent intakes, or they may reflect body stores, or a combination of these. They fulfil the need for objective assessments of nutrient adequacy, at the whole body level
- Confounding factors such as homeostatic mechanisms, acute phase effects, uneven distribution of nutrients between body compartments, can confuse interpretation, unless these modulating factors are properly understood and allowed for
- Despite these caveats, carefully-selected and properly-validated biochemical indices provide a powerful and valuable adjunct to other evidence of nutritional adequacy or inadequacy for individuals and populations. They form an essential component of nutritional research, and of public health surveillance programmes
- Clinical assessment, using signs and symptoms, such as the visual characteristics of goitre are outside the scope of this chapter

FURTHER READING

Margetts B M, Nelson M 1997 Design concepts in nutritional epidemiology, 2nd edn. Oxford University Press, Oxford

Willett W 1998 Nutritional epidemiology, 2nd edn. Oxford University Press, New York

Gibson R 1990 Principles of nutritional assessment. Oxford University Press, Oxford

World Health Organization 1995 Physical status: the use and interpretation of anthropometry. WHO Technical Report Series Number 854. WHO, Geneva

WEBSITES

Systematic reviews of health care interventions (Cochrane Collaboration)
http://www.cochrane.org/
World child growth standards
http://www.who.int/childgrowth/en/
Body mass index calculator
http://www.nhsdirect.nhs.uk/magazine/interactive/bmi/index.aspx

CHAPTER 13

Public Health Nutrition

13.1 INTRODUCTION TO PUBLIC HEALTH NUTRITION

The first sections of this chapter review briefly the extent and causes of malnutrition and some of the policy and intervention options available for reducing malnutrition. Direct nutrition interventions have a stated objective of improving nutrition, and indirect interventions or policies may affect nutrition status in important ways but do not necessarily have this as their primary goal. Adequate food supply is one of the essential factors in good nutrition. The subsequent sections describe the world food supply and past trends and future projections of the ability for supply to meet the increased demand caused by population growth and increased affluence, as well as the impact of globalization of food trade and of biotechnology on food security.

13.2 INTRODUCTION TO FOOD AND NUTRITION POLICIES AND INTERVENTIONS

Nutrition policies and interventions are designed to reduce malnutrition in populations. In this chapter the term 'malnutrition' encompasses both undernutrition (due to some combination of food, care and health deprivations) and overnutrition (due to a combination of the excess consumption of some diet components and too little physical exercise). Governments have an important role in the elimination of malnutrition because:

- many services relevant for good nutrition such as nutrition education campaigns are not provided by the private sector
- individual decisions may have a high cost for the community, eg a decision not to get immunized leading to the spread of infection
- they can help to ensure accurate information is available about a food product
- they can ensure equity of distribution such as universal salt iodization or the availability of primary health care.

Democratically elected governments have human rights obligations, including the right to adequate nutrition, and are directly accountable to the populations they serve.

The extent of various types of malnutrition differs between developing and developed countries: general undernutrition and specific vitamin and mineral deficiencies are more prevalent in developing countries, whereas chronic diseases related to poor nutrition, such as obesity, CHD, diabetes, and osteoporosis (sometimes referred to as 'overnutrition' or 'diseases of affluence') are more prevalent in developed countries. For simplicity the term 'overnutrition' is used here although it does not express the compositional imbalance of many diets in affluent countries. However, pockets of undernutrition exist in developed countries and nutrition-related chronic diseases are expanding rapidly in the developing world. Undernutrition and nutrition-related chronic diseases coexist to the greatest extent in countries undergoing rapid socioeconomic and demographic transitions such as the countries of the former Soviet Union. The challenge of balancing interventions to address under- and overnutrition is particularly great for these countries.

Good nutrition is related to access to and appropriate utilization of available food. Food supply is therefore part of the equation. The second part of the chapter therefore deals with various factors that affect world food supply and the ability of the world to provide enough food for an increasing population.

Descriptions of malnutrition are usefully classified by stage in the lifecycle. Dramatic growth failure most typically occurs between the ages of 12–18 months with a low probability of catch-up growth. The impairments in cognitive function are also largely irreversible. Hence early infant malnutrition has consequences throughout the lifecycle. Malnourished babies become malnourished adolescents and adults who are less able to learn in school and less productive in the labour market. Malnourished female babies are more likely to be malnourished girls and women who give birth to malnourished babies. Moreover the fetal origins hypothesis (see chapter 6) proposes that maternal dietary imbalances at critical periods of development in the womb can trigger adaptations that affect fetal structure and metabolism in ways that predispose the individual to chronic diseases later in life. This section reviews the extent and causes of malnutrition at different stages in the lifecycle.

Assessment of extent and worldwide distribution of malnutrition

A rough approximation of the extent, pattern and trends of the malnutrition problem can be estimated using existing data. Until recently the international organizations concentrated on documenting only nutritional status in developing countries. However, since about 2000 they have started to include the epidemiology of obesity and diet-related degenerative diseases.

Stunting (low height for age) and underweight (low weight for age) of infants in the developing world is widespread. A third of all children under the age of 5 in developing countries are stunted and underweight. In South Asia almost half are underweight, although nutritional status in all regions of the world except sub-Saharan Africa has been improving over recent decades (Table 13.1)

The proportion of adults who fall below the cut-off for underweight (BMI < 17) and above the cut-off point for obesity (BMI ≥ 30) is shown in Table 13.2. The poorest countries are therefore still grappling with underweight and the developed countries with overnutrition issues such as obesity. Despite the widespread efforts to reduce the extent of obesity and its associated diseases, their prevalence continues to increase.

Table 13.1 Percent of pre-schoolers (under-5s) that have low weight for age

Region	Percent under-fives underweight	
	1990	2000
Developing countries	32	28
East Asia/Pacific	24	16
Latin America/Caribbean	11	8
Middle East/North Africa	13	17
South Asia	55	48
Sub-Saharan Africa	32	31

Source: UNICEF 2003 (http://www.childinfo.org/eddb/malnutrition/index.htm; accessed 29 July 2003)

Table 13.2 Percent below and above BMI cut-offs: adults in 2000

	BMI < 17 (underweight)	BMI ≥ 30 (obese)
Least developed (*n* = 45)	8.9	1.8
Developing (78)	6.9	4.8
Transition (27)	2.4	17.1
Developed market (24)	1.6	20.4

Source: WHO 2002 (http://www.who.int/nut/db_bmi.htm; accessed 9 September 2002)

The major micronutrient deficiencies worldwide are iron, iodine, and vitamin A. Approximately 2 billion individuals worldwide are iron deficient, 750 million are iodine deficient and 160 million are vitamin A deficient. In developed countries certain other potential micronutrient deficiencies have become more of a concern in recent years. These include folate deficiency in women in relation to spina bifida in a small percentage of newborns, but also in men and women in relation to elevated plasma levels of homocysteine levels related to coronary heart disease.

Anaemia prevalence is used as a proxy for iron deficiency. In industrialized countries this is likely to be a close approximation, but in the developing world anaemia can occur due to factors other than iron deficiency such as malaria, other parasitic infections, current infectious diseases and other pathologies. Anaemia is a serious problem throughout the lifecycle, both in industrialized and developing countries where the prevalence is over 10% and 14% respectively. It is a particular problem for pregnant women who have high haematinic needs, with a prevalence of almost 20% in industrialized countries and almost 60% in developing countries (see chapters 5 & 8).

One of the most visible manifestations of iodine deficiency is goitre (see chapter 5) and this is used as one indicator of deficiency. The overall world prevalence of goitre is 13%, highest in the African region (20%), followed by Europe (15%), SE Asia (12%), Western Pacific (8%) and the Americas (5%)

Severe vitamin A deficiency (VAD) manifests itself clinically as night blindness and corneal xerosis (see chapter 5). Sub-clinical vitamin A deficiency in pre-school children is defined as serum retinol level $<0.7\,\mu mol/L$. While clinical signs of vitamin A deficiency are relatively rare (estimated 3 million pre-school children), subclinical deficiency, which increases the likelihood of morbidity and mortality in pre-schoolers, is estimated to be widespread (75–250 million) in developing countries only, and most likely found in South Asia and sub-Saharan Africa.

In addition to anthropometric data and patchy micronutrient status data, food balance sheet data are available for most developing countries for most years. These data are compiled by the UN's Food and Agriculture Organization (FAO) from food production, food trade and food aid flows. The foods are converted into calories and divided by population size to give the dietary energy supply (DES) in calories per capita. The DES numbers are converted to estimates of the percentages of individuals without adequate access to food: 17% in developing countries, with the highest in sub-Saharan Africa (33%), and 7% in countries in transition.

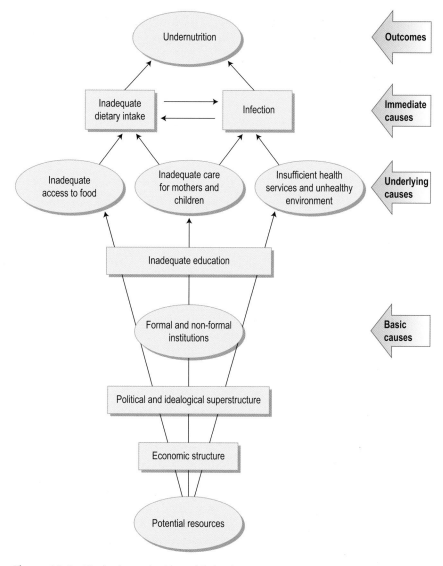

Figure 13.1 The food–care–health model of undernutrition.

Some of the factors behind the tragic decline in nutrition status in sub-Saharan Africa include: closed markets in the developed world (especially the EU) for their exports; HIV/AIDS generating a health and development crisis and undermining the ability to respond to the crisis; wars and refugee movements; military expenditure; drought; crop and livestock disease; many ecosystems making technology diffusion and adaptation difficult; under-investment in agricultural research; no economy serving as regional driver (Nigeria and South Africa's under-whelming economic performance); low levels of human capital in terms of literacy; declining terms of trade for natural resources on world markets; low population densities leading to thin infrastructure and market institutions.

Analysis of causes

Figure 13.1 summarizes the causes of undernutrition in children, but much of this scheme is also relevant to adults. The causes lie at several levels (immediate, underlying and basic) and in many sectors (agriculture, health, water, education, and employment, etc). It is important to understand the causes of malnutrition to guide the interventions needed to improve nutrition status. The following examples focus first on undernutrition, followed by similar analyses that can be made for the chronic nutrition related diseases (overnutrition).

Immediate causes

The most immediate causes of malnutrition in young children (and also adults) are poor diet and infection (see chapters 6 & 8). If the child is not able to ingest enough food, both in terms of quantity and quality that can be used for growth and development, then malnutrition occurs. Infection and an inadequate diet reinforce each other as infection reduces the intake of nutrients by diminishing appetite, inhibiting nutrient absorption, and increasing nutrient requirements for combating infection while poor diet reduces the effectiveness of the immune function.

Equivalent immediate causes of diseases of affluence are excess intake of food, eg through bottle feeding, snacking, high fat foods, and lack of exercise.

Underlying causes

Underlying causes of undernutrition include household food insecurity, poor care for mothers and children and the inadequate provision of health services and an unhealthy environment. Food security 'exists when all people, at all times, have physical and economic access to sufficient, safe, and nutritious food to meet their dietary needs and food preferences for an active and healthy life'. Household food insecurity has many interrelated causes: poor crop yields, low incomes, high food prices, low rates of exchange between food and non-food, and a lack of access to assets, including land, water, extension and credit.

Poor health services, unclean drinking water, and non-existent hygiene disposal systems all increase the likelihood of infection, particularly diarrhoea. Inadequate care for mothers and children increases the risk of infection and inadequate diet. Care includes time for resting and appropriate food during pregnancy, breast feeding and feeding of young children, psychosocial stimulation of infants, food preparation and storage practices, hygiene practices and care for children during illness, including diagnosis and health seeking behaviour.

Underlying causes for the diseases of affluence are mainly the converse, including overall food security, availability of plentiful and varied food products (although not always the most healthy), food advertising, a sedentary lifestyle at work and leisure due to labour saving devices, transport, computers, work pressures, and increased perception of risk for children in playing outside and walking or cycling to school.

Basic causes

The basic or root causes of malnutrition are essentially political and economic. There are very few instances of high levels of undernutrition (as opposed to overnutrition) above a certain GDP per capita. A 10% increase in income produces a 5% reduction in the rate of undernutrition but income growth is by no means sufficient, and there is a wide range of levels of undernutrition at a given income level. Other factors beyond income growth are obviously essential for good nutrition, such as good levels of education, social equity, and enlightened government behaviour. Good governance – by which we mean institutions that give voice to all parts of society; respect for the civil, political, economic, social and cultural rights of its citizens; and appropriate levels of investment in public goods such as safety, research, roads, health and education – is more likely to produce these conditions. Good education levels mean that individuals know how to access, assess, and use information that is helpful to the attainment of good nutrition status (such as the right types of foods to consume, what to do in the case of diarrhoea, and the optimal duration of exclusive breastfeeding). The status of women relative to men is a dimension of society and values that is crucial to the nutrition status of women and of infants.

The basic or root causes of the diseases of overnutrition are also essentially political and economic, affecting incomes, employment, work pressures, food prices, etc.

KEY POINTS

- Undernutrition is located largely in South Asia and sub-Saharan Africa; it is declining slowly in South Asia, but not in sub-Saharan Africa
- Overnutrition is present in all countries, in general is more prevalent in developed countries, but is increasing most rapidly in the developing world
- Sub-Saharan Africa is beset by multiple factors at all levels that make progress in reducing malnutrition very difficult
- The causes of undernutrition are at three levels – immediate, underlying and basic
- The immediate causes of undernutrition relate to poor food intake and infection, and of overnutrition are excess food intake of unbalanced composition, and inadequate exercise
- The underlying causes of undernutrition relate to household food insecurity, poor support for caring practices and a weak health and sanitation environment, and of overnutrition to food security, availability of wide variety of high energy foods, and an environment that discourages exercise
- The status of women is key in promoting good nutrition
- The basic causes of both under- and overnutrition are economic and political in nature

13.4 TYPES OF INTERVENTIONS

Much is known about how to combat the different forms of undernutrition. Direct interventions are those targeted specifically to improve nutrition. Those that are thought to work for malnutrition in general focus on (a) improving breastfeeding rates up to 6 months of age, (b) improving the quality and quantity of foods that complement breastfeeding beyond 6 months of age, (c) improving the quality and quantity of food consumed by adolescent girls and pregnant and lactating women, (d) supplementing diets with micronutrient capsules, fortifying foods with micronutrients during processing, (e) improving the quality of nutrition information provided to parents and caretakers, and (f) increasing the diversity of diets consumed by all individuals via home-based production of small livestock, fruit and vegetables. Efficacy trials tell us what can work under controlled conditions, and effectiveness trials and cost-effectiveness estimates tell us what works under real-life conditions.

Direct interventions

Direct interventions that are used to combat the diseases of affluence include several of the above. There is much emphasis on: providing information to the consumer including food labelling; food legislation to control composition; manufacturers voluntarily producing low fat, salt and sugar products and high fibre products with added micronutrients; encouraging physical activity; emphasizing healthy school meals; and medication for high blood pressure and obesity.

Indirect interventions

Indirect interventions are those that have an impact on nutrition, but do not have nutrition as a primary or even secondary goal, but work on the underlying causes. Indirect interventions that affect undernutrition focus on (a) lowering the price of foods to consumers via subsidies or vouchers, (b) improving access to income (more work, higher productivity), (c) improving the ability to borrow and save to smooth consumption from one period to the next, (d) improving the ability of women to make decisions that improve nutrition, (e) improving education and the ability to acquire and use information, (f) improving access to water, sanitation and preventative and curative health services, and (g) raising the productivity and nutrient content of crops and livestock. For these it is difficult to obtain a strong experimental design and we have to rely more on plausibility assessments of impact on nutrition.

Indirect interventions that are likely have an effect on the diseases of affluence include some of the above such as (d) and (e), and measures such as: taxation on some foods and beverages, a school curriculum designed to allow increased physical activity, the availability of sports facilities, cycle lanes to allow safe cycling, etc.

An extensive literature review on the efficacy of direct interventions targeting the main undernutrition outcomes in developing countries: low birth weight at term (or more precisely intrauterine growth retardation, IUGR), stunting, and the three main micronutrient deficiencies was published by

Allen & Gillespie in 2001. No such overall review has been carried out on the effectiveness of various interventions in reducing the chronic nutrition related diseases, possibly because the history of interventions is shorter. There is little information on the efficacy of approaches to overweight, obesity, and diet-related chronic disease, beyond what is known about approaches to preventing or reducing the predisposing factors of IUGR and stunting. However some systematic Cochrane reviews on interventions for the prevention and treatment of specific nutrition related conditions, such as childhood and adult obesity, diabetes, cardiovascular disease have been conducted (http://www.cochrane.org/reviews/en/index.html).

KEY POINTS

- Direct interventions are those targeted specifically at improving nutrition
- A number of direct interventions have been shown to be efficacious, effective and cost-effective in reducing undernutrition, including breastfeeding, complementary foods, vitamin supplementation and fortification, nutrition information and dietary diversification
- Direct interventions to combat overnutrition include food legislation, the manufacture of low fat, salt and sugar products and high fibre and micronutrient products, increased physical activity and the provision of healthy school meals
- Indirect interventions do not have improvements in nutrition as an explicit objective, but can have powerful indirect and supportive effects on nutrition status
- Indirect interventions relevant to undernutrition relate to agriculture, income generation and maintenance, the status of women, education, water access (quality and quantity), sanitation and health services (preventive and curative)
- Indirect interventions relevant to overnutrition include taxation, school curricula and facilities for physical activity
- More is known about the efficacy and effectiveness of interventions for undernutrition than overnutrition as they have been evaluated over a longer period.

13.5 THE EVOLUTION OF THINKING ABOUT FOOD AND NUTRITION SECURITY AND NUTRITION-RELEVANT INTERVENTIONS AND POLICY

Before the 1970s most of the international nutrition focus was on malnutrition in developing countries and control of nutrient deficiencies in developed countries.

1970s concerns

The 1970s saw an increased interest in nutrition policy for developed countries, with the growing realization that existing legislation – which was based on food purity and the prevention of adulteration, as well as control of deficiencies – was not adequate to deal with the changing nature of nutrition problems such as chronic nutrition-related diseases. Several government advisory, professional and consumer bodies in the USA, UK and other countries recommended appropriate dietary goals with the common theme of reducing fat, sugar and salt intake and increasing the intake of dietary fibres, fruit and vegetables. In contrast to policies related to undernutrition that promote increased consumption of nutrients, the advice to reduce the intake of certain nutrients appeared to be a threat to some sectors of the food industry. There was considerable opposition to the advice and arguments about the validity of the evidence on which the recommendations were based. Additional constraints to updating food and nutrition policy included legislation designed to prevent adulteration and maintain quality as previously perceived, such as minimum fat levels in milk and premiums on animals with high fat content. However, the proposals were gradually accepted and incorporated into government policies, while industry recognized new opportunities in the production of foods high in fibre and low in fat, salt and sugar.

Norway was the first developed country to have an integrated Food and Nutrition Policy as promoted in the World Food Conference in 1974. The UK and other European countries subsequently developed food and nutrition policies within their health and agriculture sectors. For example, in the UK explicit nutritional goals were set for the first time in the 1992 government health policy 'The Health of the Nation' which focused on five key areas for action: coronary heart disease and stroke; cancers; mental illness; HIV/AIDS and sexual health; and accidents – the first two of which are diet related. The diet and nutrition targets for 2005 with a baseline of 1990 were to reduce: the average % food energy from saturated fats by at least 35% (to no more than 11% food energy); the average % food energy from total fat by at least 12% (to no more than about 35% food energy); the % of men and women aged 16–64 who are obese by at least 25% and 35% respectively (to no more than 6% of men and 8% of women); and the % of men drinking more than 21 units of alcohol per week and women drinking more than 14 units per week by 30% (to 18% of men and 7% of women).

By concentrating on these targets it was expected that the associated dietary changes and reduction in obesity would have beneficial consequences for such diseases as cancer, osteoarthritis, and diabetes. A Nutrition Task Force was set up to oversee implementation of action, promote coordination and cooperation between interested parties, and establish mechanisms for monitoring and evaluating progress. On a regional basis, the WHO European Region prepared The First Action Plan for Food and Nutrition Policy 2000–2005, which included a Food and Nutrition Task Force.

1980s concerns

The 1980s saw greater recognition of the notion that micronutrients play a more general role in child survival (beyond deficiency diseases) and led to the promotion in developing countries of small-scale home gardening, capsule distribution and fortification programmes. Such programmes had been in use for several decades in developed countries, such as providing land for kitchen garden allotments, and the provision of supplements to children and mothers, during the world wars, and the fortification of white flour with vitamins and minerals from that period. Compulsory fortification of margarine with vitamins A and D has existed in the UK since the 1967 Margarine Regulations came into force in 1971.

The 1980s formalized the notion of food insecurity as being not just about lack of access to food today, but also about the risk of losing access to food tomorrow. The risk of losing access was debilitating and also led to actions fashioned to cope with that risk, but which had very high costs – such as short-termism on the issues of natural resource mining, the over-diversification of income sources and the uneconomic storage of food at the household level. Finally, in the 1980s the importance of the triumvirate of food–care–health for nutrition became to be accepted. Interactions became clearer: poor quality drinking water could undermine household food security; without adequate care for mothers, children could not be breastfed; without time to undertake health-seeking behaviour, preventive (and often curative) health care would not be accessed.

1990s concerns

Food safety became a major concern in the 1990s, particularly in the developed countries. European consumers in particular, having lost faith in the science establishment due to their initial assurances about the lack of danger to human health of BSE ('mad cow disease'), have become extremely cautious about the safety of the food they purchase. They are able and willing to pay a premium for assurances about the food production and processes used. In the UK this distrust also led to a revision in government structure through the Food Standards Act 1999, by which agricultural and consumer food interests, which had been combined within the Ministry of Agriculture Fisheries and Food (MAFF), were separated into the Food Standards Agency (FSA) (www.fsa.org) to champion consumer interests, and the Department for the Environment Food and Rural Affairs to look after agriculture (www.defra.org). A similar body was established within the European Union in 2002, the European Food Safety Authority (www.efsa.eu.int). In the United States, food and nutrition are regulated by the Food and Drug Administration (www.fda.gov). The capacity required to adhere to the new food safety expectations have made it harder for developing country exporters to gain market share in the developed world, harming their own food security through constraints on export opportunities.

Another concern is about genetically modified (GM) foods. To date, GM foods have realized benefits largely for producers in terms of higher productivity, and lower costs. Despite no obvious benefits to consumers other than perhaps lower prices, those in the US have been consuming GM soybean products for most of the 1990s. But European consumers and many in the US are concerned that the food safety and environmental safety issues related to GM foods have not been adequately researched.

Also, in the 1990s awareness increased that pockets of food poverty still existed in developed countries, following the increased economic inequality that occurred in the 1980s in the UK and other countries, partly due to government cutbacks in welfare programmes. This led to reports and actions to relieve the constraints of the poor. This echoed a similar period in the United States in the 1960s about 'Hunger in America' which resulted in new welfare programmes.

Finally, the right to food – first formalized in the 1948 Universal Declaration of Human Rights, and then confirmed in milestones such as the 1966 Covenants on Civil and Political Rights and on Economic, Social and Cultural Rights, the 1989 Convention on the Rights of the Child, and the 1996 World Food Summit hosted by FAO – has come of age in the 1990s. The concepts are that governments have a duty to respect, protect, facilitate and fulfil if necessary the rights of the individual to secure adequate food and nutrition.

Current concerns and emerging issues

Globalization, namely the rapidly increasing levels of global food trade, financial flows, labour flows and information flows, present opportunities to be seized and risks to be managed in the pursuit of improved nutrition. Governments have to invest in infrastructure and market institutions that allow them to take advantage of new opportunities and they have to design and implement safety net programmes that protect and compensate those who stand to lose from more open markets.

Urbanization is progressing rapidly throughout the world. The poor in urban areas are at equal risk of undernutrition as the poor in rural areas, perhaps more so since they have little access to the means to produce their own food. Interventions that work in rural areas cannot be assumed to work as well in urban areas without re-design. This is because the main differences in urban areas – a reliance on food purchase, the large numbers of mothers working away from home, and water and air pollution from waste and fuels – make nutrition more susceptible to loss of regular employment, food price fluctuation, the quantity and quality of child care for low-income working mothers, and illnesses caused from environmental contaminants.

The aging of the populations of all countries, a result of lower infant mortality rates and lower birth rates, places new pressure on efforts to finance undernutrition efforts adequately through public finance due to the new demands for spending on overnutrition-related issues such as diabetes and heart disease. In most of the world life expectancy is on the rise, but in sub-Saharan Africa, due to HIV/AIDS, it is on the decline, along with a decline in nutritional status.

The main emerging issue in the developed countries is the continued increase in obesity, in both adults and children, with concomitant increases in related diseases such as diabetes. In the UK it has been recognized that this cannot be tackled only on the nutrition front, and the UK government task forces associated with the first explicit nutrition policy in 1992 included an activity task force. Increasing research refines the association between various food factors with aspects of health and so determines policy. For example, the USA has already undertaken folate fortification of flour and the UK is considering doing so.

13.6 INTRODUCTION TO FOOD SUPPLY

The previous sections have outlined the extent of malnutrition throughout the world, its causes, and interventions used to improve nutrition. One of the essential factors is food supply and the following sections review food supply in relation to population growth in the past and predictions for the future, as well as factors that affect supply.

At the 1996 World Food Summit, high-level representatives of 186 nations and the European Union, including over 100 heads of state and government, agreed to the Rome Declaration on World Food Security, which states:

> We consider it intolerable that more that 800 million people throughout the world, and particularly in developing countries, do not have enough food to meet their basic nutritional needs. This situation is unacceptable. Food supplies have increased substantially, but constraints on access to food, instability of supply and demand, as well as natural and man-made disasters, prevent basic food needs from being fulfilled.

These problems persist. Although access to food is the critical problem and absolute food shortages are much less of a concern today than in the past, many analysts continue to worry that human population growth will outpace the earth's ability to produce adequate food supplies. This concern, voiced by Thomas R. Malthus in 1798, remains a preoccupation two centuries later, notwithstanding the successful role of science, technology, and public policy in addressing this dilemma in the 20th century. Growing demand for animal products in the developing world further fuels concern about overburdening the earth's 'carrying capacity'. Will technological and institutional innovation continue to allow food production to keep pace with population growth and rising food demand, as well as the environmental costs that this will entail?

Definitions related to food security

According to one widely accepted definition: 'Food security exists when all people, at all times, have physical and economic access to sufficient, safe, and nutritious food to meet their dietary needs and food preferences for an active and healthy life.'

This definition is in keeping with the principle that everyone has a right to adequate food, to be free from hunger, and to enjoy general human dignity, enshrined in the International Bill of Human Rights. Food insecurity, then, is the absence of food security. Hunger, a condition in which people lack the basic food intake to provide them with the energy and nutrients for fully productive, active lives, is an outcome of food insecurity. Famine is at the extreme end of food insecurity, a catastrophic disruption of the social, economic, and institutional systems that provide for food production, distribution, and consumption. Contemporary famines stem less from crop failure than from the political and financial failures of governments to prevent famine and respond effectively. The emergence of 'new-variant famines', in which HIV/AIDS interacts with violence, natural disaster, and/or political–economic failure, means that the margin for coping and recovery has narrowed greatly among vulnerable people, especially in sub-Saharan Africa.

The availability of adequate food is a necessary condition for achieving food security, but it is not sufficient. Of equal importance are access to food and appropriate utilization of food. Even when food supplies are satisfactory, food insecurity may persist because people lack access, whether by means of production, purchase, public social safety net programmes, private charity, or some combination of these, to available food. In addition, people may fail to consume sufficient quantities of food or a balanced diet even when supplies are ample.

13.7 WORLD FOOD SUPPLY

Past crises and their resolution

Scholars and policy makers alike have long worried about how to balance food supplies with the demands of a rapidly growing population. There have been periodic 'food crises' over the last century where there was widespread concern that the world was running out of food. All have been characterized by rapidly increasing food prices making it hard for consumers to buy adequate quantities and quality of food. The most recent was in 2008, ascribed to shifts in policies of the largest food producers such as the US and EU away from supporting food production, which was creating excesses, to biofuel and the increase in oil prices. The most analysed was the food crisis in the late 1960s and early 1970s when analysts wrote off much of Asia as 'a hopeless basket case' and the threat of famine gripped West and Central Africa, Ethiopia, and Bangladesh.

The Green Revolution

In fact, food availability rose dramatically between 1970 and 1997, as farmers in Asia, Latin America and throughout the world widely adopted high-yielding varieties of cereals, and governments, especially in Asia, implemented policies that supported agricultural development. The use of high yielding varieties and the associated package of irrigation and fertilizers has been designated the 'Green Revolution'. By 2002, developing-country cereal harvests were triple those of 40 years earlier, while the population was a little over twice as large. However, in sub-Saharan Africa calorie availability per person remained below minimum requirements and was barely above the threshold in South Asia.

The Green Revolution also had environmental benefits as increased yields alleviated the need to clear new land in order to boost production, thereby conserving biodiversity and limiting atmospheric releases of carbon that can cause global warming. At the same time, widespread planting of high-yielding varieties of cereal crops in some instances has contributed to environmental problems, such as increased soil salinity and lowered water tables in irrigated areas; water, air, and soil degradation resulting from excessive agricultural input use; and human health problems due to heavy pesticide use. There is some evidence that increased cereal output has come at the expense of pulses and vegetables that could improve dietary quality. In contrast to cereals, there has been little research to develop yield-increasing technology for other crops, such as roots and tubers. However, the Green Revolution is one example of the ability of suitable agricultural policies and technology to address food needs.

Future supply outlook

According to projections to the year 2020 by the International Food Policy Research Institute (IFPRI), aggregate global food supplies are expected to remain adequate, despite the growth in the world population – which is expected to increase by nearly 30% between 2000 and 2025, from 6.1 billion to 7.9 billion. Daily calorie availability per person is projected to exceed minimum requirements in all regions, although only barely so in sub-Saharan Africa.

Constraints on production

Commercial agriculture by definition produces a large proportion of the world food trade, largely in cereals, but much of the total world food production is by small farmers in developing countries who face many problems in their struggle for sustainable livelihoods. These include socioeconomic, political, agro-ecological, and health constraints.

Among the socioeconomic and political limitations on food production are public policies and investments that are biased against poor farmers and consumers, women, and less-favoured areas; inadequate infrastructure; inequitable access to land and other critical resources; poorly functioning and poorly integrated markets; and lack of access to credit and technical assistance.

Agro-ecological constraints include low soil fertility and lack of access to plant nutrients, along with variable weather and acid, salinated, and waterlogged soils that contribute to low yields, production risks, and natural resource degradation. Losses to pests reduce potential farm output value by 50%. Unless properly managed, fresh water may well emerge as the key constraint on global food production. Although there is disagreement among scientists and policy makers over global climate change, there is consensus that it is leading to higher average temperatures and sea levels and to less stable weather patterns, with the probability of more frequent and severe droughts and flooding. Many of the poorest countries are extremely vulnerable. Drier soils and heat could also reduce crop production in some parts of the North American 'breadbasket'. Agriculture accounts for about 20% of the 'greenhouse gases' that lead to warming, but increased levels of carbon dioxide, which contribute to global warming, also lead to improvements in plant growth.

Health constraints include infectious disease, which has a significant bearing on food production, especially in sub-Saharan Africa. About 36 million people are currently living with HIV/AIDS, two-thirds of them in sub-Saharan Africa, and it is spreading dramatically in Asia. It has contributed to labour shortages, a decline in the transfer of farmer knowledge across generations, weaker collective action, weaker property rights, a declining asset base, breakdown of social bonds, loss of livestock, and reliance on crops that are easier to produce but less nutritious and economically valuable. Because malaria often strikes during harvest time, it also threatens food output. New cultivation technologies and varieties need to be developed that do not rely so much on labour, yet allow crops to remain drought-resistant and nutritious.

13.8 WORLD FOOD DEMAND

Food demand derives primarily from income growth, population growth and urbanization. When people move to cities, their lifestyles become more sedentary, and women experience higher opportunity costs on their time. As a result, urban dwellers tend to shift consumption to foods that require less preparation time, and to more meat, milk, fruit, vegetables, and processed foods. IFPRI projects a 49% increase in cereal demand in developing countries between 1997 and 2020. There will be an increased demand for meat and the feed to produce it. The United States and European Union will boost their exports to fill in the gap.

13.9 GLOBALIZATION, INTERNATIONAL TRADE AND FOOD SECURITY

Globalization is the term applied to the growing integration of global markets for goods, services and capital, resulting in part from technological developments in transportation, information, and communications. The volume of the global cereal trade, the most important agricultural commodity, more than doubled during 1967–97, led by developing-country imports of wheat for food and maize for feed. Developed countries (mainly the United States, European Union, and Australia) heavily dominate world export sales, along with a handful of developing countries (mainly Argentina, with India, Thailand, and Vietnam lagging far behind).

The World Trade Organization (WTO) was established in 1994 from the General Agreement on Tariffs and Trade (GATT) with the aim to liberalize world trade. With the strong encouragement of aid donors many developing countries have responded to the WTO Agreement on Agriculture and have liberalized food and agricultural trade. But the developed countries have not reciprocated, instead maintaining barriers to high-value imports from developing countries such as beef, sugar, groundnuts, dairy products, and processed goods. Developed countries' own domestic farm subsidies, such as those of the European Union (EU) Common Agricultural Policy (CAP), which exceed six times the level of development assistance, have depressing effects on world prices, making developed-country exports cheaper than domestic produce and export crops in many developing countries. The effect of current trade agreements is likely to be adverse for most African countries whose share of world agricultural trade continues to decline rapidly.

Another aspect of food globalization is the expansion of developed-country supermarkets (particularly European chains) in developing countries. Issues related to this development include whether poor farmers will be able to meet quality standards and whether large-scale food marketing will meet the needs of poor consumers in terms of both affordability and accessibility.

13.10 THE POTENTIAL OF MODERN AGRICULTURAL BIOTECHNOLOGY FOR FOOD SECURITY

Agricultural research that is publicly funded and generally carried out by national government agencies or international organizations played a critical role in the success of the Green Revolution. The public sector has funded virtually all of the research on so-called 'orphan crops', ie crops widely consumed by poor people but for which markets are poorly developed and offer little profit potential, eg cassava, varieties of beans such as cowpeas, and coarse grains such as millet. The private sector, in contrast, focuses on agricultural research for which there is a market and profit potential, eg hybrid maize, soybeans, and fruits and vegetables that are traded internationally.

Rapid changes in the organization of agricultural research, and the proprietary nature of the agricultural sciences, are placing an increasing share of agricultural research and the ownership of new technologies in the private domain, raising concerns about the extent to which agricultural research and development will help eliminate hunger for the world's poor people in the decades to come. Public investment in agricultural research that can improve small farmers' productivity in developing countries is especially important for food security. Nevertheless, between 1990 and 2000, donors' support for international agricultural research centres declined about 10% in real terms.

Modern agricultural biotechnology offers many potential benefits to developing countries. These include help to: achieve the productivity gains needed to feed a growing global population; introduce resistance to pests and diseases without high-cost purchased inputs; heighten crop tolerance to adverse weather such as drought and soil conditions such as salinity; improve the nutritional value of some foods with, for example, higher levels of vitamin A or iron; and enhanced durability of products during harvesting or shipping – as well as the production of edible vaccines. These could reduce the need to cultivate new lands, help conserve biodiversity, and reduce reliance on pesticides, thereby reducing farmers' crop protection costs and benefiting both the environment and public health.

Except for limited work on rice and cassava, little GM crop research currently focuses on the productivity and nutrition of poor people. In 2002, North America accounted for 72% of GM crop plantings, with the United States alone accounting for 66%. Additional public and philanthropic resources are needed in support of the appropriate research in developing countries.

Successful adaptation of GM crop technology for the benefit of poor farmers and consumers in developing countries will require the establishment of appropriate institutions to assess and manage public health and environmental risks. Developing countries that wish to adopt GM crop technology will need to enact and enforce an appropriate intellectual property rights regime. Poor farmers in developing countries often rely on seed saved from the current year's harvest for planting their next crop. Private companies that have developed GM seeds generally subject them to patents or other forms of intellectual property rights protection. Thus, developing countries need legislation that can balance the desire of seed companies to profit from their innovations with the continuing ability of poor farmers to save, reuse, and exchange seed.

Given consumer resistance to GM food in the European Union and Japan, developing countries that rely on those markets for agricultural exports would either need to avoid using biotechnology, or would have to adopt and manage a system to differentiate and label GM and non-GM foods. A large share of the food imported by developing countries originates in the United States, and these importing countries must decide whether they wish to insist on product differentiation and labelling in the case of imported food. Rejection of GM crops in Europe and Japan may make such crops cheaper for developing country importers that are willing to purchase them.

13.11 CONCLUSIONS

Accelerated progress toward sustainable food security will depend upon the willingness of developing and developed country governments, international aid agencies, non-governmental organizations, business and industry, and individuals to back their anti-hunger rhetoric with action, resources, and changes in behaviour and institutions.

KEY POINTS

- Food security requires more than just adequate food availability; it is also a matter of access to the food that is available and of its appropriate utilization
- Famine is at the extreme end of food insecurity, a catastrophic disruption of the social, economic, and institutional systems that provide for food production, distribution, and consumption
- Projections to the year 2020 indicate that food supplies will remain adequate
- There have been periodic 'food crises' with fears that food supply cannot balance the demands of rapid population growth
- Technological and institutional innovation has permitted food production to more than keep pace with population growth
- Food demand derives from income growth, population growth and urbanization

- Small-scale farmers face many constraints, including lack of access to productive resources, natural resource degradation, and health crises
- Unless developed countries reduce their agricultural subsidies and open their markets to developing country exports, the potential of globalization to contribute to food security will mostly go unrealized
- Agricultural research focused on poor countries, including biotechnology, has a critical role to play in efforts to attain food security

FURTHER READING

ACC/SCN (United Nations Standing Committee on Nutrition) 2004 Fifth report on the world nutrition situation. SCN, Geneva

Allen L H, Gillespie S R 2001 What Works? A Review of the Efficacy and Effectiveness of Nutrition Interventions. ACC/SCN Nutrition Policy Paper No. 19. Asian Development Bank. Nutrition and Development Series No. 5. SCN, Geneva

FAO 2002 The State of Food Insecurity in The World 2002. FAO, Rome, Accessible at http://www.fao.org/docrep/005/y7352e/y7352e00.htm

Lancet 2008 Vol. 371 Series on Maternal and Child Undernutrition

WEBSITES

Food and Agriculture Organization (FAO)
www.fao.org
World Health Organization (WHO)
www.who.org
Cochrane reviews
www.cochrane.org/reviews/en/index.html
UN Standing Committee for Nutrition (SCN)
www.unscn.org
UK Department for Environment and Rural Affairs (DEFRA)
www.defra.org
International Food Policy Research Institute (IFPRI)
www.ifpri.org
UK Food Standards Agency (FSA)
www.fsa.org
US Food and Drug Administration (FDA)
www.fda.gov

13.11 Conclusions

Appendix 1: Glossary

acetyl CoA An important molecule in metabolism, acetyl CoA plays a role in many biochemical reactions. The main one is to transport carbon atoms within the acetyl group to the tricarboxylic cycle to be used in energy production

achlorhydria Deficiency of hydrochloric acid in gastric digestive juice

acrylamide A chemical that can be generated when the amino acid asparagine is heated above 100°C in the presence of sugars

additive Any compound not commonly regarded or used as a food which is added to foods as an aid in manufacturing or processing, or to improve the keeping properties, flavour, colour, texture, appearance, or stability of the food, or as a convenience to the consumer. The term excludes vitamins, minerals, and other nutrients added to enrich or restore nutritional value. Herbs, spices, hops, salt, yeast, or protein hydrolysates, air and water are usually excluded from this definition

adenosine triphosphate (ATP) The coenzyme that acts as an intermediate between energy-yielding (catabolic) metabolism (the oxidation of metabolic fuels) and energy expenditure as physical work and in synthetic (anabolic) reactions. *See* energy metabolism

adipocyte A fat-containing cell in adipose tissue

adipose tissue Body fat storage tissue, distributed under the skin, around body organs and in body cavities – composed of cells that synthesize and store fat, releasing it for metabolism in fasting. Also known as white adipose tissue, to distinguish it from the metabolically more active brown adipose tissue, which is involved in heat production to maintain body temperature. The energy yield of adipose tissue is 34–38 MJ (8000–9000 kcal) per kg

adulteration The addition of substances to foods etc. in order to increase the bulk and reduce the cost, with intent to defraud the purchaser

aerobic (1) Aerobic microorganisms (aerobes) are those that require oxygen for growth; obligate aerobes cannot survive in the absence of oxygen. The opposite are anaerobic organisms, which do not require oxygen for growth; obligate anaerobes cannot survive in the presence of oxygen. (2) Aerobic exercise is physical activity that requires an increase in heart rate and respiration to meet the increased demand of muscle for oxygen, as contrasted with maximum exertion or sprinting, when muscle can metabolize anaerobically

AIDS Acquired immune deficiency syndrome; *see* HIV

albumin (albumen) A group of relatively small water-soluble proteins: ovalbumin in egg-white, lactalbumin in milk; plasma or serum albumin is one of the major blood proteins, which transports certain metabolites including non-esterified fatty acids in the bloodstream. Serum albumin concentration is sometimes measured as an index of protein energy malnutrition. Often used as a non-specific term for proteins (eg albuminuria is the excretion of proteins in the urine)

alcohol Chemically, alcohols are compounds with the general formula $C_nH_{(2n11)}OH$. The alcohol in alcoholic beverages is ethyl alcohol (ethanol, C_2H_5OH)

aldosterone A steroid hormone secreted by the adrenal cortex; controls the excretion of salts and water by the kidneys

allergen A chemical compound, commonly a protein, which causes the production of antibodies, and hence an allergic reaction

allergy Adverse reaction to foods caused by the production of antibodies

amino acids The basic units from which proteins are made. Chemically compounds with an amino group ($-NH_3^+$) and a carboxyl group ($-COO^-$) attached to the same carbon atom

amylases Enzymes that hydrolyse starch. α-Amylase (dextrinogenic amylase or diastase) acts to produce small dextrin fragments from starch, while β-amylase (maltogenic amylase) liberates maltose, some free glucose, and isomaltose from the branch points in amylopectin. Salivary and pancreatic amylases are α-amylases

anaemia A shortage of red blood cells, leading to pallor and shortness of breath, especially on exertion. Most commonly due to a dietary deficiency of iron, or excessive blood loss. Other dietary deficiencies can also result in anaemia, including deficiency of vitamin B_{12} or folic acid (megaloblastic anaemia), vitamin E (haemolytic anaemia), and rarely vitamin C or vitamin B_6

anaerobes Microorganisms that grow in the absence of oxygen. Obligate anaerobes cannot survive in the presence of oxygen, facultative anaerobes grow in the presence or absence of oxygen

angina (angina pectoris) Paroxysmal thoracic pain and choking sensation, especially during exercise or stress, due to partial blockage of a coronary artery (blood vessel supplying the heart), as a result of atherosclerosis

anorexia nervosa A psychological disturbance resulting in a refusal to eat, possibly with restriction to a very limited range of foods, and often accompanied by a rigid programme of vigorous physical exercise, to the point of exhaustion. The result is a very considerable loss of weight, with tissue atrophy and a fall in basal metabolic rate. It is especially prevalent among adolescent girls; when body weight falls below about 45 kg there is a cessation of menstruation

anthropometry Body measurements used as an index of physiological development and nutritional status; a non-invasive way of assessing body composition. Weight for age provides information about the overall nutritional status of children; weight for height is used to detect acute malnutrition (wasting); height for age to detect chronic malnutrition (stunting). Mid-upper arm circumference provides an index of muscle wastage in undernutrition. Skinfold thickness is related to the amount of subcutaneous fat as an index of over- or undernutrition

antibody Immunoglobulin which specifically counteracts an antigen or allergen (see allergen)

antigen Any compound that is foreign to the body (eg bacterial, food, or pollen proteins or complex carbohydrates) which, when introduced into the circulation, stimulates the formation of an antibody

antioxidant A substance that retards the oxidative rancidity of fats in stored foods. Many fats, and especially vegetable oils, contain naturally occurring antioxidants, including vitamin E, which protect them against rancidity for some time

antioxidant nutrients Highly reactive oxygen radicals are formed during normal metabolism and in response to infection and some chemicals. They cause damage to fatty acids in cell membranes, and the products of this damage can then cause damage to proteins and DNA. A number of different mechanisms are involved in protection against, or repair after, oxygen radical damage, including a number of nutrients, especially vitamin E, carotene, vitamin C, and selenium. Collectively these are known as antioxidant nutrients

apoptosis In multicellular organisms, a series of biochemical events leading to a characteristic cell morphology and death. It is signalled by the nuclei in normally functioning human and animal cells when the cell's health or age dictates.

arm, chest, hip index (ACH index) A method of assessing nutritional status by measuring the arm circumference, chest diameter, and hip width

ascorbic acid Vitamin C, chemically L-xyloascorbic acid, to distinguish it from the isomer D-araboascorbic acid (isoascorbic acid or erythorbic acid), which has only slight vitamin C activity

asthma Chronic inflammatory disease of the airways which renders them prone to narrow too much. The symptoms include paroxysmal coughing, wheezing, tightness and breathlessness. Asthma may be caused by an allergic response or may be induced by non-immunological mechanisms

atherosclerosis Degenerative disease in which there is accumulation of lipids, together with complex carbohydrates and fibrous tissue (atheroma) on the inner wall of arteries. This leads to narrowing of the lumen of the arteries

atrophy Wasting of normally developed tissue or muscle as a result of disuse, ageing or undernutrition

basal metabolic rate (BMR) The energy cost of maintaining the metabolic integrity of the body, nerve and muscle tone, respiration and circulation. For children it also includes the energy cost of growth. Experimentally, BMR is measured as the heat output from the body, or the rate of oxygen consumption, under strictly standardized conditions, 12–14 hours after the last meal, completely at rest (but not asleep) and at an environmental temperature of 26–30°C, to ensure thermal neutrality

bile Alkaline fluid produced by the liver and stored in the gall bladder before secretion into the small intestine (duodenum) via the bile duct. It contains the bile salts, bile pigments (bilirubin and biliverdin), phospholipids, and cholesterol

bilirubin, biliverdin The bile pigments, formed by the degradation of haemoglobin

binge–purge syndrome A feature of the eating disorder bulimia nervosa, characterized by the ingestion of excessive amounts of food and the excessive use of laxatives

biotin A vitamin, sometimes known as vitamin H, required for the synthesis of fatty acids and glucose, among other reactions, and in the control of gene expression and cell division

blood sugar Glucose; normal concentration is about 5 mmol (90 mg)/L, and is maintained in the fasting state by mobilization of tissue reserves of glycogen and synthesis from amino acids. Only in prolonged starvation does it fall below about 3.5 mmol (60 mg)/L. If it falls to 2 mmol (35 mg)/L there is loss of consciousness (hypoglycaemic coma)

body mass index (BMI) An index of fatness and obesity. The weight (in kg) divided by the square of height (in metres). The acceptable (desirable) range is 20–25. Above 25 is overweight, and above 30 is obesity. Also called Quetelet's index

bulimia nervosa An eating disorder, characterized by powerful and intractable urges to overeat, followed by self-induced vomiting and the excessive use of purgatives

cachexia The condition of extreme emaciation and wasting seen in patients with advanced cancer and AIDS. Due partly to an inadequate intake of food and mainly the effects of the disease in increasing metabolic rate (hypermetabolism) and the breakdown of tissue protein

calorie A unit of energy used to express the energy yield of foods and energy expenditure by the body; the amount of heat required to raise the temperature of 1 g of water through 1°C (from 14.5 to 15.5°C). Nutritionally the kilocalorie (1000 calories) is used (the amount of heat required to raise the temperature of 1 kg of water through 1°C), and is abbreviated as either kcal or Cal to avoid confusion with the cal. The calorie is not an SI unit, and correctly the Joule is used as the unit of energy, although kcal is widely used. 1 kcal = 4.18 kJ; 1 kJ = 0.24 kcal

calorimetry The measurement of energy expenditure by the body. Direct calorimetry is the measurement of heat output from the body, as an index of energy expenditure, and hence requirements

carbohydrate The major food source of metabolic energy, the sugars and starches. Chemically they are composed of carbon, hydrogen, and oxygen in the ratio $C_n:H_{2n}:O_n$

carboxypeptidase An enzyme secreted in the pancreatic juice which hydrolyses amino acids from the carboxyl terminal of proteins

carcinogen A substance that can induce cancer

caries Dental decay caused by attack on the tooth enamel by acids produced by bacteria that are normally present in the mouth

carnitine A derivative of the amino acid lysine, required for the transport of fatty acids into mitochondria for oxidation

carotenes The red and orange pigments of plants; all are antioxidant nutrients. Three are important as precursors of vitamin A: α-, β- and γ-carotene

catabolism Those pathways of metabolism concerned with the breakdown and oxidation of fuels and hence provision of metabolic energy. People who are undernourished or suffering from cachexia are sometimes said to be in a catabolic state, in that they are catabolizing their body tissues, without replacing them

catalase An enzyme that splits hydrogen peroxide to yield oxygen and water; an important part of the body's antioxidant defences

cereal Any grain or edible seed of the grass family which may be used as food; eg wheat, rice, oats, barley, rye, maize, and millet. Collectively known as corn in the UK, although in the USA corn is specifically maize

cholecalciferol Vitamin D

cholecystokinin Hormone that stimulates gall bladder and pancreatic secretion

cholesterol The principal sterol in animal tissues, an essential component of cell membranes and the precursor of the steroid hormones. Not a dietary essential, since it is synthesized in the body

chromosome Collection of genes packaged with histone proteins found in the nucleus of cells; humans have 23 pairs

chronic energy deficiency A term recently introduced to describe adult malnutrition.

Commonly defined by wasting or a low body mass index (*see also* protein energy malnutrition – PEM)

coagulation A process involving the denaturation of proteins, so that they become insoluble; it may be effected by heat, strong acids and alkalis, metals, and other chemicals. The final stage in blood clotting is the precipitation of insoluble fibrin, formed from the soluble plasma protein fibrinogen

cobalamin Vitamin B_{12}

coeliac disease Intolerance of the proteins of wheat, rye, barley and sometimes oats; specifically, the gliadin fraction of the protein gluten. The villi of the small intestine are severely affected and absorption of food is poor. Stools are bulky and fermenting from unabsorbed carbohydrate, and contain a large amount of unabsorbed fat (steatorrhoea)

colitis Inflammation of the large intestine, with pain, diarrhoea and weight loss; there may be ulceration of the large intestine (ulcerative colitis)

collagen Insoluble protein in connective tissue, bones, tendons, and skin of animals and fish; converted into the soluble protein, gelatine, by moist heat

Committee on Medical Aspects of Food Policy (COMA) Previous name for the permanent Advisory Committee to the UK Department of Health, now called the Scientific Advisory Committee on Nutrition (SACN)

C-reactive protein A marker of inflammation, CRP can rise up to 50,000-fold in acute conditions such as cancer, tuberculosis, rheumatoid arthritis and myocardial infarction

creatine A derivative of the amino acids glycine and arginine, important in muscle as a store of phosphate for resynthesis of ATP during muscle contraction and work (*see* ATP)

cretinism Underactivity of the thyroid gland (hypothyroidism) in children, resulting in poor growth, severe mental retardation and deafness

Crohn's disease Chronic inflammatory disease of the bowel, of unknown origin, also known as regional enteritis, since only some regions of the gut are affected

cystic fibrosis A genetic disease due to a failure of the normal transport of chloride ions across cell membranes. This results in abnormally viscous mucus, affecting especially the lungs and secretion of pancreatic juice, hence impairing digestion

deoxyribonucleic acid (DNA) The genetic material in the nuclei of all cells. A linear polymer composed of four kinds of deoxyribose nucleotide, adenine, cytosine, guanine and thymidine (A, C, G and T), linked by phosphodiester bonds, that is the carrier of genetic information. In its native state DNA is a double helix

Department of the Environment, Food and Rural Affairs (DEFRA) website http://www.defra.gov.uk

dermatitis A lesion or inflammation of the skin; many nutritional deficiency diseases include more or less specific skin lesions, but most cases of dermatitis are not associated with nutritional deficiency, and do not respond to nutritional supplements

dextrose   Alternative name for glucose. Commercially the term 'glucose' is often used to mean corn syrup (a mixture of glucose with other sugars and dextrins) and pure glucose is called dextrose

diabetes insipidus   A metabolic disorder characterized by extreme thirst, excessive consumption of liquids and excessive urination, due to failure of secretion of the antidiuretic hormone

diabetes mellitus   A metabolic disorder involving impaired metabolism of glucose due to either failure of secretion of the hormone insulin (insulin-dependent or type I diabetes) or impaired responses of tissues to insulin (non-insulin-dependent or type II diabetes)

dietary fibre   Material mostly derived from plant cell walls which is not digested by human digestive enzymes; a large proportion consists of non-starch polysaccharides

dietary reference values (DRV)   A set of standards of the amounts of each nutrient needed to maintain good health. People differ in the daily amounts of nutrients they need; for most nutrients the measured average requirement plus 20% (statistically 2 standard deviations) takes care of the needs of nearly everyone and in the UK this is termed reference nutrient intake (RNI), elsewhere known as recommended daily allowances or intakes (RDA or RDI), population reference intake (PRI), or dietary reference intake (DRI). This figure is used to calculate the needs of large groups of people in institutional or community planning. Obviously some people require less than the average (up to 20% or 2 standard deviations less). This lower level is termed the lower reference nutrient intake, LRNI (also known as the minimum safe intake, MSI, or lower threshold intake LTI). This is an intake at or below which it is unlikely that normal health could be maintained. If the diet of an individual indicates an intake of any nutrient at or below LRNI then detailed investigation of his/her nutritional status would be recommended. For energy intake only a single dietary reference value is used, the average requirement, because there is potential harm (of obesity) from ingesting too much

dietitian (UK), dietician (US)   One who applies the principles of nutrition to the feeding of individuals and groups; plans menus and special diets; supervises the preparation and serving of meals; instructs in the principles of nutrition as applied to selection of foods

digestibility   The proportion of a foodstuff absorbed from the digestive tract into the bloodstream, normally 90–95%. It is measured as the difference between intake and faecal output, with allowance being made for that part of the faeces that is not derived from undigested food residues (shed cells of the intestinal tract, bacteria, residues of digestive juices)

disaccharides   Sugars composed of two monosaccharide units; the nutritionally important disaccharides are sucrose, lactose, and maltose. *See* carbohydrate

diverticular disease   Diverticulosis is the presence of pouch-like hernias (diverticula) through the muscle layer of the colon, associated with a low intake of dietary fibre and high intestinal pressure due to straining during defecation. Faecal matter can be trapped in these diverticula, causing them to become inflamed, causing pain and diarrhoea, the condition of diverticulitis

eicosanoids   Compounds formed in the body from long-chain polyunsaturated fatty acids (eicosaenoic acids, mainly arachidonic acid), formed by cyclo-oxygenase or lipoxygenase, including the prostaglandins, prostacyclins, thromboxanes, and leukotrienes, all of which act as local hormones and are involved in inflammation, platelet aggregation, and a variety of other functions

electrolytes   Chemically salts that dissociate in solution and will carry an electric current; clinically used to mean the mineral salts of blood plasma and other body fluids, especially sodium and potassium

emaciation   Extreme thinness and wasting, caused by disease or undernutrition

endocrine glands   Ductless glands that produce and secrete hormones. Some respond directly to chemical changes in the bloodstream; others are controlled by hormones secreted by the pituitary gland, under the control of the hypothalamus

energy   The ability to do work. The SI unit of energy is the joule, and nutritionally relevant amounts of energy are kilojoules (kJ, 1000 J) and megajoules (MJ, 1,000,000 J)

energy metabolism   The various reactions involved in the oxidation of metabolic fuels (mainly carbohydrates, fats, and proteins), to provide energy (linked to the formation of ATP (adenosine triphosphate) from ADP (adenosine diphosphate) and phosphate ions)

epidemiology   the study of the distribution and causes of disease in populations

ergocalciferol   Vitamin D_2

essential fatty acids (EFA)   Polyunsaturated fatty acids of the n-6 (linoleic acid) and n-3 (linolenic acid) series, which are essential dietary components because they cannot be synthesized in the (human) body. They are essential components of cell membranes; they are also precursors of prostaglandins, prostacyclins and related hormones and signalling molecules

European Food Safety Authority (EFSA)   website http://www.efsa.ei.int

European Society for Parenteral and Enteral Nutrition (ESPEN)   website http://www.espen.org

famine   A catastrophic disruption of the social, economic, and institutional systems that provide for food production, distribution, and consumption

fasting   Going without food. The metabolic fasting state begins some 4 hours after a meal, when the digestion and absorption of food is complete and body reserves of fat and glycogen begin to be mobilized

fat   Chemically, fats (or lipids) are substances that are insoluble in water but soluble in organic solvents such as ether, chloroform, and benzene, and are actual or potential esters of fatty acids. The term includes triacylglycerols (triglycerides), phospholipids, waxes, and sterols. In more general use the term 'fats' refers to the neutral fats which are triacylglycerols, mixed esters of fatty acids with glycerol; *see* fatty acids

fatty acids Organic acids consisting of carbon chains with a carboxyl group at the end. The nutritionally important fatty acids have an even number of carbon atoms. In addition to their accepted names, fatty acids can be named by a shorthand giving the number of carbon atoms in the molecule (eg C18), then a colon and the number of double bonds (eg C18:2), followed by the position of the first double bond from the methyl end of the molecule as n- or ω (eg C18:2 n-6, or C18:2 ω6)

fibre, dietary *See* dietary fibre

fluorosis Damage to teeth (white to brown mottling of the enamel) and bones caused by an excessive intake of fluoride

Food and Agriculture Organization of the United Nations (FAO) Founded in 1943; headquarters in Rome. Its goal is to achieve freedom from hunger worldwide. According to its constitution the specific objectives are 'raising the levels of nutrition and standards of living … and securing improvements in the efficiency of production and distribution of all food and agricultural products'; website http://www.fao.org

Food and Drug Administration (FDA) US government regulatory agency; website http://www.fda.gov; website for FDA consumer magazine http://www.fda.gov/fdac

food chain The chain between green plants (the primary producers of food energy) through a sequence of organisms in which each eats the one below it in the chain, and is eaten in turn by the one above. Also used for the chain of events from the original source of a foodstuff (from the sea, the soil, or the wild) through all the stages of handling until it reaches the table

food, foodstuffs Any solid or liquid material consumed by a living organism to supply energy, build and replace tissue, or participate in such reactions. Defined by the FAO/WHO Codex Alimentarius Commission as a substance, whether processed, semi-processed, or raw, which is intended for human consumption and includes drink, chewing gum, and any substance that has been used in the manufacture, preparation, or treatment of food but does not include cosmetics, tobacco, or substances used only as drugs. Defined in EU directives as products intended for human consumption in an unprocessed, processed, or mixed state, with the exception of tobacco products, cosmetics, and pharmaceuticals

Food and Nutrition Information Center (FNIC) Located at the National Agricultural Library, part of the US Department of Agriculture; website http://www.nal.usda.gov/fnic

food science The study of the basic chemical, physical, biochemical, and biophysical properties of foods and their constituents, and of changes that these may undergo during handling, preservation, processing, storage, distribution, and preparation for consumption

food security When all people, at all times, have physical and economic access to sufficient, safe, and nutritious food to meet their dietary needs and food preferences for an active and healthy life. Food security requires more than just adequate food availability; it is also a matter of access to the food that is available and appropriate utilization

Food Standards Agency (FSA) Permanent advisory body to UK Parliament through Health Ministers, established in 2000 to protect the public's health and consumer interests in relation to food; website http://www.food.gov.uk

food technology The application of science and technology to the treatment, processing, preservation and distribution of foods. Hence the term food technologist

fructose Also known as fruit sugar or laevulose. A six-carbon monosaccharide sugar (hexose) differing from glucose in containing a ketone group (on carbon-2) instead of an aldehyde group (on carbon-1)

fruitarian A person who eats only fruits, nuts, and seeds; an extreme form of vegetarianism

functional foods Foods eaten for specified health purposes because of their (rich) content of one or more nutrients or non-nutrient substances which may confer health benefits

gene Physical and functional unit of heredity. It is the entire DNA sequence necessary for the synthesis of a functional polypeptide or RNA molecule; *see* DNA, RNA

gene expression Overall process by which information encoded by a gene is converted to an observable phenotype, usually in the form of a protein

genome The complete genetic information of an organism

genomics The study of the structure and function of genes

glucagon A hormone secreted by the α-cells of the pancreas which causes an increase in blood glucose by increasing the breakdown of liver glycogen and stimulating gluconeogenesis

gluconeogenesis The synthesis of glucose from non-carbohydrate precursors, such as glycerol, lactate, and a variety of amino acids

glucose A six-carbon monosaccharide sugar (hexose), with the chemical formula $C_6H_{12}O_6$, occurring free in plant and animal tissues and formed by the hydrolysis of starch and glycogen. Also known as dextrose, grape sugar and blood sugar

glucosinolates Substances occurring widely in plants of the genus *Brassica* (eg broccoli, Brussels sprouts, cabbage); broken down by the enzyme myrosinase to yield, among other products, the mustard oils that are responsible for the pungent flavour (especially in mustard and horseradish). There is evidence that the various glucosinolates in vegetables may have useful anti-cancer activity, since they increase the rate at which a variety of potentially toxic and carcinogenic compounds are conjugated and excreted

gluten The protein complex in wheat, barley, rye and to a lesser extent oats, which gives dough the viscid property that holds gas when it rises. There is none in oats, barley, or maize.

It is a mixture of two proteins, gliadin and glutelin. Allergy to, or intolerance of, gliadin gluten is coeliac disease

glycaemic index The ability of a carbohydrate to increase blood glucose, compared with an equivalent amount of glucose. Glycaemic load is the product of multiplying the amount of carbohydrate in the food by the glycaemic index

glycogen The storage carbohydrate in the liver and muscles, a branched polymer of glucose units

glycogenolysis The breakdown of glycogen to glucose for use as a metabolic fuel and to maintain the normal blood concentration of glucose in the fasting state. Stimulated by the hormones glucagon and adrenaline

glycolysis The first sequence of reactions in glucose metabolism, leading to the formation of two molecules of pyruvic acid from each glucose molecule

goitre Enlargement of the thyroid gland, seen as a swelling in the neck; may be hypothyroid, with low production of hormones, euthyroid (normal levels of the hormones) or hyperthyroid

goitrogens Substances found in foods (especially *Brassica* spp. but including also groundnuts, cassava, and soya bean) which interfere with the synthesis of thyroid hormones (glucosinolates) or the uptake of iodide into the thyroid gland (thiocyanates), and hence can cause goitre, especially when the dietary intake of iodide is marginal

Gomez classification One of the earliest systems for classifying protein energy malnutrition in children, based on percentage of expected weight for age: over 90% is normal, 76–90% is mild (first degree) malnutrition, 61–75% is moderate (second degree) malnutrition and less than 60% is severe (third degree) malnutrition

gout Painful disease caused by accumulation of crystals of uric acid in the synovial fluid of joints; may be due to excessive synthesis and metabolism of purines, which are metabolized to uric acid, or to impaired excretion of uric acid

green revolution A process in which cereal crop yields increased as a result of farmer adoption of high yielding varieties bred at international agricultural research centres and adapted to local conditions at national agricultural research institutions. Planting of these varieties has coincided with expansion of irrigated area and fertilizer use

growth hormone Somatotrophin, a peptide hormone secreted by the pituitary gland that promotes growth of bone and soft tissues. It also reduces the utilization of glucose, and increases breakdown of fats to fatty acids; because of this it has been promoted as an aid to weight reduction, with little evidence of efficacy. Sometimes abbreviated to HGH (human growth hormone); growth hormone from other mammals differs in structure and activity

haem The iron-containing pigment which forms the oxygen-binding site of haemoglobin and myoglobin. It is also part of a variety of other proteins, collectively known as haem proteins, including the cytochromes; *see* haemoglobin

haemochromatosis Iron overload; excessive absorption and storage of iron in the body, commonly the result of a genetic defect. In most cases it is caused by a recessive gene ie it can only be passed on if both parents are carriers of the gene predisposing to the disorder. Around one in seven people in northern Europe are carriers of the recessive gene. Homozygotes are susceptible to iron toxicity from high absorption of dietary iron which can lead to tissue damage (including liver cancer, heart disease and diabetes) and bronze coloration of the skin. Sometimes called bronze diabetes. The disorder is usually treated by regular venesection, a procedure similar to blood donation, where around 500 ml of blood is removed

haemoglobin The red haem-containing protein in red blood cells which is responsible for the transport of oxygen and carbon dioxide in the bloodstream

halal Food conforming to the Islamic (Muslim) dietary laws. Meat from permitted animals (in general grazing animals with cloven hooves, and thus excluding pig meat) and birds (excluding birds of prey). The animals are killed under religious supervision by cutting the throat to allow removal of all blood from the carcass, without prior stunning. Food that is not halal is haram

health foods Substances the consumption of which is advocated by various reform movements, including vegetable foods, whole grain cereals, food processed without chemical additives, food grown on organic compost, supplements such as bees' royal jelly, lecithin, seaweed, etc., and pills and potions. Numerous health claims are made but rarely is there evidence to support these claims

heat of combustion Energy released by complete combustion, as for example, in the bomb calorimeter. Values can be used to predict energy physiologically available from foods only if an allowance is made for material not completely oxidized in the body

histamine The amine formed by decarboxylation of the amino acid histidine. Excessive release of histamine from mast cells is responsible for many of the symptoms of allergic reactions. It also stimulates secretion of gastric acid, and administration of histamine provides a test for achlorhydria; *see* achlorhydria

homeostasis (homeostatic) The control of concentration of key components (in blood etc.) to ensure constancy and physiological normalization of their concentrations

homocysteine A sulphur amino acid formed as an intermediate in the metabolism of methionine; it is demethylated methionine. Normally present at only low concentration (eg less than 10 mM in serum or plasma). High blood concentrations of homocysteine (occurring as a result of poor folic acid, vitamin B_6, and B_{12} status and in certain other dietary and medical situations) have been implicated in the development of atherosclerosis, heart disease, and stroke

human immunodeficiency virus (HIV) The virus which causes AIDS (acquired immune deficiency syndrome). In many developing countries this virus is acquired by heterosexual intercourse, and may also be acquired 'vertically', either at the time of birth or in breast milk (around 25 to 30% of all vertical transmission by breastfeeding mothers). The level of access to specific treatment is still much lower in poor countries.

hunger A condition in which people lack the basic food intake to provide them with the energy and nutrients for fully productive, active lives; it is an outcome of food insecurity

hyperalimentation Provision of unusually large amounts of energy, either intravenously (parenteral nutrition) or by nasogastric or gastrostomy tube (enteral nutrition)

hypercalcaemia, idiopathic Elevated plasma concentrations of calcium believed to be due to hypersensitivity of some children to vitamin D toxicity. There is excessive absorption of calcium, with loss of appetite, vomiting, constipation, flabby muscles, and deposition of calcium in the soft tissues and kidneys. It can be fatal in infants

hypercholesterolaemia Abnormally high blood concentrations of cholesterol. Generally considered to be a sign of high risk for atherosclerosis and ischaemic heart disease

hyperglycaemia Elevated plasma concentration of glucose, caused by a failure of the normal hormonal mechanisms of blood glucose control

hyperinsulinism Excessive secretion of insulin, resulting in hypoglycaemia

hyperlipidaemia (hyperlipoproteinaemia) A variety of conditions in which there are increased concentrations of lipids in plasma: phospholipids, triacylglycerols, free and esterified cholesterol, or unesterified fatty acids

hypertension High blood pressure; a risk factor for ischaemic heart disease, stroke, and kidney disease. May be due to increased sensitivity to sodium

hypocalcaemia Low blood calcium, leading to vomiting and uncontrollable twitching of muscles if severe; may be due to underactivity of the parathyroid gland, kidney failure, or vitamin D deficiency

hypoglycaemia Abnormally low concentration of plasma glucose; may result in loss of consciousness – hypoglycaemic coma

immunoglobulin A member of a family of proteins from which antibodies are derived. There are five main classes in humans known as IgM, IgG, IgA, IgD and IgE

index of nutritional quality (INQ) An attempt to provide an overall figure for the nutrient content of a food or a diet. It is the ratio between the percentage of the reference intake of each nutrient and the percentage of the average requirement for energy provided by the food

insulin Polypeptide hormone that regulates carbohydrate metabolism

interferon One of a family of naturally occurring proteins produced by the cells of the immune system, attacking viruses, bacteria, tumours and other foreign substances

International Network of Food Data Systems (INFOODS) Created to develop standards and guidelines for collection of food composition data, and standardized terminology and nomenclature; website http://www.fao.org/infoods

International Union of Food Science and Technology (IUFoST) website http://www.iufost.org

International Union of Nutritional Sciences (IUNS) website http://www.iuns.org

intrinsic factor A protein secreted in the gastric juice which is required for the absorption of vitamin B_{12}; impaired secretion results in pernicious anaemia

irritable bowel syndrome (IBS) Also known as spastic colon or mucous colitis. Abnormally increased motility of the large and small intestines, leading to pain and alternating diarrhoea and constipation; often precipitated by emotional stress

ischaemic heart disease or coronary heart disease Group of syndromes arising from failure of the coronary arteries to supply sufficient blood to heart muscles; associated with atherosclerosis of coronary arteries

joule The SI (Système Internationale) unit of energy; used to express energy content of foods

Keys score Method of expressing the lipid content of a diet, calculated as $1.35 \times (2 \times \%$ energy from saturated fat $- \%$ energy from polyunsaturated fat$) + 1.5 \times \sqrt{}$(mg cholesterol/1000 kcal)

Kjeldahl determination Widely used method of determining total nitrogen in a substance by digesting with sulphuric acid and a catalyst; the nitrogen is reduced to ammonia which is then measured. In foodstuffs most of the nitrogen is protein, and the term crude protein is the total 'Kjeldahl nitrogen' multiplied by a factor of 6.25 (since most proteins contain 16% nitrogen)

kosher The selection and preparation of foods in accordance with traditional Jewish ritual and dietary laws. Foods that are not kosher are traife. The only kosher flesh foods are from animals that chew the cud and have cloven hoofs, such as cattle, sheep, goats, and deer; the hindquarters must not be eaten. The only fish permitted are those with fins and scales; birds of prey and scavengers are not kosher. Moreover, the animals must be slaughtered according to ritual, without stunning, before the meat can be considered kosher

kwashiorkor (from the Ga language of West Africa) A disease which occurs frequently in young (weanling) children in some developing countries where weaning foods are of poor quality, and is characterized by oedema (swelling due to extracellular fluid accumulation), failure to thrive, abnormal hair appearance (dyspigmentation), often enlarged liver and increased mortality risk. Associated especially with poor diets that are low in protein and other nutrients, and also with frequent infections; *see* protein energy malnutrition

lactose The carbohydrate of milk, sometimes called milk sugar, a disaccharide of glucose and galactose

laxative Or aperient, a substance that helps the expulsion of food residues from the body. If strongly laxative it is termed purgative or cathartic. Dietary fibre and cellulose function because they retain water and add bulk to the contents of the intestine; Epsom salts (magnesium sulphate) also retain water; castor oil, and drugs such as aloes, senna, cascara, and phenolphthalein irritate the intestinal mucosa. Undigested carbohydrates such as lactulose and sugar alcohols are also laxatives

legumes Members of the family Leguminosae, consumed as dry mature seeds (grain legumes or pulses) or as immature green seeds in the pod. Legumes include the groundnut, *Arachis hypogaea*, and soya bean, *Glycine max*, grown for their oil and protein, the yam bean *Pachyrrhizus erosus*, and African yam bean *Sphenostylis stenocarpa*, grown for their edible tubers as well as seeds

leptin Hormone secreted by adipose tissue that acts to regulate long-term appetite and energy expenditure by signalling the state of body fat reserves

leucocytes White blood cells, normally 5000–9000/mm^3; includes polymorphonuclear neutrophils, lymphocytes, monocytes, polymorphonuclear eosinophils, and polymorphonuclear basophils. A 'white cell count' determines the total; a 'differential cell count' estimates the numbers of each type. Fever, haemorrhage, and violent exercise cause an increase (leucocytosis); starvation and debilitating conditions a decrease (leucopenia)

lipids, plasma Triacylglycerols, free and esterified cholesterol and phospholipids, present in lipoproteins in blood plasma. Chylomicrons consist mainly of triacylglycerols and protein; they are the form in which lipids absorbed in the small intestine enter the bloodstream. Very low-density lipoproteins (VLDL) are assembled in the liver and exported to other tissues, where they provide a source of lipids. Lipid-depleted VLDL becomes low-density lipoprotein (LDL) in the circulation; it is rich in cholesterol and is normally cleared by the liver. High-density lipoprotein (HDL) contains cholesterol from LDL and tissues
that is returned to the liver. *See also* hypercholesterolaemia; hyperlipidaemia

low birthweight (LBW) Used as shorthand to describe babies born at weight less than 2.5 kg. Average birthweight is close to 3.5 kg (WHO reference mean). LBW can result from delivery before term (preterm) or from intrauterine growth retardation (IUGR) due to many causes including fetal undernutrition

lower reference nutrient intake (LRNI) Set 2 standard deviations below the EAR for a nutrient. Intakes of nutrients below this point will almost certainly be inadequate for most individuals; *see* reference nutrient intake

malnutrition Disturbance of form or function arising from deficiency or excess of one or more nutrients

marasmic kwashiorkor The most severe form of protein energy malnutrition in children, with weight for height less than 60% of that expected, and with oedema and other symptoms of kwashiorkor

marasmus An old term still in common use in Anglophone developing countries. The adjective (marasmic) described abnormally small and thin infants. As noun and adjective the term was later used by nutritionists to define a weight less than 60% of the reference mean weight for age. This definition is still used in resource-poor areas where stature is not measured. Now the term protein energy malnutrition (PEM) is more commonly used

menarche The initiation of menstruation in adolescent girls, normally occurring between the ages of 11 and 15. The age at menarche has become younger in Western countries, possibly associated with a better general standard of nutrition, and is later in less-developed countries

metabolic equivalent (MET) Unit of measurement of heat production by the body; 1 MET = 50 kcal/hour/m^2 body surface area

metabolism The processes of interconversion of chemical compounds in the body. Anabolism is the process of forming larger and more complex compounds, commonly linked to the utilization of metabolic energy. Catabolism is the process of breaking down larger molecules to smaller ones, commonly oxidation reactions linked to release of energy. There is approximately a 30% variation in the underlying metabolic rate (basal metabolic rate) between different individuals, determined in part by the activity of the thyroid gland

micronutrients Vitamins and minerals, which are needed in very small amounts (micrograms or milligrams per day), as distinct from fats, carbohydrates, and proteins which are macronutrients, since they are needed in considerably greater amounts

mid-upper-arm-circumference (MUAC) A rapid way of assessing nutritional status, especially applicable to children; *see* anthropometry

Ministry of Agriculture, Fisheries and Food (MAFF) Former UK Ministry now replaced by DEFRA and FSA

monosaccharides Group name of the simplest sugars, including those composed of three carbon atoms (trioses), four (tetroses), five (pentoses), six (hexoses), and seven (heptoses). The units from which disaccharides, oligosaccharides, and polysaccharides are formed

mutagen Compound that causes mutations and may be carcinogenic

National Center for Health Statistics (NCHS) standards Tables of height and weight for age used as reference values for the assessment of growth and nutritional status of children, based on data collected by the US National Center for Health Statistics in the 1970s. The most comprehensive such set of data, and used in most countries of the world

National Health and Nutrition Examination Survey (NHANES) Conducted by the National Center for Health Statistics (NCHS), Centers for Disease Control and Prevention, designed to collect information about the health and diet of people in the United States

net dietary protein energy ratio (NDpE) A way of expressing the protein content of a diet or food taking into account both the amount of protein (relative to total energy intake) and the protein quality. It is protein energy multiplied by net protein utilization divided by total energy. If energy is expressed in kcal and the result expressed as a percentage, this is net dietary protein calories per cent, NDpCal%

net protein ratio/retention (NPR) Weight gain of a test animal plus weight loss of a control animal fed a non-protein diet per gram of protein consumed by the test animal

net protein utilization (NPU) The proportion of nitrogen intake that is retained, ie the product of biological value and digestibility

net protein value (NPV) A way of expressing the amount and quality of the protein in a food; the product of net protein utilization and protein content per cent

neural tube defect Congenital malformations of the brain (anencephaly) or spinal cord (spina bifida) caused by the failure of the closure of the neural tube in early embryonic development

niacin The generic descriptor for two compounds that have the biological activity of the vitamin: nicotinic acid and its amide, nicotinamide. In the USA, niacin is used specifically to mean nicotinic acid, and niacinamide for nicotinamide

nicotinamide adenine dinucleotide and its phosphate (NAD, NADP) The coenzymes derived from niacin. Involved as hydrogen acceptors in a wide variety of oxidation and reduction reactions

nitrogen conversion factor Factor by which nitrogen content of a foodstuff is multiplied to determine the protein content; it depends on the amino acid composition of the protein. For wheat and most cereals it is 5.8; rice, 5.95; soya, 5.7; most legumes and nuts, 5.3; milk, 6.38; other foods, 6.25. In mixtures of proteins, as in dishes and diets, the factor of 6.25 is used. 'Crude protein' is defined as N 36.25

non-starch polysaccharides (NSP) Those polysaccharides other than starches, found in foods. They are the major part of dietary fibre and can be measured more precisely than total dietary fibre; include cellulose, pectins, glucans, gums, mucilages, inulin, and chitin (and exclude lignin); *see* dietary fibre

nutrition surveillance Monitoring the state of health, nutrition, eating behaviour, and nutrition knowledge of the population for the purpose of planning and evaluating nutrition policy. Especially in developing countries, monitoring may include factors that may give early warning of nutritional emergencies

nutritional genomics (nutrigenomics) The field encompassing the interactions between nutrients and the genome and gene products, the function of gene products, and the identification and understanding of the genetic basis for individual and population differences in the response to diet

obesity Excessive accumulation of body fat. A body mass index above 30 is considered to be obese (and above 40 grossly obese)

oedema Excess retention of fluid in the body; may be caused by cardiac, renal, or hepatic failure or by starvation (famine oedema)

oestrogens are steroid hormones principally secreted by the ovaries, which maintain female characteristics

Office of Dietary Supplements (ODS) Office of the US National Institutes of Health; website http://dietary-supplements.info.nih.gov

oncogene a protein encoding gene, which, when deregulated, plays a role in the onset and development of cancer. Genetic mutations that result in oncogene activation increase the chance of a normal cell developing into a tumor cell.

omophagia Eating of raw or uncooked food

organic Chemically, a substance containing carbon in the molecule (with the exception of carbonates and cyanide). Substances of animal and vegetable origin are organic; minerals are inorganic. The term organic foods refers to 'organically grown foods', meaning plants grown without the use of (synthetic) pesticides, fungicides, or inorganic fertilizers, and prepared without the use of preservatives

osteoporosis Degeneration of the bones with advancing age due to loss of bone mineral and protein as a result of decreased secretion of hormones (oestrogens in women and testosterone in men)

para-aminobenzoic acid (PABA) Essential growth factor for microorganisms. It forms part of the molecule of folic acid and is therefore required for the synthesis of this vitamin. Mammals cannot synthesize folic acid, and PABA has no other known function; there is no evidence that it is a human dietary requirement. Not normally present in human diets, can be used to validate 24 h urine collections, because an oral dose, given at each of three meal-times, is rapidly and quantitatively excreted in the urine

pareve (parve) Jewish term for dishes containing neither milk nor meat. Orthodox Jewish law prohibits mixing of milk and meat foods or the consumption of milk products for 3 hours after a meat meal

PARNUTS EU term for foods prepared for particular nutritional purposes (intended for people with disturbed metabolism, or in special physiological conditions, or for young children). Also called dietetic foods

pentosuria The excretion of pentose sugars in the urine. Idiopathic pentosuria is an inherited metabolic disorder almost wholly restricted to Ashkenazi (North European) Jews, which has no adverse effects. Consumption of fruits rich in pentoses (eg pears) can also lead to (temporary) pentosuria

pescetarian Vegetarian who will eat fish, but not meat

phase I metabolism reactions The first phase of metabolism of foreign compounds (xenobiotics), involving metabolic activation. These reactions occur mainly in the liver but also in the small intestine and lungs and comprise the microsomal or mixed function oxidase system, NADPH-dependent enzymes and cytochrome P450 proteins. Generally regarded as detoxication reactions, but may in fact convert inactive precursors into metabolically active compounds, and be involved in activation of precursors to carcinogens

phase II metabolism reactions The second phase of the metabolism of foreign compounds, in which the activated derivatives formed in phase I metabolism are conjugated with amino acids, glucuronic acid or glutathione, to yield water-soluble derivatives that are excreted in urine or bile

phospholipids Glycerol esterified to two molecules of fatty acid, one of which is commonly polyunsaturated. The third hydroxyl group is esterified to phosphate and one of a number of water-soluble compounds, including serine (phosphatidylserine), ethanolamine (phosphatidylethanolamine), choline (phosphatidylcholine, also known as lecithin), and inositol (phosphatidylinositol)

physical activity level (PAL) Total energy cost of physical activity throughout the day, expressed as a ratio of basal metabolic rate. Calculated from the physical activity ratio for each activity, multiplied by the time spent in that activity

physical activity ratio (PAR) Energy cost of physical activity expressed as a ratio of basal metabolic rate

pica An unnatural desire for foods; alternative words are cissa, cittosis, and allotriophagy. Also a perverted appetite (eating of earth, sand, clay, paper, etc.)

plaque (1) Dental plaque is a layer of bacteria in an organic matrix on the surface of teeth, especially around the neck of each tooth. May lead to development of gingivitis, periodontal disease and caries. (2) Atherosclerotic plaque is the development of fatty streaks in the walls of blood vessels

polysaccharides Complex carbohydrates formed by the condensation of large numbers of monosaccharide units, eg starch, glycogen, cellulose, dextrins, inulin. On hydrolysis the simple sugar is liberated

polyunsaturated fatty acids Long-chain fatty acids containing two or more double bonds, separated by methylene bridges: $-CH_2-CH=CH-CH_2-CH=CH-CH_2-$

ponderal index An index of fatness, used as a measure of obesity: the cube root of body weight divided by height. Confusingly, the ponderal index is higher for thin people, and lower for fat people

prion The infective agent(s) responsible for Creutzfeldt-Jakob disease, kuru and possibly other degenerative diseases of the brain in human beings, scrapie in sheep, and bovine spongiform encephalopathy (BSE). They are simple proteins, and unlike viruses, do not contain any nucleic acid. Transmission occurs by ingestion of infected tissue

probiotics Preparations of live microorganisms added to food (or used as animal feed), claimed to be beneficial to health by restoring microbial balance in the intestine. The organisms commonly involved are lactobacilli, bifidobacteria, streptococci, and some yeasts and moulds, alone or as mixtures

protein All living tissues contain proteins; they are polymers of amino acids, joined by peptide bonds. There are 21 main amino acids in proteins, and any one protein may contain several hundred or over a thousand amino acids, so an enormous variety of different proteins occur in nature. Generally a polymer of relatively few amino acids is referred to as a peptide (eg di-, tri-, and tetrapeptides); oligopeptides contain up to about 50 amino acids; larger molecules are polypeptides or proteins

protein efficiency ratio (PER) Weight gain per weight of protein eaten

protein energy malnutrition (PEM) A spectrum of disorders, especially in children, due to inadequate feeding. Used to describe children who are wasted or underweight due to insufficient intake of macronutrients. In fact PEM is commonly associated with multiple micronutrient deficiencies. Marasmus is severe wasting and can also occur in adults; it is the result of a food intake inadequate to meet energy expenditure. Kwashiorkor affects only young children and includes severe oedema, fatty infiltration of the liver, and a sooty dermatitis; it is likely that deficiency of antioxidant nutrients and the stress of infection may be involved. Emaciation, similar to that seen in marasmus, occurs in patients with advanced cancer and AIDS; in this case it is known as cachexia; *see* chronic energy deficiency

protein–energy ratio The protein content of a food or diet expressed as the proportion of the total energy provided by protein (17 kJ (4 kcal)/g). The average requirement for protein is about 7% of total energy intake; average Western diets provide about 14%

protein quality A measure of the usefulness of a dietary protein for growth and maintenance of tissues, and, in animals, production of meat, eggs, wool, and milk. It is only important if the total intake of protein barely meets the requirement. The quality of individual proteins is unimportant in mixed diets, because of complementation between different proteins

protein retention efficiency (PRE) The net protein retention converted to a % scale by multiplying by 16, then becoming numerically the same as NPU

proteome The protein complement of a cell, tissue or organism translated from its genomic DNA sequence

proteomics The study of the proteome, particularly of structure and function

proximate analysis Analysis of foods and feeding-stuffs for nitrogen (for protein), ether extract (for fat), crude fibre and ash (mineral salts), together with soluble carbohydrate calculated by subtracting these values from the total (carbohydrate by difference). Also known as Weende analysis, after the Weende Experimental Station in Germany, which in 1865 outlined the methods of analysis to be used

P/S ratio The ratio between polyunsaturated and saturated fatty acids. In Western diets the ratio is about 0.6; it is suggested that increasing it to near 1.0 would reduce the risk of atherosclerosis and coronary heart disease

QUAC stick Quaker arm circumference measuring stick. A stick used to measure height which also shows the 80th and 85th centiles of expected mid-upper arm circumference. Developed by a Quaker Service Team in Nigeria in the 1960s as a rapid and simple tool for assessment of nutritional status

quantitative ingredients declaration (QUID) Obligatory on food labels in EU since February 2000; previously legislation only required declaration of ingredients in descending order of quantity, not specific declaration of the amount of each ingredient present

reference intakes (of nutrients) Amounts of nutrients greater than the requirements of almost all members of the population, determined on the basis of the average requirement plus twice the standard deviation, to allow for individual variation in requirements and thus cover the theoretical needs of 97.5% of the population

reference man, woman An arbitrary physiological standard; defined as a person aged 25, weighing 65 kg, living in a temperate zone of a mean annual temperature of 10°C. Reference man performs medium work, with an average daily energy requirement of 13.5 MJ (3200 kcal). Reference woman is engaged in general household duties or light industry, with an average daily requirement of 9.7 MJ (2300 kcal)

reference nutrient intake (RNI) Defined by COMA (Committee on Medical Aspects of Food Policy for the UK Department of Health), most recently in 1991, as being the amount of each nutrient that is sufficient to meet the needs of the majority (mean 12 standard deviations) of healthy people in a defined population, or subgroup of it. Approximately equivalent (in concept, but not necessarily in magnitude) to the US or WHO RDAs (recommended dietary amounts)

reference standards (international reference standard)/growth standards These refer to databases recording the linear and ponderal growth of healthy children. They include anthropometric data collected on suitably large samples, and analysed with precise specifications to provide a useful basis for reference

riboflavin Vitamin B_2

ribonucleic acid (RNA) A linear single-stranded polymer composed of four types of ribose nucleotide, adenine, cytosine, guanine, thymine (A, C, G and U), linked by phosphodiester bonds and formed by the transcription of DNA. The three types of cellular RNA – rRNA, tRNA and mRNA – play different roles in protein synthesis

rickets Malformation of the bones in growing children due to deficiency of vitamin D, leading to poor absorption of calcium. In adults the equivalent is osteomalacia. Vitamin D resistant rickets does not respond to normal amounts of the vitamin but requires massive doses. Usually a result of a congenital defect in the vitamin D receptor, or metabolism of the vitamin; it can also be due to poisoning with strontium

saliva Secretion of the salivary glands in the mouth: 1–1.5 litres secreted daily. A dilute solution of the protein mucin (which lubricates food) and the enzyme amylase (which hydrolyses starch), with small quantities of urea, potassium thiocyanate, sodium chloride, and bicarbonate

satiety The sensation of fullness after a meal

Schilling test A test of vitamin B_{12} absorption and status

Scientific Advisory Committee on Nutrition (SACN) providing expert advice to the UK Food Standards Agency and Department of Health

scurvy Deficiency of vitamin C leading to impaired collagen synthesis, causing capillary fragility, poor wound healing and bone changes

sitapophasis Refusal to eat as expression of mental disorder

sitology Science of food

sitomania Mania for eating, morbid obsession with food; also known as phagomania

sitophobia Fear of food; also known as phagophobia

skinfold thickness Index of subcutaneous fat and hence body fat content. Usually measured at four sites: biceps (midpoint of front upper arm), triceps (midpoint of back upper arm), subscapular (directly below point of shoulder blade at angle of 45 degrees), supra-iliac (directly above iliac crest in mid-axillary line); *see* anthropometry

staple food The principal food, eg wheat, rice, maize, etc., which provides the main energy source for communities

starch Polysaccharide, a polymer of glucose units; the form in which carbohydrate is stored in the plant; it does not occur in animal tissue

statins A family of related drugs used to treat hypercholesterolaemia. They act by inhibiting hydroxymethylglutaryl CoA reductase (HMG CoA reductase), the first and rate-limiting enzyme of cholesterol synthesis

stroke Also known as cerebrovascular accident (CVA); damage to brain tissue by hypoxia due to blockage of a blood vessel as a result of thrombosis, atherosclerosis or haemorrhage

stunting Reduction in the linear growth of children, leading to lower than expected height for age, generally resulting in lifelong short stature. A common effect of protein energy malnutrition, and associated especially with inadequate protein intake

sugar alcohols Also called polyols, chemical derivatives of sugars that differ from the parent compounds in having an alcohol group (CH_2OH) instead of the aldehyde group (CHO); thus mannitol from mannose, xylitol from xylose, lacticol from lactulose (also sorbitol, isomalt, and hydrogenated glucose syrup). Several occur naturally in fruits, vegetables, and cereals. They range in sweetness from equal to sucrose to less than half. They provide bulk in foods such as confectionery (in contrast to intense sweeteners), and so are called bulk sweeteners. They are slowly and incompletely metabolized, and are tolerated by diabetics, and provide less energy than sugars: they are less cariogenic than sucrose

sweeteners Four groups of compounds are used to sweeten foods: (1) the sugars, of which the commonest is sucrose (2) bulk sweeteners, including sugar alcohols (3) synthetic non-nutritive sweeteners (intense sweeteners), which are many times sweeter than sucrose (4) various other chemicals such as glycerol and glycine (70% as sweet as sucrose), and certain peptides

taste The tongue can distinguish five separate tastes: sweet, salt, sour (or acid), bitter, and savoury (sometimes called umami, from the Japanese word for a savoury flavour), due to stimulation of the taste buds. The overall taste or flavour of foods is due to these tastes, together with astringency in the mouth, texture, and aroma

thermogenesis Increased heat production by the body, either to maintain body temperature (by shivering or non-shivering thermogenesis) or in response to intake of food and stimulants such as coffee, nicotine and certain drugs

thiamin Vitamin B_1

transgenics the integration of a gene from one species into the genomic DNA of another organism

triacylglycerols Sometimes called triglycerides; lipids consisting of glycerol esterified to three fatty acids (chemically acyl groups). The major component of dietary and tissue fat. Also known as saponifiable fats, since on reaction with sodium hydroxide they yield glycerol and the sodium salts (or soaps) of the fatty acids

triglycerides *See* triacylglycerols

United Nations Children's Fund (UNICEF) originally the United Nations International Children's Emergency Fund; website http://www.unicef.org

US Department of Agriculture (USDA) Created as an independent department in 1862; website http://www.usda.gov

US Recommended Daily Allowances (USRDA) Reference intakes used for nutritional labelling of foods in the USA

vegans Those who consume no foods of animal origin. (Vegetarians often consume milk and/or eggs.)

vitamers Chemical compounds structurally related to a vitamin, and converted to the same overall active metabolites in the body. They thus possess the same biological activity

vitamin Thirteen organic substances that are essential in very small amounts in food

waist:hip ratio Simple method for describing the distribution of subcutaneous and intra-abdominal adipose tissue

weaning foods Foods specially formulated for infants aged between 3 and 9 months for the transition between breast- or bottle-feeding and normal intake of solid foods

Wellcome classification A system for classifying protein energy malnutrition in children based on percentage of expected weight for age and the presence or absence of oedema. Between 60 and 80% of expected weight is underweight in the absence of oedema, and kwashiorkor if oedema is present; under 60% of expected weight is marasmus in the absence of oedema, and marasmic kwashiorkor if oedema is present

wholefoods Foods that have been minimally refined or processed, and are eaten in their natural state. In general nothing is removed from, or added to, the foodstuffs in preparation. Wholegrain cereal products are made by milling the complete grain

World Food Programme (WFP) Part of the Food and Agriculture Organization of the United Nations; intended to give international aid in the form of food from countries with a surplus; website http://www.wfp.org

World Health Organization (WHO) Headquarters in Geneva; website http://www.who.in

FURTHER READING

Bender DA 2004 Oxford dictionary of food and nutrition. Oxford University Press, Oxford

Bender DA, Bender AE 1999 Benders' dictionary of nutrition and food technology, 7th edn. Soodhead Publishing, Cambridge

On-line Medical Dictionary: http://cancerweb.ncl.ac.uk/omd/index.html

Appendix 2: Dietary Reference Values

The following tables summarize the dietary reference values (DRVs) for energy and nutrients, for the United Kingdom (see also chapters 4 and 5). Information has been taken from: Department of Health (1991) Dietary Reference Values for Food Energy and Nutrients for the United Kingdom (HMSO, London). For most nutrients the reference nutrient intake (RNI) is given, which is 2 standard deviations from the estimated average intake for a particular age group. An intake above the RNI would therefore satisfy the requirements of almost all people in that age group.

For some nutrients there is not enough information available on which to base the setting of an RNI and in these cases a 'safe intake' is given.

Table A1   Dietary reference values for energy for males and females

Age	EAR[1]			
	males		females	
	(MJ/day)	(kcal/day)	(MJ/day)	(kcal/day)
0–3 months	2.28	545	2.16	515
4–6 months	2.89	690	2.69	645
7–9 months	3.44	825	3.20	765
10–12 months	3.85	920	3.61	865
1–3 years	5.15	1230	4.86	1165
4–6 years	7.16	1715	6.46	1545
7–10 years	8.24	1970	7.28	1740
11–14 years	9.27	2220	7.92	1845
15–18 years	11.51	2755	8.83	2110
19–50 years	10.60	2550	8.10	1940
51–59 years	10.60	2550	8.00	1900
60–64 years	9.93	2380	7.99	1900
65–74 years	9.71	2330	7.96	1900
75+	8.77	2100	7.61	1810
Pregnancy			+0.80[2]	+0.80[2]
Lactation			+1.9–2.0	+1.9–2.0

[1]EAR = estimated average requirement

[2]Last trimester

Dietary reference values for energy are given as MJ/day and kcal/day, and values for fat and carbohydrate are expressed as percentage of total energy intake (or percentage of food energy, which excludes alcohol).

Table A2 Dietary reference values for protein (g/day)

Age	EAR[1]	RNI[2]
0–3 months	–	12.5
4–6 months	10.6	12.8
7–9 months	11.0	13.7
10–12 months	11.2	14.9
1–3 years	11.7	14.5
4–6 years	14.8	19.7
7–10 years	22.8	28.3
Males		
11–14 years	33.8	42.1
15–18 years	46.1	55.2
19–50 years	44.4	55.5
50+ years	42.6	53.3
Females		
11–14 years	33.1	42.1
15–18 years	46.1	55.2
19–50+ years	44.4	55.5
50+ years	42.6	53.3
Pregnancy		+6
Lactation		+11

[1]EAR = Estimated average requirement
[2]RNI = reference nutrient intake

Table A3 Dietary reference values for fat and carbohydrate for adults as a percentage of daily total energy intake (percentage food energy)

| | UK | | |
	Individual minimum	Population average[1]	Individual maximum
Saturated fatty acids		10 (11)	
Cis-polyunsaturated		6 (6.5)	10
Fatty acids			
n-3	0.2		
n-6	1.0		
Cis-monounsaturated		12 (13)	
Fatty acids			
Trans fatty acids		2 (2)	
Total fatty acids		30 (32.5)	
Total fat		33 (35)	
Non-milk extrinsic sugars	0	10 (11)	
Intrinsic milk sugars and starch		37 (39)	
Total carbohydrate		47 (50)	
Non-starch polysaccharide (g/day)	12	18	24

[1]Total energy intake assumes 5% alcohol; food energy (in parenthesis) excludes alcohol

Table A4 Dietary reference values for fat-soluble vitamins

Age	RNI		UK safe intakes	
	Vitamin A (μg retinol equivalents)	Vitamin D (μg)	Vitamin E (mg α tocopherol/ g PUFA)	Vitamin K (μg)
0–6 months	350	8.5	0.4	10
7–12 months	350	7.0	0.4	10
1–3 years	400	7.0	0.4	–
4–6 years	400	0[1]	0.4	–
7–10 years	500	0[1]	0.4	–
Males				
11–14 years	600	0[1]		
15–50+ years	700	0[1]	>4	1 μg/kg body weight
65+ years		10		
Females				
11–14 years	600	0[1]		
15–50+ years	600	0[1]	>3	1 μg/kg body weight
65+ years		10		
Pregnancy	+100	+10		1 μg/kg body weight
Lactation	+350	+10		

[1] *If exposed to the sun*

Table A5 Reference nutrient intakes for water-soluble vitamins

Age	Thiamin (B₁) (mg)	Riboflavin (B₂) (mg)	Niacin (mg)	Pyridoxine (B₆) (mg)	Folate (μg)	Cyanocobalamin (B₁₂) (μg)	Ascorbate (C) (mg)
0–6 months	0.2	0.4	3	0.2	50	0.3	25
7–12 months	0.3	0.4	5	0.3–0.4	50	0.4	25
1–3 years	0.5	0.6	8	0.7	70	0.5	30
4–6 years	0.7	0.8	11	0.9	100	0.8	30
7–10 years	0.7	1.0	12	1.0	150	1.0	30
Males							
11–14 years	0.9	1.2	15	1.2	200	1.2	35
15–50+ years	0.9	1.3	16–18	1.4–1.5	200	1.5	40
Females							
11–14 years	0.7	1.1	12	1.0	200	1.2	35
15–50+ years	0.8	1.1	12–14	1.2	200	1.5	40
Pregnancy	+0.1[1]	+0.3	–	–	+100	–	+10
Lactation	+0.2	+0.5	–	–	+60	+0.5	+30

[1] *For last trimester only*

Table A6 Reference nutrient intakes for minerals

Age	Calcium (mg)	Phosphorus (mg)	Magnesium (mg)	Iron (mg)	Zinc (mg)	Copper (mg)	Selenium (μg)	Iodine (μg)
0–3 months	525	400	55	1.7	4.0	0.2	10	50
4–6 months	525	400	60	4.3	4.0	0.3	13	60
7–9 months	525	400	75	7.8	5.0	0.3	10	60
10–12 months	525	400	80	7.8	5.0	0.3	10	60
1–3 years	350	270	85	6.9	5.0	0.4	15	70
4–6 years	450	350	120	6.1	6.5	0.6	20	100
7–10 years	550	450	200	8.7	7.0	0.7	30	110
Males								
11–14 years	1000	775	280	11.3	9.0	0.8	45	130
15–18 years	1000	775	280	11.3	9.5	1.0	70	140
19–50 years	700	550	300	8.7	9.5	1.2	75	140
50+ years	700	550	300	8.7	9.5	1.2	75	140
Females								
11–14 years	800	625	280	14.8	9.0	0.8	45	130
15–18 years	800	625	300	14.8	7.0	1.0	60	140
19–50 years	700	550	270	14.8	7.0	1.2	60	140
50+ years	700	550	270	8.7	7.0	1.2	60	140
Pregnancy	–	–	–	–	–	–	–	–
Lactation	+550	+440	+50	–	+6.0	+0.3	+15	–

Table A7 Reference nutrient intakes for sodium, potassium and chloride

Age	Sodium (mg)	Potassium (mg)	Chloride (mg)
0–3 months	210	800	320
4–6 months	280	850	400
7–9 months	320	700	500
10–12 months	350	700	500
1–3 years	500	800	800
4–6 years	700	1100	1100
7–10 years	1200	2200	1100
Males and females			
11–14 years	1600	3100	2500
15–50+ years	1600	3500	2500

Table A8 UK safe intake for biotin and pantothenic acid

Age	Biotin (μg)	Pantothenic acid (mg)
0–6 months	–	1.7
7–12 months	–	1.7
1–3 years	–	1.7
4–10 years	–	3.7
Males and females		
10–50+ years	10–20	3–7

Appendix 3: Bibliography

GENERAL NUTRITION REFERENCE BOOKS

Bender D 2005 A dictionary of food and nutrition, 2nd edn. Oxford University Press, Oxford

Byrom S 2002 Pocket guide to nutrition and dietetics. Churchill Livingstone, Edinburgh

Coultate T P 2002 Food: the chemistry of its components, 4th edn. Royal Society of Chemistry, London

Department of Health 1991 Dietary reference values of food energy and nutrients for the UK. Report on Health and Social Subjects no 41. DoH, London

Fieldhouse P 1995 Food and nutrition – customs and culture, 2nd edn. Thomas Nelson, London

Food Standards Agency 1995 Manual of nutrition, 10th edn. HMSO, London

MacBeth H 1997 Food preferences and taste: continuity and change. Berghahn Books, Oxford

Food Standards Agency 2002 McCance and Widdowson's The composition of foods, 6th edn. Royal Society of Chemistry, London

Nestle M 2002 Food politics: how the food industry influences food and nutrition. University of California Press, Los Angeles

Webster-Gandy J, Madden A, Holdsworth M (eds) 2006 The Oxford handbook of food and nutrition. Oxford University Press, Oxford

Vaughan J G, Geissler C A 1997 The new Oxford book of food plants, rev. edn 2009. Oxford University Press, Oxford

INTERNATIONAL ORGANIZATION PUBLICATIONS

Energy

UNU/WHO/FAO 2004 Human energy requirements. Report of a joint FAO/WHO/UNU expert consultation 17–24 October 2001, Rome, Italy. UNU/WHO/FAO, Rome

World Health Organization 2005 Human energy requirements. Scientific background papers of the joint FAO/WHO/UNU Expert consultation 17–24 October 2001, Rome, Italy. Public Health Nutrition Vol 8 (7A) Oct 2005, special issue

Nutrients

Food and Agriculture Organization/World Health Organization 2007 Joint FAO/WHO scientific update on carbohydrates in human nutrition. European Journal of Clinical Nutrition Vol 61 (suppl 1)

World Health Organization 1993 Global prevalence of vitamin A deficiency. WHO, Geneva

World Health Organization 2007 Iodine deficiency in Europe – a continuing public health problem. WHO, Geneva

World Health Organization 2007 Protein and amino acid requirements in human nutrition. Report of a joint FAO/WHO/UNU Expert consultation. WHO Technical Report Series no. 935. WHO, Geneva

World Health Organization/Food and Agriculture Organization 2004 Vitamin and mineral requirements in human nutrition, 2nd edn. WHO, Geneva

Fetal development

World Health Organization 2002 Programming of chronic disease by impaired fetal nutrition. Evidence and implications for policy and intervention strategies. WHO, Geneva

World Health Organization 2003 Promoting optimal fetal development: report of a technical consultation. WHO, Geneva

Child feeding

World Health Organization 2002 Nutrient adequacy of exclusive breast feeding for the term infant during the first six months of life. WHO, Geneva

World Health Organization 2003 Global strategy for infant and young child feeding. WHO, Geneva

World Health Organization 2005 Guiding principles on feeding non-breast-fed children 6–24 months of age. WHO, Geneva

Older people

World Health Organization 2002 Keep fit for life. Meeting the nutritional needs of older people. WHO, Geneva

Chronic diseases

World Health Organization 2002 Diet, nutrition and the prevention of chronic diseases. Report of a joint WHO/FAO expert consultation. WHO, Geneva

World Health Organization 2004 Diet, nutrition, and the prevention of chronic diseases: scientific background papers of the joint WHO/FAO expert consultation 2002. Public Health Nutrition vol 7 (1 A) Feb 2004, special issue

World Health Organization 2004 Global strategy on diet, physical activity and health. Final strategy document and resolution. WHO, Geneva

World Health Organization 2004 Obesity: preventing and managing the global epidemic. Report of a WHO consultation. WHO, Geneva

World Cancer Research Fund/American Institute of Cancer Research 2007 Food, nutrition, physical activity and the prevention of cancer: a global perspective. AICR, Washington DC

Anaemia

Badham J, Zimmermann M B, Kraemer K (eds) 2007 The guidebook: nutritional anaemia. Sight and Life Press, Basel, Switzerland

International Nutritional Anaemia Consultation Group 1998 Guidelines for the use of iron supplements to prevent and treat iron deficiency anaemia. WHO/UNICEF, Washington

Kraemer K, Zimmermann M B (eds) 2007 Nutritional anemia. Sight and Life Press, Basel, Switzerland

World Health Organization 2008 World prevalence of anaemia 1993–2005. WHO global database on anaemia. WHO, Geneva

Malnutrition

World Health Organization 2004 Severe malnutrition: report of a consultation to review current literature. WHO, Geneva

HIV/AIDS

World Health Organization 2003 Nutrient requirements for people living with HIV/AIDS. Report of a technical consultation. WHO, Geneva

Child growth standards

World Health Organization 2006 WHO child growth standards. WHO, Geneva

World Health Organization 2006 Comparison of World Health Organization (WHO) Child Growth Standards and the National Center for Health Statistics/WHO international growth reference: implications for child health programmes. Public Health Nutrition 9:941–947

World Health Organization 2007 Development of a WHO growth reference for school aged children and adolescents. Bulletin of WHO 85:660–667

SOME USEFUL WEBSITES FOR NUTRITION INFORMATION

UK

British Nutrition Foundation (includes sections on healthy eating, educational materials, publications): *www.nutrition.org.uk*

British Dietetic Association (includes section on food facts): *www.bda.uk.com*

Department for Environment, Food and Rural Affairs (pages on food & drink, sustainable development, farming, fisheries, etc): *www.defra.gov.uk*

Department of Health (includes government nutrition policy and programmes): *www.doh.gov.uk*

Food Standards Agency (sections on nutrition, safety & hygiene, labelling and packaging, GM & Novel Foods, BSE, etc): *www.food.gov.uk*

Institute of Food Research (includes science publications and briefs): *www.ifr.ac.uk*

Rowett Research Institute (includes educational material and publications): *www.rowett.ac.uk*

European

European Union (gateway to EU, includes subjects such as agriculture, consumers, food safety, public health, etc): *http://europa.eu*

European Food Safety Authority: *www.efsa.eu.int*

USA

Food and Drug Administration (includes topics such as food safety, nutrition, etc): *www.fda.gov*

Food and Nutrition Information Center (subjects includes dietary guidance, lifecycle nutrition, diet and disease, food composition, etc): *http://fnic.nal.usda.gov*

United States Department of Agriculture (includes Children's Research Center, Human Nutrition Research Center: *www.usda.gov*

International

Sight and Life (publications re micronutrient deficiencies): *www.sightandlife.org*

International Council for Control of Iodine Deficiency Disorders: *www.iccidd.org*

World Health Organization (re international health including nutrition, links to regional offices): *www.who.int*

Food and Agriculture Organization (re world food situation, includes food balance sheets showing consumption in individual countries): *www.fao.org*

World Food programme (information on food aid): *www.wfp.org*

United Nations Children's Fund (information on children's health including nutrition): *www.unicef.org*

International Food Policy Research Institute (publications on food and nutrition): *www.ifpri.org*

Standing Committee for Nutrition (organization to promote cooperation among UN agencies to end malnutrition, publications on state of nutrition and interventions): *www.unscn.org*

Medical dictionaries

Several online medical dictionaries define terms and give examples of their use, including:

- *cancerweb.ncl.ac.uk/omd/*
- *www.online-medical-dictionary.org/*
- *www.nlm.nih.gov/medlineplus/mplusdictionary.html*

Index

Hypothalamus
  hunger–satiety centres, 19, 20
  water balance regulation, 73, 74
Hypothermia, elderly people, 130
Hypothyroidism, endocrine obesity, 167
Hypoventilation syndrome, 165

I

Ileal brake, 211
Immobility, weight gain, 167
Immune function, 89, 92, 94
  elderly people, 129
  gastrointestinal tract, 207
  iron, 99–100, 187
  zinc, 102
Immune system maturation, 111
Immunoglobulins, 26, 207
  breast milk, 112, 113
  placental transfer, 122
Incidence, definition, 234, 235
'Indigestible/unavailable' polysaccharides, 46
Indirect calorimetry, 17
Individual level dietary assessment, 245–246
  prospective methods, 245
  retrospective methods, 245, 246, 247
  strengths/limitations of measurements, 246
Infant formula, 114, 125, 126
  composition, 112, 113, 114
  cow's milk allergy management, 222
  digestion/absorption, 112
  specialized, 114
*Infant Formula and Follow-on Formula
  Regulations*, 114
Infant measuring board, 248
Infants, 109–110
  breastfeeding, 112–113
  cow's milk intake, 116
  food intake, 111
  formula feeding, 114, 125, 126
  gastrointestinal function development, 112
  immunological development, 111–112
  nutrition, 112–116, 176
    relationship to adult health (Barker
      hypothesis), 111
  renal function development, 112
  undernutrition, 260
  vitamin supplementation, 114
  weaning (complementary feeding), 114–115
Infections
  negative nitrogen balance, 61
  role in undernutrition, 260
Infectious agents, cancer associations, 158
Infertility, obesity association, 120, 125, 163,
  165
Inflammatory bowel disease, 193, 215
  see also Crohn's disease; Ulcerative colitis
Information bias, 236
Information provision, nutritional, 262
Insulin, 92, 102, 105
  diabetes pathophysiology, 150
    type 1, 150, 151
    type 2, 151, 152
  fat metabolism regulation, 58
  functions, 50, 52
  protein synthesis regulation, 63
  secretion, 47, 50, 51
Insulin resistance, 55
  diabetes type 2, 152, 154
  metabolic syndrome, 164
  pregnanct women, 122
Insulin therapy, 155, 167

Insulin-like growth factors, 192
Intestinal biopsy, 221
Intestinal bypass, 171
Intestinal motility, 211, 213
Intracellular fluid, 6
Intrauterine growth retardation, 124, 175, 188
Intrinsic factor, 85
Iodine, 26, 103–104
  absorption, 104
  deficiency, 103–104
    worldwide extent, 258
  dietary requirements, 104
  dietary sources, 104
  excess, 104
  functions, 103
  metabolism, 104
  nutrition status monitoring, 252
    intake estimation, 253
  status assessment, 104
  tissue distribution, 104
  transport, 104
  vegetarian diet, 34
Iodothyronine deiodinase, 105
Ionizing radiation, cancer associations, 159
Iron, 99–102
  absorption, 101
    vitamin C enhancement, 86, 100, 101, 118
  antioxidant activity, 99
  bioavailability, 100–101
  cereals/cereal products, 24
  deficiency, 100, 129
    children/adolescents, 34, 118
    elderly people, 132
    worldwide extent, 258
  dietary requirements, 102
  food sources, 100
  forms in food, 100
  functions, 7, 99–100
  homeostasis, 101
  overload, 99, 100
  status assessment, 102, 186
  supplements, 185, 187–188
    athletes, 140
    pregnant women, 188
  transferrin receptors gene expression
    regulation, 228
  transport, 101
  vegetarian diet, 34, 35
Iron deficiency anaemia, 99, 100, 140, 184, 185,
  186–187
  children/adolescents, 118, 187
  coeliac disease, 215
  cognitive development impairment, 187
  Crohn's disease, 216
  immune function effects, 187
  prevention, 188
  treatment, 187–188
Irritable bowel syndrome, 218–220, 221, 222
  clinical features, 219
  dietary treatment, 220
Ischaemic heart disease *see* Coronary heart
  disease
Isoflavones, 161, 197
Isoleucine, 63
Isomaltose, 212
Isoniazid, 82
Isoprostanes, 253
Isothiocyanates, 160

J

Joule (J), 12

INDEX

311